Mapping Medical Modernity

Histories and Ecologies of Health
Robert Peckham, *Editor*

MAPPING MEDICAL MODERNITY

Urban Space and Public Health in Tokyo, 1868–1920

SUSAN L. BURNS

UNIVERSITY *of* PITTSBURGH PRESS

Published by the University of Pittsburgh Press, Pittsburgh, Pa., 15260

Printed on acid-free paper
10 9 8 7 6 5 4 3 2 1

Cataloging-in-Publication data is available from the Library of Congress

Hardcover: 978-0-8229-4888-9
Paperback: 978-0-8229-6799-6

Cover art: Detail from Miyamae Kenji, ed., *Kaisei kubun Tōkyō saizu: zen* (Tokyo: Tsutsumi Kichibei, 1881). https://lapis.nichibun.ac.jp/chizu/map_detail.php?id=001084862. Courtesy of the International Research Center for Japanese Studies.

Cover design: Alex Wolfe

Publisher: University of Pittsburgh Press, 7500 Thomas Blvd., 4th floor, Pittsburgh, PA 15260, United States, www.upittpress.org

EU Authorized Representative: Easy Access System Europe, Mustamäe tee 50, 10621 Tallinn, Estonia, gpsr.requests@easproject.com

CONTENTS

ACKNOWLEDGMENTS

Much of this book was written during the academic year of 2021–2022, during the COVID-19 pandemic, with the support of a National Endowment for the Humanities (NEH) fellowship and a research leave granted by the University of Chicago. Although the isolation of the lockdown period was challenging, the pandemic era proved to be a stimulating time to think about public health, medicine, and urban space. After reading this book in manuscript form, my colleague Faith Hillis remarked that it was "haunted" by the pandemic, and I think this is true. The outbreak, the many deaths it caused, and the political and social tensions that followed revealed the difficulty of forging public health policies that are effective, compassionate, and equitable. In the years since the pandemic, trust in public health policy and institutions has continued to erode. I hope that this book might contribute to discussions about the politics of public health and its social impact.

My writing of this book during that solitary COVID year was aided greatly by the support of friends, family, and colleagues. As always, I am profoundly grateful to my daughter Hannah Tomio. Although she faced her own struggles in starting a challenging PhD program during COVID, she was always just a phone call or text away, and she never seemed to tire of hearing about Tokyo, hospitals, doctors, and disease. Thanks as well to Ollie, Charlie, and Sascha, who offered their own quiet support. I am grateful to Amanda Seaman, who read chapters of the work and offered helpful advice, to Suzanne Gottschang, who invited me to workshop parts of the project at Smith College, and to my colleague Hoyt Long, who organized a series of workshops devoted to digital humanities, where I presented my early attempts at mapping using geographic information systems (GIS). Ken Daimaru's invitation to be a visiting professor at the University of Paris Cité in April 2024 allowed me to present parts of this work to European colleagues, and I benefited greatly from their feedback, including that of Marta Hanson who introduced me to the concept of "healthscaping." The members of the UChicago Kuzushiji Reading Group, especially our leader Hiroyoshi Noto, aided me greatly in reading the archival materials referenced in this book. Thanks as well to Faith Hillis and the students of her methods seminar who read the manuscript as I was in the midst of revisions and offered much needed feedback.

Finally, and most importantly, I owe a huge debt to my research assistants, Mark Chen and Yoko Nabeshima, whose tireless work in compiling spread sheets with hundreds, at times thousands, of data points facilitated the GIS analysis featured in the book. Their patience, diligence, and goodwill were invaluable.

While the NEH supported the writing of this study, much of the research was accomplished with the aid of research funds from the Center for East Asian Studies, which funded my yearly summer research trips to Japan. I am also immensely grateful to the staff of the Tokyo Metropolitan Archives, who were always kind, patient, and efficient during my many visits. I am also deeply appreciative of the support of William Hammell, my editor at the University of Pittsburgh Press, and Robert Peckham, the editor of the series Histories and Ecologies of Health. Finally, I am grateful to the two anonymous reviewers whose comments greatly aided me in revising the book.

Mapping Medical Modernity

Introduction

Medical Modernization and the Healthscaping of Tokyo

As the coronavirus pandemic began in the spring of 2020, it soon exposed the vulnerability of urban communities to outbreaks of disease, even in the twenty-first century. Population density, disparities in income and living conditions, constraints on the availability of medical care, cleavages among diverse communities of residents, and the fallibility of public health policies in the face of a new disease led to the rapid spread of the COVID-19 virus and spiraling rates of infection and death in cities as diverse as Wuhan, Rome, Lima, and New York. The devastating effects of disease on urban space, residents, and everyday life is of course not a new development. Indeed, as the epidemiologist Sandro Galea recently commented, "It is hard to think of the impact that epidemics have on society without thinking of them through the lens of cities, and conversely, it is hard to think of cities without understanding how epidemics have shaped their growth over the centuries."[1]

Historical research on cities around the world offers support for Galea's observation. The past two decades have seen the publication of many monographs on public health in cities like Mexico City, London, Buenos Aires, Shanghai, San Francisco, and Los Angeles, among others.[2] Several of these works explore the impact of a specific disease such as plague, cholera, tuberculosis, or yellow fever on urban residents and the resulting efforts at social management. To that end, these studies examine the development of new policies to control the spread of disease, including efforts to establish new institutions such as quarantine hospitals and sanitoriums. Other works focus more broadly on efforts to improve health, such as the establishment of housing codes, the creation of public parks, and the development of new infrastructure consisting of drainage systems, sewers, and waterworks.

Despite their geographic and thematic diversity, these works share a concern for the period from the mid-nineteenth century to the early twentieth century, a time that saw both the rapid growth of cities around the world and a new political will to invest in medical institutions and public health, as health was reimagined as a key indicator of modernity and national strength, power, and influence. This was particularly the case for cities in countries outside of Europe and North America, which were dealing with the threat of imperialist encroachment (such as Shanghai) or seeking to overcome their colonial pasts (such as Mexico City). But even in cities in Europe and the US, efforts to improve public health were always political in nature and were mediated by the racial, ethnic, and socioeconomic tensions that were shaping these expanding urban spaces.

Mapping Medical Modernity draws inspiration from and seeks to contribute to this literature by exploring the process of medical modernization in Tokyo from the 1870s to about 1920. The focus on a single city is a departure from recent works on the social history of medicine in Japan, still a relatively new area of research. William Johnston's history of tuberculosis, Alexander Bay's study of beriberi, and my own work on leprosy are all framed by the boundaries of the nation-state rather than a specific locale, even though regional variations and the urban-rural divide are important—indeed, defining—aspects of Japan's modernity.[3]

The transformation of health care in the city is an essential but largely overlooked part of the history of modern Tokyo. The handful of monographs aimed at general readers that deal wholistically with the history of Japan's modern capital, including Edward Seidensticker's two-volume work published in the 1990s and more recent works by Keiko Packard and Stephen Mansfield, do not address public health or the many ways in which medical reforms reshaped the city.[4] Other aspects of Tokyo's history have received some scholarly attention: recent monographs have examined the role of Christian churches in the city, the function of expositions and museums, and the establishment of Ueno zoological park and its place in national and imperial culture.[5] The only work that gives some attention to public health is Sally Hastings's *Neighborhood and Nation in Tokyo*, which examines the impact of national policies on a working-class Tokyo neighborhood after 1905.[6] I argue, however, that the period before 1905 was more significant for shaping the city and the lives of its residents.

In exploring the history of medicine and public health in Tokyo, *Mapping Medical Modernity* takes a granular approach to the city while also seeking to be attentive to the larger national and international contexts that were shaping policy decisions. Like many national capitals, Tokyo was a distinctive kind of city. Scott Campbell, a scholar of urban planning, has stated that capital cities "are far more heterogeneous than other kinds of cities." He notes that while every capital city hosts the government apparatus of the country in question, not every capital is to the same degree also a center of population, finance, industry, education, and culture.[7] Until 1868, Edo, as Tokyo was then known, was an early modern castle town, albeit the largest and most prosperous in the country. It was an administrative center and home to the political elite of the day, the Tokugawa shoguns and their vassals, as well as merchants and artisans and a large and heterogeneous population of marginalized people that included entertainers, day laborers, and so-called outcast people. Five decades later, Tokyo was not only the political capital of Japan and its expanding empire but also the industrial, commercial, cultural, and educational center of both. The city drew visitors from around the world who came as tourists, diplomats, students, and for economic pursuits. Many were from elsewhere in Asia, and they looked to the city and Japan for inspiration for their own nationalistic dreams.

Tensions between local, national, and international concerns are central to the story of medical modernization in Tokyo. Until 1889, the urban space of Tokyo was subsumed within Tokyo-fu (Tokyo Prefecture), which included six rural districts and was under the direction of the appointed prefectural governor. But from the 1870s the urban wards of the prefecture became objects of intense concern for officials within the central government. In 1874 the authority of the prefectural government was challenged when many aspects of city life came under the control of the newly created Tokyo Metropolitan Police (Keishichō, hereafter TMP), which was under the direction of the Home Ministry, although financed by prefectural taxes. The TMP's duties encompassed not only the maintenance of social order but also the policing of entertainment (including prostitution), public health, and many aspects of the built environment. Over time its authority expanded, and the TMP became involved in surveilling political activism and the nascent labor movement. Clashes between the TMP and Tokyo officials would shape both the evolution of public health policy and the responses of Tokyo residents who often resisted the heavy-handed tactics of the TMP.

International tensions, in what was the age of high imperialism in East Asia, also reverberated in Tokyo, shaping priorities and policies and affecting the lives of Tokyo residents. In the 1850s the Tokugawa shogunate, under duress, signed a series of "unequal treaties" with the US and many European countries that gave foreign nationals extraterritoriality and fixed import and export tariffs. The new government inherited these treaties, the terms of which soon became a hot-button domestic issue in this era of growing nationalism. Although the government made multiple efforts to revise the treaties, it was only in 1911 that the last of their terms was abolished. As a result, public health policies too were constrained by international pressure. A case in point is the government's attempt in 1877 to establish a system of maritime quarantine in nearby Yokohama, the largest and most prosperous of the treaty ports, to prevent the introduction of cholera via ships coming from regions where the disease was present. When the British consul complained that this was an unnecessary infringement on his country's treaty rights, the government backed down and, in the aftermath, turned of necessity from attempting to control the introduction of the disease to Japan to regulating traffic into and activities within the city to stop its spread.

In exploring the history of medical and public health reform in Tokyo, *Mapping Medical Modernity* draws upon a large body of Japanese scholarship. While the first wave of historical works on public health was largely celebratory, casting medical modernization as one of the crowning achievements of the modern state, recent work by scholars such as Kojima Kazutaka and Kasahara Hidehiko is more nuanced in exploring the struggles and missteps that accompanied the formation of national policy.[8] At the center of their work is Nagayo Sensai, a physician who became the head of the national government's Medical Affairs Bureau, the predecessor of the Hygiene Bureau, in 1874. He was one of the architects of the Medical Policy (Isei), an ambitious plan for reform that sought to remake medical care in Japan with profound implications for Tokyo. It addressed medical education and licensing, the pharmaceutical industry, and the creation of a public health system. An advocate of the Anglo-American approach to public health, which gave localities considerable autonomy, Nagayo pushed back, with growing futility, against the centripetal tendencies of the new government.

While I have learned much from this body of scholarship, my concern is less the struggles among elite officials over national policy than the impact of policies on the city and the lives of those who lived within it. The central government responded to the Medical Policy by designating the country's three largest cities—Tokyo, Osaka, and Kyoto—as testing grounds for the planned reforms. Of these, Tokyo proved to be the most contentious and arguably the most important site of reform, as tensions emerged between local needs and national aspirations. My work is particularly indebted to two scholars whose research centers on Tokyo, Kitahara Itoko and Ishizuka Hiromichi.[9] Although Kitahara focused on efforts to provide health care to the poor and Ishizuka was concerned with the relationship between disease, health, and the built environment, both gave much needed attention to the impact of public health on the city and its residents. The depth of their empirical research and their attention to marginalized Tokyo residents who were often the intended objects of public health policy have shaped my own approach. Important too is Kobayashi Takehiro's study of public health in Kyoto, which, like the research of Kitahara and Ishizuka, prompted me to think beyond the conventional focus on the nation-state that has shaped so much work on Japan.[10]

Mapping Medical Modernity is based on extensive archival research in the Tokyo Metropolitan Archives, which houses prefectural and municipal records, but it draws as well on a large and heterogeneous body of print sources including scientific, medical, and police reports, medical journals, personal memoirs, literary works, and products of the popular press, including newspapers, magazines, and guidebooks to the city. One particularly important resource was the statistical data collected and published annually from 1882 until 1943 in the *Tokyo Prefectural Statistical Handbook* (*Tōkyō-fu tōkeisho*), which always included a section on "hygiene" (*eisei*).[11] Organized by the fifteen wards and the rural districts that made up the prefecture, the handbook offers a window onto the changing landscape of health and health care in its detailing of rates of disease, numbers of medical professionals and the nature of their training, numbers of hospitals, rates of death, births, stillbirths, and more. This information was compiled with the support of private practice doctors, who by statute were required to participate in the collection of data and its submission to ward officials.

Certainly, these data contain blinders, gaps, contradictions, and even perhaps some degree of purposeful obfuscation. Information was gathered at the level of the ward, the administrative boundaries of which were developed for reasons other than the promotion of public health, and these are often unwieldly units for exploring health and its management within the city.[12] In this period, the fifteen wards varied greatly in topography, no less than in

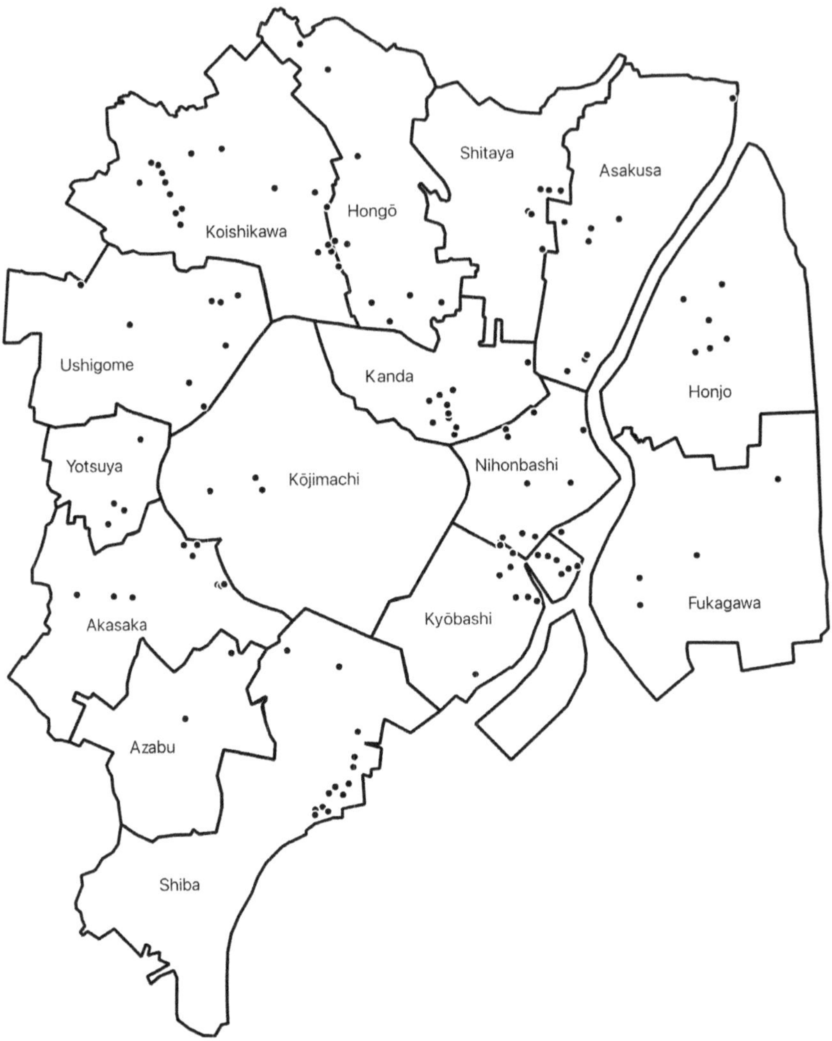

Figure I.1. Slum neighborhoods in Tokyo by ward, ca. 1890. This map was created using information from N. A., "Kyūmin ibun," *Kokumin shinbun*, June 15–16, 18, 20, 1890, reprinted in Nakagawa, *Meiji Tōkyō kasō seikatsushi*, 31–36. Kure Ayatoshi, "Tōkyō-fuka hinmin no jōkyō," *Sutachisuchikku zasshi* 57 (1891), reprinted in Nakagawa, *Meiji Tōkyō kasō seikatsushi*, 77–89.

population, infrastructure, and social class; and many wards encompassed a mix of wealthy and poor residents, and private, rental, and public landholdings. In 1890, for example, Kōjimachi, the area surrounding the imperial palace that had once been home to the high-ranking vassals of the shogun, contained three "blocks" (*machi*, the administrative unit below the ward), where crudely constructed and crowded tenement housing predominated (see fig. I.1). Similarly, Kanda, the "hospital district" of the city, was home to nine such blocks.[13] Officials and others would single out these areas for particularly scrutiny, suggesting that the prevailing unhygienic conditions within them threatened the health of their more prosperous, hygienic, and industrious neighbors, but the fact that we have no information on administrative units below the level of the ward makes it difficult to evaluate such claims.

In addition, it goes without saying that people did not live their lives constrained by the administrative borders of the ward.[14] Gender, age, and social class shaped patterns of movement around the city: poor women and their children were likely more bound to the area of their residences than upper-middle-class men. To be sure, the situation evolved over time. Initially, the lack of public transportation and the expense of alternative means of transportation (most notably, the rickshaw), as well as the fact that many small-scale manufacturers and merchants lived and worked in the same or adjacent spaces, meant that many people's living arrangements were far more spatially constrained than we might imagine today. However, as the streetcar system took form beginning with the first horse-drawn tram in 1880, people began to traverse the city in new ways, making the administrative boundaries based on residence perhaps less relevant. Capturing patterns of movement of any individual is impossible, but to the degree possible I have sought to understand the impact of new modes of transportation on the movement of people in the city.

There are other issues with the statistical data as well. For one thing, the categories of data changed several times over the course of their publication, complicating efforts at longitudinal analysis. But more significant is what went unrecorded. Syphilis is a telling case of the gaps in available data. Intense concern about syphilis in the city made it one of the first objects of public health policy, but no attempt was made to survey its spread among the general population until 1916. Instead, city officials and the TMP relentlessly tracked rates of infection among Tokyo's licensed prostitutes who had to submit to regular examinations as part of the licensing procedure, reflecting the assumption that prostitutes were responsible for infecting their clients—but the reverse was just as likely.

Although the data in the handbook and in other sources has these limitations, the compilation of this wealth of information on medical practitioners, institutions, patients, and rates of infectious diseases over many years makes it possible to adopt what the sociologist Mark Gottdiener, building on the work of Henri Lefebvre, has termed a "sociospatial perspective."[15] Efforts to prevent and combat sickness and disease did not occur in a vacuum but reflected and responded to the material and social aspects of the urban environment. To conceptualize the intimate relationship between the urban environments and health, I follow the historians, anthropologists, and others working on health and medicine in adopting the term "healthscape" to capture the complex relationship between urban environments, individuals, institutions, and policies that unfolded within the city. As deployed by the sociologist of health Adele E. Clark, "healthscape" derived from Arujun Appadurai's use of "scapes" (ethno, media, techno, finance, and ideo) to describe forms of cultural flow. In her use, "healthscape" referred to the regimes of representation that shaped how health, illness, health care, and medicine were known and understood. According to Clarke, "healthscapes are kinds of assemblages . . . infrastructures of assumptions, as well as people, things, places, images."[16]

In this formulation, a healthscape is an aspect of the social imaginary rather than the objective reality of the physical landscape and the built environment, but others have used it to examine empirically defined places. Medical and health geographers have long focused on specific sites, locales, and regions to explore the distribution of diseases, access to sanitation, the distribution of health providers and services, and the like. Writing in 1992, the cultural and health geographer Wilbert Gesler coined the term "therapeutic landscape" and argued that it was necessary to explore the social, symbolic, and affective associations that led some places to be viewed as hygienic and healthy, while others were not.[17]

Reflecting the interest in both the material space and the process that lead to the association of some places with health and well-being and others with the obverse, some urban historians working on medicine and public health have used the concept of "healthscaping" to explore the ideas, practices, theories, and objectives that animated individuals, communities, health professionals, and municipal governments to manage and reorder urban space with the aim of producing healthy cities and citizens. The "Healthscaping Urban Europe" project is an example of this kind of work. It brings together historians and archeologists to explore how residents of Europe's medieval and early modern cities "thought about and pursued population-level health."[18] The historian Guy Geltner, a member of the project, has expanded on this definition, writing that healthscaping refers to "the physical, social, legal, administrative, and political process of managing the built and natural environment to promote wellbeing."[19]

I use "healthscape" in Geltner's sense, but I add to the factors he mentions, the rising influence of medical capitalism. Before 1868, Edo's shogunal authorities and their commoner counterparts, the city elders, played only a small role in regulating medicine or promoting health by supporting a limited number of institutions intended to aid the most vulnerable city residents. In contrast, Tokyo's civil authorities were initially deeply concerned with developing policies that would extend medical care and modern medical knowledge to the populace, including the poor. By the early 1880s, however, the straitened finances of the prefecture and organized opposition from the city's doctors brought an end to such efforts. As a result, few charitable or publicly funded provisions were made for low-cost medical care, and doctors and hospitals competed for fee-paying patients.

To analyze and visualize the impact of the reforms and medical capitalism on the city, *Mapping Medical Modernity* makes extensive use of geographic information system (GIS) analysis to create the maps that are an important part of this work. Using data from sources such as the *Tokyo Prefectural Statistical Handbook*, newspapers, guidebooks, and archival sources and the open access software QGIS, I use mapping to explore the evolving and complex relationships that unfolded among pathogens, medical facilities, the natural and built environments, and, of course, the people who lived and worked within the city. The ability to create layers of different kinds of data makes it possible to discern relationships that otherwise go undetected. For example, mapping the location of hospitals and the ratio of doctors to population by ward brings into focus the emergence of what might be termed "health-care deserts" in Tokyo by the 1890s. Tracing rates of cholera infection brings into sharp relief the relationship of the disease with the natural topography of the city and the decaying infrastructure of its water supply.

Mapping also aids us in understanding the city as it existed in the late nineteenth century. This book was written in Chicago, a city that has retained a good deal of its nineteenth-century footprint and much of its early twentieth-century residential housing in some neighborhoods. In contrast, little of the Tokyo of this era remains. Much of the city was destroyed in the 1923 earthquake and later because of Allied bombing during the Pacific War, and the process of rebuilding, as well as the expansion of the city via land reclamation and the incorporation of formally rural areas, have obscured even the urban footprint of the city as it once existed.

To understand the city as it existed in the late nineteenth and early twentieth centuries, I have made use of historical maps that are dense with various kinds of information. Early modern maps of Edo, like the base map of Plate 1, used family crests (*kamon*) to designate the site of warrior residences, color coding to show the areas held by religious institutions, and careful demarcation to indicate the neighborhoods in which commoners resided. Meiji period maps (1868–1912) of Tokyo are even more jam-packed with information: wards, blocks, and the numbered subunits of the blocks are depicted, as are roads, trolley lines, and train tracks. Many maps incorporate a rich array of symbols to show features such as markets, temples, shrines, paddy fields, schools, bridges, military installations, and more. While this work uses mapping to explore the impact of public health and medical modernization on the spatial organization of the city, it is also concerned with space at scales smaller than any administrative unit. A case in point is the growing concern that cholera brought to the proximity of human waste to people, residences, and sources of water, as what had once been seen as a valuable commodity and an inescapable part of urban life was newly viewed as a source of deadly disease.

While *Mapping Medical Modernity* explores the formation of the modern healthscape of Tokyo, it is attentive as well to the city's residents and their agency in the reform process. Too often histories of medicine and public health adopt a top-down approach, in part because of the limits of sources that allow us access to the experiences of ordinary people. Indeed, writing almost four decades ago, the medical historian Roy Porter called for a "medical history from below" that makes patients, families, and communities an integral part of historical research on medicine, disease, and health.[20] To understand and incorporate the experience of Tokyo residents, I draw upon a variety of sources, including petitions to city officials, newspapers and other kinds of reportage, and literary works and memoirs.

In incorporating the perspective of patients and families, my concern is not only to provide a fuller picture of the process of medical reform but also to understand the place of ordinary subjects within the new politics of health that emerged in this period. Here, I am influenced by Dora B. Weiner's work *The Citizen-Patient in Revolutionary and Imperial Paris*.[21] Weiner explored the emergence of a new political concern for citizens' health and the central paradox that shaped the process of medical reform in Paris: while patients were expected to be docile recipients of expert knowledge from hygienists, doctors, and officials, they were simultaneously imagined as citizens, who were endowed with inalienable rights, including a right to health. As a result, the right to health care carried with it new "duties." Citizens were expected to be self-reliant and industrious in their pursuit of health, and they were faulted for their perceived failure to embrace this new "politics of health," even if poverty and other social conditions mitigated against it. In writing about the social significance attached to illness, the historian Sander Gilman has observed that "the infected person is never value-neutral."[22]

Although the concept of "citizen" that was operative in revolutionary and postrevolutionary Paris did not have the same powerful ideological value in late nineteenth-century Tokyo, the 1870s saw the emergence of a new conviction that improving the health of ordinary people was both a social and governmental responsibility and a means to establish the legitimacy of the new state. This commitment to ensuring accessible medical care was ultimately short-lived, and its demise ushered in the era of medical capitalism. The stance that health was a requirement for full civic participation remained unchanged and indeed grew stronger over time. Under the TMP, the goal of public health shifted from "protecting" the health of individual residents to "policing" their bodies for the benefit of society and the nation. As a result, poor health was transformed from an unfortunate but all too common aspect of urban life into a source of shame and stigma.

Mapping Medical Modernity is organized into six chapters. The first three trace the formation of policy and transformation of the city over the course of the nineteenth century. Chapter 1 examines the healthscape of the early modern city of Edo, focusing on the limited provisions for health care provided by the city magistrates and their commoner counterparts and the nature of the early modern medical marketplace upon which most of the city's residents relied. It also explores the crucial last two decades of shogunal rule, which saw both the creation of new medical institutions and the collapse of the early modern medical marketplace. Chapter 2 turns to the post-1868 period and the emergence of new political concern for health as a governmental responsibility and the subsequent development of the Medical Policy, a master plan for institutionalizing so-called Western medicine and creating a functioning system of public health. The second half of the chapter turns to Tokyo, one of three cities designated as "test sites" for the Medical Policy. It explores the situation in the city in the 1870s, the problems that would shape efforts to implement the Medical Policy, and experimentation with a new administrative system designed to improve health in the city.

Chapter 3 examines the establishment of the new medical infrastructure in Tokyo, including doctors trained in "Western medicine" and the formation of hospitals, a new site of medical care. At the center of the chapter is the short-lived Tokyo Prefectural Hospital, a groundbreaking institution that sought to provide low-cost health care to the city's residents at the hands of the first generation of modern physicians, midwives, and nurses, while also improving the skills of the city's private physicians. Unfortunately, this effort to create a system of community health care would prove short-lived due to the prefecture's financial constraints and protests from private physicians. In the aftermath of the prefectural hospital's closing, a highly stratified system of privatized care soon emerged. While a host of private hospitals and clinics competed for paying patients, a very small number of charity institutions served the city's poor and working classes.

In contrast to the first three chapters, chapters 4 through 6 are topical in nature, with each focusing on a particular disease that became an object of new institutions and policies. While much of the literature on public health in Japan has centered on cholera and other acute infectious diseases, the first efforts to prevent and control an infectious disease focused instead on syphilis, the topic of chapter 4. Syphilis was a familiar disease that had plagued the city for centuries, but it now assumed new importance as a threat to male health, in particular. Inspired by policies used in several European countries, local authorities instituted a licensing system for prostitutes in the early 1870s. To obtain a license, women in the sex trade were required to submit to regular examinations for syphilis and to agree to confinement for treatment if they were found to be infected. It soon became apparent that this system was not effective. As cases of syphilis increased among the city's residents, private hospitals and clinics, claiming expertise in the treatment of sexually transmitted infections, proliferated.

Chapter 5 takes up another overlooked aspect of public health policy in this era, concern for the mentally ill. Amid the disorder of the 1870s, the mentally ill were increasingly viewed as a threat to public safety and social order, which led to the establishment of the Tokyo Prefectural Asylum in Ueno Park, a profound innovation for a country in which the "mad" were traditionally confined within their homes. Eventually, the asylum was relocated to the more sparsely populated Sugamo area of Koishikawa Ward, on the outskirts of the city. Private hospitals were soon established in the area around the prefectural institution, which was renamed Sugamo Hospital. Although the private hospitals accepted some paying patients, their financial viability depended primarily on *itaku kanja*, patients who were committed involuntarily by the Tokyo Metropolitan Police.

Chapter 6 explores the crisis posed by repeated outbreaks of cholera in Tokyo and the local government's failed attempts to control them. Although early evidence suggested that the city's aging aqueduct system was responsible for the spread of contaminated water, neither the local nor central government was willing to commit the funds needed to undertake this kind of expensive infrastructure project. Unlike syphilis and mental illness, which could be regarded as issues of immoral or marginalized people, cholera posed a new kind of threat, one to which all Tokyo residents were vulnerable. The knowledge that cholera was spreading via the water supply, which was susceptible to contamination by human waste, confirmed the interconnectedness of city residents, and this led to new criticism of the poor, whose unhygienic living conditions were frequently cited as responsible for the spread of the disease. Amid intermittent struggles between the prefectural government and the Tokyo Metropolitan Police, the policies that emerged unfairly targeted the city's poor and working-class residents for conditions that were beyond their control.

In conclusion, *Mapping Medical Modernity* makes two intertwined arguments. First, it demonstrates that the ambitious plan for medical reform had only limited success in improving health in the city. The government's unwillingness to commit adequate funding to public health, the authoritarian stance embraced by the TMP, and resistance on the part of city residents, private physicians, and others meant that, while sickness and disease were newly stigmatized, many of the city's residents benefited little (and in some cases suffered greatly) from the stratified system of medical care that had emerged by the early twentieth century. While private for-profit clinics and hospitals proliferated in the city, their fees were high, leaving the poor no option but to rely on private philanthropy or on teaching institutions, where they were offered little privacy, respect, or compassion.

This outcome notwithstanding, medical modernization and public health led to the reconfiguration of urban space in enduring ways. Before 1868, Edo was a city organized around notions of status, with specific areas of the city designated for use by warriors, commoners, and outcast people. By the turn of the century, public health measures and medical capitalism had changed the city and the lives of those within it. Writing on the history of public health in Tianjin, China's third largest city and a treaty port, the historian Ruth Rogaski coined the term "hygienic modernity" to explain that health and sanitation had become linked to new ideas about modernity, race, and nation.[23] Although Tokyo differed from Tianjin in important ways—it was the capital of a new sovereign state and aspiring empire—hygienic modernity captures how health was now mediated by new ideas about class, gender, and prerogatives of the nation-state.

Problematic "populations," including syphilis-transmitting prostitutes and people with mental illness, were pushed to the margins of the city with the aim of safeguarding morality and social order within the city proper. And while pockets of poverty endured around the city, these areas and their residents were stigmatized as vectors of disease that threatened the health of the city's productive residents. By 1920, the healthscaping process had transformed health into a crucial attribute of the modern Japanese subject and reshaped the imperial capital.

1

Medical Edo

The Healthscape of the Early Modern Metropolis

The medical modernization of Tokyo that began in the 1870s was mediated by the existing healthscape of the early modern city of Edo. In the decades that followed, some aspects of the healthscape were preserved, others were dismantled, and new institutions, practitioners, and policies took form. This chapter explores the provisions for health care that shaped urban life during the 250 years of shogunal rule. By the early nineteenth century, Edo had become an important center of medical care, home to many physicians and several medical institutions that received shogunal support. The impact of these developments is the subject of debate. Writing in the 1990s, the historian Susan Hanley argued that the health of the Japanese people before modernity was on a par with or superior to Americans and Europeans in the same period.[1] More recent research, however, casts the situation in Edo in less rosy terms. The historical demographer Murakoshi Kazunori used the genealogies of the roughly two hundred daimyo (senior vassals of the shogun) who resided in Edo to explore infant and child mortality, a key population health indicator. He argues that while infant mortality among these families, the most privileged of Edo's residents, was lower in the city than in the other castle towns in the seventeenth century, it increased significantly over time, reaching 396 per 1,000 live births by the early nineteenth century, more than double the rate in the late seventeenth century. Childhood mortality (ages one to five) also increased over the eighteenth and nineteenth centuries, albeit less dramatically. Murakoshi speculates that the rising rates of infant and childhood mortality were due to increasingly poor conditions within the city as the population grew.[2]

Murakoshi's research raises important questions about the densely populated urban environment of Edo, its impact on the health of city residents, and the availability of medical care. In 1700 Edo was still a relatively new city with a history of only about a century, but it was already one of the largest cities in the world. Its estimated population of about one million made it significantly larger than Beijing, London, and Paris at the time. The city would continue to grow with some scholars speculating that population may have reached as much as two million by 1860.[3] It was, however, quite compact: the outskirts of the city were within ten kilometers of the various gates of Edo Castle, which stood in the city's center. A relatively healthy adult could then traverse the length or breadth of the city on foot in a matter of hours. As in other cities of the early modern world, urban life was highly stratified, although in this case by conceptions of status rather than by class, race, or ethnicity. The natural topography of the area was used to reinforce the emergent status system imposed by the Tokugawa state, most notably the division between samurai and commoners. The highlands in the western part of the city were designated for warrior residences, while the lowlands of the eastern city were largely populated by commoners.

Plate 1 represents the elevation of the city today. Although the physical environment of the city has changed over the course of several centuries—landfill has caused elevated lowlands, waterways have been filled or diverted, and highlands, leveled—it is still possible to discern the topographical divide that once shaped city life. Edo Castle and the adjacent areas that were reserved for warriors of rank occupied some of the highest land in city, while the areas devoted primarily to commoner residences (Nihonbashi, Kyōbashi, Fukagawa, Honjo, and parts of Shiba) were established on low-lying land. Outcast people, including members of the officially recognized beggar fraternity (*hinin*) and those who engaged in stigmatized occupations (*eta*), were confined to a particularly low-lying area of what would later become Asakusa Ward. As plate 2 illustrates, population density also diverged along this topographical divide. About 66 percent of the total area of the city was utilized by warrior households in the eighteenth century, although warriors made up only about 30 percent of the city's population. In contrast, the burgeoning commoner population was limited to less than 20 percent of the city's area, with the remainder held by temples and shrines.[4] As a result, neighborhoods occupied primarily by commoners were densely populated, with as many as 55,000 people living in one square kilometer, more than four times the density of the parts of the city that were primarily occupied by warriors.[5]

The topographical divides and the differing degrees of population density that accompanied them had an impact on the health of city residents in several ways. For one thing, the residents of the low areas were disproportionately vulnerable to natural and man-made disasters. Situated near or below sea level, these areas were threatened by the many floods that occurred in this era. In July and August, heavy summer rains and the storm surges and high tides that accompanied typhoons often caused the many rivers (the Sumida, Edo, Kanda, Tone, and Ara) that ran through the city and neighboring areas to swell. Although the shogunate actively engaged in river management to control flooding, its efforts were not entirely successful, and major floods occurred in 1680, 1704, 1721, 1723, 1735, 1742, 1749, 1780, 1786, 1802, 1846, and 1856. In August 1680, for example, heavy rains followed by a storm surge caused heavy flooding in Honjo and Fukagawa, which resulted in the deaths of an estimated seven hundred people and the destruction of more than three thousand residences.[6] Commoner neighborhoods, where wooden houses and shops were crowded together, were also vulnerable to the many fires that swept through Edo. At least fifteen significant fires took place in Edo between 1601 and 1855, and no less than six of these began in commoner neighborhoods. In 1760, for example, fire broke out in a shop in Kanda. It quickly spread, eventually jumping the Sumida River and causing considerable damage in Honjo and Fukagawa.[7]

Disasters then threatened the lives of Edo residents, but more importantly for this work, so too did a variety of pathogens. Repeated outbreaks of epidemic diseases, most notably smallpox and measles, spread quickly in the crowded commoner neighborhoods. The medical historian Fujikawa Yū documented thirteen outbreaks of measles and six of smallpox between 1607 and 1862.[8] Gastrointestinal diseases too were commonplace, even before cholera was introduced in Japan in the early nineteenth century. Some were likely caused by intestinal parasites, which entered the human body via a reliance on human waste as fertilizer for food crops. It is worth noting that parasitic diseases continued to be a public health issue well into the postwar era, when mass screening and treatment brought a rapid decline in the number of cases.[9]

Other outbreaks of gastrointestinal disease probably resulted from the contamination of the city's water supply. To supply the city with drinking water, a system of aqueducts was constructed in the late sixteenth and early seventeenth centuries. The first of these dated from the 1590s. Known as the

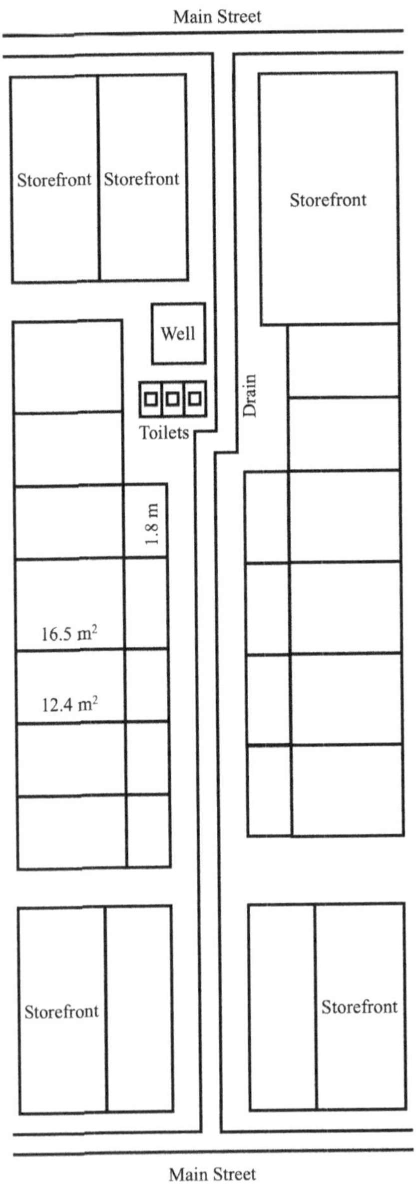

Figure 1.1. The layout of a typical backstreet "longhouse" complex in Edo and early Tokyo. Note the proximity of the well to the communal toilets. Diagram by Hannah Tomio, adapted from image available at https://www.token.co.jp/estate/history/edo/.

Kanda aqueduct, it moved water from Inokashira Pond, located twenty kilometers outside of the city center, through open channels until it reached a weir at Sekiguchi in Koishikawa. From there the water entered a system of underground wooden and bamboo pipes that provided water to Koishikawa, Ushigome, Kanda, and Nihonbashi, before finally being discharged into the Sumida River. As Edo's population grew, the Kanda aqueduct could no longer supply enough water for city residents, and construction began in the 1650s on a second aqueduct. This was the Tamagawa aqueduct, which moved water from the Tama River through forty-three kilometers of open conduits into the city. At Yotsuya, the water moved underground to Akasaka, Azabu, Shiba, Kōjimachi, and Kyōbashi, before being discharged into the Sumida River. Edo residents accessed water through a system of wells that were connected to the aqueducts.

Large swaths of the city, however, did not have access to this water. The aqueduct system never extended to the area east of the Sumida River, leaving residents to rely on water dealers and the brackish groundwater accessible via wells in these low-lying areas. Significantly, some of the warrior residents of the city's highlands were in a similar situation, since engineering knowledge at the time could not solve the issue of how to bring aqueduct water to the most elevated areas of the city. They, too, then had to rely on water dealers, whose water was of unknown origin and quality. What the city's elite could avoid, however, was the likely contamination of aqueduct water due to the proximity of wells and toilets. While samurai elites lived in large estates, many commoners resided in so-called longhouses (*nagaya*), one-story wooden structures that were divided into small single-room apartments. These buildings were typically sandwiched between parallel streets lined with the homes and businesses of more prosperous city residents, and residents shared communal toilets and a well (see fig. 1.1). The toilets were quite simple: waste was collected in underground wooden, earthenware, or ceramic containers and removed from the containers through an opening in the floors. The proximity of the toilets to the wells (and often to community garbage dumps as well) meant that drinking water could easily be contaminated.

In cities across Europe in the early modern period, repeated episodes of bubonic plague over the course of several centuries gave rise to many of the strategies now associated with modern public health systems, including the use of quarantine, cordon sanitaire, and even attempts at what we now call contact tracing.[10] In Edo, however, the situation was different. Although the shogunate would eventually provide financial support to a limited number of medical facilities, for the most part, residents relied on the medical marketplace made up of profit-driven private doctors, itinerant practitioners of various types, pharmacies, and faith-based healing offered by shrines and temples. This situation began to change in the final decades of shogunal rule as the new threat of cholera, the growing popularity of "Western medicine," and the outbreak of civil war threatened the medical culture of the time.

Governance and Health Care in Edo

Responsibility for managing the commoner areas of the growing city was in the hands of the two city magistrates, who were selected from among the high-ranking direct retainers of the shogun. Aided by a skeleton force of only 120 lower-ranking samurai officials each, the magistrates were primarily concerned with maintaining law and order. They investigated crimes, determined punishments, and managed the city's jail.[11] Much of the management of other aspects of urban life in the commoner areas was in the hands of the three city elders (*machidoshiyori*), members of three prominent commoner families who had forged a relationship with the shogunate in the early days of the city. Their work was supported by the more than two hundred *machi* headmen (*machi nanushi*), the lowest level of urban officials. A *machi* was the basic unit of the city and consisted of the lots along both sides of a block-long section of a street. These were typically demarcated by gates that were closed at night, and access to the machi was controlled by guards, who were tasked with keeping out troublemakers. Initially Edo was made up of about three hundred machi but as the city grew so did their number. By the mid-eighteenth century there were 1,678 machi. Each of the machi headmen was responsible for multiple machi, from as few as three to ten or more. Below them were the *ienushi*, who were in charge of a single machi.[12]

This network of commoner officials played an important role in managing the everyday life of the city's commoners, including matters that affected the health of the populace. They were responsible for ensuring the removal of household garbage and other waste and organizing appropriate aid to people who were sick, injured, elderly, and destitute. They played an important role in maintaining the city's water supply. The aqueduct system required upkeep to continue operating smoothly. Failure to clean and dredge the open canals led to flooding in the city, while the pipe system required regular monitoring and repair lest brackish groundwater and other contaminants enter the water supply.[13] Commoner officials were also involved in providing aid during outbreaks of epidemic disease. For example, in 1803, when a measles epidemic in Edo led to spiraling prices for medicines and the foods believed to aid recovery, the magistrates ordered the town elders to crack down on merchants who engaged in price gouging.[14]

Beyond these efforts, however, Edo's authorities, commoner and samurai alike, generally treated sickness and disease as private concerns and left them to individuals and families to manage. There were important exceptions to this general rule. The city magistrates exercised some oversight of institutions that were established over time to provide a safety net of sorts for the city's most vulnerable residents (see plate 3). For much of the early modern period, these were limited to the *tame* or "holding places" managed by the city's beggar fraternity, the Yōjōsho, an infirmary for the city's poor, and the Igakukan or "Medical Institute," a shogunate-supported medical school. In the late 1850s, concerned commoners created a vaccination clinic for smallpox, which eventually received shogunal support as well.

Of these, the *tame* was not a medical facility per se, although it was responsible for providing medical care to its residents. Four outcast "huts" (*hiningoya*) in Edo, in Asakusa, Fukagawa, Shinagawa, and Yoyogi, housed members of the city's beggar fraternity, which comprised people who, because of their birth, disability, or some other reason, were reduced to outcast status. Although traditionally termed "huts," the areas were distinguished from commoner neighborhoods primarily by the thatched roofs of the structures within them, since sumptuary laws forbade outcast people from living in homes with ceramic roof tiles.[15] Each of the "huts" had its own head man, and two of these, Kurumazenshichi of Asakusa and Matsuemon of Shinagawa, also oversaw a *tame*, a set of buildings enclosed by walls that were located near the "huts." The *tame* housed a heterogeneous population of the city's sick and vulnerable people. Both were initially established in 1687, and their operation was made the responsibility of the beggar fraternity. Like other status groups in this period, fraternity members were allowed certain privileges (in this case, the right to beg) but in return were required to perform certain kinds of public service. The management of the *tame* and its residents was one of the primary roles of the beggar fraternity.

By the eighteenth century, the *tame* in Asakusa was located in an area of the city to which stigmatized people and practices were relegated by design (see plate 4). Nearby was Yoshiwara, the brothel district; the Kozukahara execution ground; the "eta village," where the leatherwork industry, a lucrative but stigmatized occupation, was relegated; and Saruwakachō, the theater district, the site of an immensely popular but officially disdained form of entertainment. This spatial organization notwithstanding, it was not sickness itself that was stigmatized, but its association with poverty, criminality, lack of familial ties, or some combination of these factors.

Combining the function of a prison hospital, orphanage, poorhouse, and hospice, the two *tame* housed seriously ill prisoners from the city's jail, as well as ordinary commoners who were elderly, infirm, or disabled and without family support, orphaned and abandoned children, and travelers and homeless people who fell ill. They were also used to house those suffering from *ranshin* ("disordered heart"), the term used to describe people with mental illness and others whose socially aberrant behavior was a cause for concern, although in some cases *ranshin* sufferers were also confined in the city's jail.[16] As the Asakusa *tame* expanded after 1700, it included a structure reserved for female patients and dedicated spaces for sufferers of "disordered heart." Although the *tame* was involved in providing medical care to those in their charge, no doctors were on staff. Instead, medical care was provided by commoner doctors who came once a day to examine the sick and prescribe medicines. The actual preparation and administration of medicines was the responsibility of one of the fraternity members who staffed the *tame*, known as the *tame kusuri yaku* (medical official).[17] The number of those cared for in the *tame* was quite small, especially when considered as a ratio of the population of the city. In 1770, for example, the two *tame* cared for a total of 847 people over the course of twelve months.[18]

Unlike the *tame*, another shogunate-supported institution, the Seyakuin (charity infirmary), also known as the Yōjōsho (institute for health cultivation), was a thoroughly medical institution. Writing in 1889, one author declared it to be "a point of origin for the national hospital of this era," noting that "the intent of both institutions was the same, in spite of other differences great and small."[19] The assertion that the Yōjōsho was akin to a public hospital is problematic, but it was an innovative institution in its time. It was proposed by a commoner doctor named Ogawa Shōsen. In July 1721, the reform-minded eighth shogun Tokugawa Yoshimune ordered that a suggestion box be established near one of the gates of Edo Castle three days each month, and notices were posted around the city inviting residents to submit proposals to improve life within the city. A few months later, Ogawa submitted a proposal to establish a new facility to provide medicines and medical care to the city's working poor. He argued that many in Edo lacked the resources to buy medicines, and lived alone, without a spouse, children, or other relatives to care for them when they fell ill.[20]

This was no doubt true, and Ogawa's proposal came at an opportune moment, amid growing concern within the shogunate about the large number of migrants in the city, many of whom eked out a living as day laborers or by other kinds of casual work. An illness could quickly reduce these marginalized city residents to destitution and transform them into *mushuku hinin* or "homeless beggars" who were not part of the beggar fraternity, making them a troubling population for Edo's officials.[21] Yoshimune ordered the city magistrates to meet with Ogawa to discuss his proposal. According to the plan that emerged from these discussions, the new institution was to be staffed by low-ranking doctors in service to the shogunate (*yoriai'i* and *kobunshin'i*). They would treat patients from late morning to early afternoon each day, while town doctors who lived nearby were to be "on call" at other times in case an emergency arose. Patients would be provided with a set of clothes, according to the season, and with bedding and other supplies as needed. The clinic was to be funded and managed by the town magistrates, who would purchase necessary supplies, provide security, transport patients to the facility, and pay for the funerals of those who died while in care.[22]

The shogunate had its own interests in mind in making such generous provisions: the new institution offered an opportunity to demonstrate its commitment to "benevolent rule," the ideological position that prompted other forms of public relief, such as distributions of rice to the poor during times of famine. Based on Confucian notions of governance, the concept of "benevolent rule" required both the shogun and the daimyo to help those in need directly but also to encourage those below them to do the same. In keeping with this conception of benevolence, certain costs were made the responsibility of the city elders, including the rent for the land the facility stood on, which was adjacent to the shogunate's medicinal garden in Koishikawa.[23] The garden had been established in 1684, after a smaller garden created in Azabu forty years earlier was relocated to this larger site of about 15,000 hectares. In this period, the shogunate was concerned about the mounting cost of importing expensive raw drugs from elsewhere in Asia, a trade that was draining Japan of hard currency.[24] In an attempt to develop domestic sources, the garden was used to experiment with the cultivation of medicinal herbs that were native to other parts of Asia and to identify indigenous substitutes. The location of the clinic, adjacent to the garden in an area dotted with daimyo mansions, was a pleasant one, although far from the crowded commoner neighborhoods (see plate 3).

The Yōjōsho opened just a few months after Ogawa submitted his proposal. It was initially housed in a *nagaya*, a one-story rectangular wooden structure with a thatched roof and comprising three wards, one for women and two for men, as well as an examination room for outpatients, a kitchen, and offices for staff.[25] The day-to-day management of the new institution was in the hands of twelve samurai officials from the magistrates' office. The medical staff consisted initially of two practitioners of *hondō* or internal medicine, but by the following year, the number of doctors had grown to five and included two experts in "external medicine" (*geka*), who treated wounds and other injuries, and a specialist in eye diseases. Among the other employees were two women who worked as nurses, as well as cooks, cleaners, and guards.[26]

At the planning stage, to forestall concerns that the new institution would be overwhelmed with patients, a burdensome admissions procedure was put in place. Those seeking care were to apply to the head of the local machi, who was then to investigate the circumstances of the potential patient and make a recommendation to the magistrates' office on whether the person in question qualified for admission. Initially, it seems that some machi officials were disinclined to do this, either because of the work involved or perhaps because they feared it would cast them in a bad light by suggesting that they were unable to manage the situation on their own.[27] In addition, rumors swirled around the new, unfamiliar facility, which may have discouraged potential patients. It was said that patients were to be used as test subjects for the herbs being grown in the medicinal garden and that people would be treated only with domestic ginseng, generally regarded as inferior to that imported from the Korean peninsula. Reflecting the newness of institutionalized medical care, it was rumored that the nursing staff was recruited from among the outcasts, suggesting that initially some people conflated the Yōjōsho with the *tame*. The city magistrates responded by ordering the machi headman to stamp out such rumors, but they also streamlined the admission process. Patients were allowed to go directly to the clinic for care and, if necessary, an investigation into their circumstances could take place after the fact.[28]

These efforts paid off, and the number of patients began to grow. In time, four new wards were constructed and the capacity of the hospital eventually tripled to 150 beds. Initially, patients were limited to no more than a two-month stay, at which point their case was presumed to be hopeless and they were discharged, but eventually the maximum stay was extended to twelve months.[29] As the number of inpatients increased, the Yōjōsho ended the practice of treating outpatients, although exceptions were made for some groups. For example, patients with leprosy were not admitted to the facility but were treated as outpatients.[30] However, the focus on inpatients, many of whom were chronically ill, meant that the impact of the Yōjōsho, like the *tame*, was limited. In the early nineteenth century, it was providing care for only 500–800 people a year.[31]

In addition to the *tame* and the Yōjōsho, a third official institution offered medical care to Edo residents. This was the Igakukan or "medical institute," a medical school that was funded by the shogunate from 1791. The school had its origins in a private medical academy known as the Seijukan, which was founded in 1765 by Taki Motokata, a medical official of the shogunate. It received a degree of shogunal support from the time of its founding, presumably because it was performing a public service by providing medical training. The shogunate granted Taki a plot of land in Sakuma-chō in Kanda on which to build his school, and it subsequently ordered commoner doctors to make "donations" to fund the school.[32] At first, Taki's school offered medical instruction to would-be doctors from different status groups, including commoners, low-ranking shogunal doctors, and the sons of medical officials.[33] The education on offer was relatively broad, although wholly within the textual traditions of Chinese medicine. There were lectures on both "ancient medicine" (that is, Han-era medical classics) and the "latter-day school," which focused on Chinese medical knowledge from the twelfth to the fourteenth centuries. The "latter-day school" had been the dominant form of medical knowledge in Japan until the seventeenth century, when "ancient medicine," which focused less on abstract theory and more on empirically based treatments, began to attract a growing number of adherents. In addition, students received training in *honzōgaku*, the study of materia medica.[34]

The "bureaucratization" of the school, as Machi Senjurō has termed the shogunate's decision to fund it fully in 1791, was prompted by several factors. For one thing, donations notwithstanding, the Seijukan struggled financially and seemed unlikely to survive without a new funding source. In addition, there was growing concern at this time about the proliferating number of poorly trained doctors who, in the words of one observer, "forgot about virtue and cared only about profit."[35] Political concerns were involved as well. Matsudaira Sadanobu, then the chief official of the shogunate, wanted to restore the moral authority of the government. His predecessor, Tanuma Okitsugu, had become notorious for fostering a culture of corruption that Matsudaira sought to counter by, among other things, making the shogunate a patron of education. However, official support of the medical school fundamentally changed its mission. For the next four decades, it was solely concerned with training medical officials, and it was not until 1832 that commoner doctors were again allowed to attend its lectures.[36]

One aspect of the medical school that did not change after 1791 was the effort to provide students with some clinical training, a practice that brought them into contact with commoner residents of the city. The building that housed the Seijukan included a ten-tatami room (approximately fifteen square meters in area) known as the "patient examination room," where patients were treated six days a month. In 1793, two years after the shogunate took over the institution, an attempt was made to put the Yōjōsho, which had to this point been administered by the town magistrates, under the direction of the Medical Institute. The aim of this plan was threefold: to improve the quality of care at the Yōjōsho, to reduce the costs of its operation, and to strengthen the clinical training of Medical Institute students. Problems soon became apparent, however. The Medical Institute's leadership was committed to the text-based study of medicine to which clinical training was an adjunct, and it was ill-prepared for the transition from operating a small outpatient clinic a few days a month to managing an institution with more than a hundred resident patients who required daily care. In addition, the financial arrangement proposed, which would have shifted the cost of medicines provided to Yōjōsho patients to the Medical Institute, was also unappealing from the perspective of the Taki family. In the end, the planned merger was abandoned.[37]

Clinical education at the Medical Institute continued, albeit on a limited basis. After a fire in 1806 destroyed the Sakuma-chō structure, the school was rebuilt in Shitaya and the new facilities included both a patient waiting room (interestingly, termed a *tame* in some sources) and an examination room.[38] On clinic days, five or six student doctors took turns examining, diagnosing, and treating patients under the guidance of their instructors. According to one source, "patients were few in number and the atmosphere was one of a school."[39] Although case notes were compiled detailing the symptoms and treatments of patients, only fourteen examples survive. These suggest that most patients were adults and residents of tenement housing in nearby neighborhoods in Kanda, Hongō, and Koishikawa, although some patients came from outside the city. The ailments treated were varied in nature and included paralysis, eye disorders, menstrual difficulties, and even one case of a toothache.[40]

Edo's Medical Marketplace

The *tame*, Yōjōsho, and Medical Institute clinic were the only "public" medical institutions in the city, and they provided care annually to only 2,000–3,000 of the city's 650,000 or more commoner residents. As a result, most people in Edo relied instead on what I will call the "medical marketplace" for their medical treatments. This term was adopted by Anglophone historians in the 1980s to described the diversity of commercialized forms of medical care available in early modern England and elsewhere, including physicians, surgeons, apothecaries, and others, but it also describes the situation in early modern Japan and certainly in Edo.[41] Over the course of the early modern period, a flourishing new medical culture emerged in Japan, and it quickly became an integral part of daily life, first in cities and later in villages. The rapid expansion of print culture played an important role in promoting interest in medicine among both would-be doctors and the public. In the seventeenth century an extraordinary profusion of medical texts began to be published, including medical treatises, commentaries, dictionaries, formularies, collections of case notes, and health manuals, contributing to the diffusion of medical knowledge to aspiring doctors and patients alike. Significant too was the emergence of new opportunities for medical education: established doctors in villages, cities, and towns began to take on students, making medical training available as never before. But other less quantifiable factors were also involved: the rising standard of living in this era of relative peace and prosperity, the new commodity culture, and the tensions of the status system, which prompted the ambitious or disgruntled to pursue different occupations and other social roles.

We can learn much about Edo's medical marketplace from the texts that were circulated to help the city's residents navigate it. Three directories of the city's doctors were published between 1819 and 1825. Taken together, the *A Directory of Physicians in Edo in This Era* (*Edo kinsei ika jinmeiroku*, 1819), *A Directory of Physicians* (*Ika jinmei roku*, 1820), and *A Directory of Physicians in Edo in This Era* (*Edo kinsei ika jinmeiroku*, 2nd ed., 1825) provide information on 2,192 doctors, including their names, addresses, and medical specialties.[42] These works were not exhaustive, as their authors readily admitted. In the preface to the 1819 inaugural volume, which had 542 entries, the authors Takei Shūsaku and Inaba Katsudō asked doctors whose names were omitted to contact them so they could be included in the planned second edition. Similar sentiments were expressed by Shiratsuchi Ryūhō, the editor of the four-volume 1820 work, although this edition contained an additional 1,503 names.

Of the 2,192 doctors listed in the directories, 56 resided outside the city itself: 19 in post-stations such as Hachiōji, Senju, and Shinagawa, which stood along the highways that provided access to Edo, and the others in villages in what are now Chiba, Saitama, and Ibaragi Prefectures. However, even if we exclude the doctors who lived outside of Edo, the city was awash with doctors. Although doctors were scattered widely around Edo, most were clustered in densely populated areas west of the Sumida River such as Kanda, Nihonbashi, and Kyōbashi (see plate 5). In contrast, low-lying Fukagawa, west of the Sumida, had comparatively few doctors. This pattern is important: it would persist into the early twentieth century. Today, the World Health Organization (WHO) recommends a minimum of one doctor per one thousand in population. Although it is difficult to discern Edo's true population at any given moment, if we use the conventional figure of one million, Edo had a ratio of 2.175 doctors per thousand in population, more than double the WHO guideline. And since the directories omitted many casual or itinerant practitioners in favor of more elite doctors, the actual number of doctors may have been much higher.

Many of those listed in the directories were "domanial doctors" (*han'i*)—that is, doctors in the employ of one of the daimyo. More than half of the city's doctors were employed as domanial doctors, and 60 percent of these resided on the grounds of one of their employer's estates, a pattern reflected in plates 5 and 6. The white dots are used to show the location of domanial doctors, many of whom lived in parts of the city where warrior residences predominated. For example, roughly 11 percent of the city's doctors resided in the area outside the inner moat of Edo Castle, known as Kōjimachi, a part of the city reserved for warrior residences, and a similar percentage resided in Shiba, where many daimyo families maintained a second (or third) residence.

As their listings in the physician directories suggest, many domanial doctors pursued extra income through a sideline private practice. A case in point is the physician and scholar Sugita Genpaku. Sugita was born in Edo as the son of a domanial doctor in service to the Sakai family, lords of Obama Domain (now part of Fukui province). He followed his father's path and was employed by the Sakai lord beginning in 1752, and he continued in this position until his retirement in 1807. Initially, he attended to family members in their residence near Edo Castle and later in their *naka yashiki* (secondary residence) in Hamamatsu-chō. Although at times he lived on the grounds of one or another of the domanial estates, for most of his life, he also maintained his own residence, first in Nihonbashi and later in Hamamatsu.[43] In the late eighteenth century, Sugita gained fame for his leading role in the pioneering translation of *Ontleedkundige Tafelen*, a Dutch version of a German anatomical text authored by Johann Adam Kulmus. With only a rudimentary knowledge of Dutch at the outset, Sugita and his colleagues labored for three years on the work they called *Kaitai shinsho* (A New Book of Anatomy).[44] Published in 1774, it spurred new interest in "Dutch medicine," as European medicine was then known.

Sugita was also a busy practicing physician. His diary, which covers the years from 1787 to 1804, when his fame was at its height, reveals that his position as domanial doctor notwithstanding, he spent much of his time treating private patients. In the 1780s and early 1790s, he generally devoted four to six days a month attending to members of the Sakai family, but after about 1794 his official duties were limited to a day or two per month. In contrast, throughout this period, he saw on average between thirty-three and fifty-two private patients each month, typically at a pace of two or three patients a day over the course of thirteen to twenty-one days of the month.[45]

The prevalence of domanial doctors like Sugita in Edo was one of the characteristics of its medical marketplace, but there were many commoner doctors as well. In plates 5 and 6, the residences of commoner doctors are indicated by black dots. It is not much of an exaggeration to say that there was a doctor in every machi of the commoner neighborhoods east of the castle. The organization of the directories—medical specialty first, then location, then name—seems to have been designed to aid readers in locating a physician close to them.[46] The 1820 work was in fact divided into four volumes covering the northern, southern, eastern, and western parts of the city, respectively.

That said, the location of a doctor's residence may not have been as significant as this organization implies. Sugita's diary reveals that at times he traveled considerable distance to see patients who were scattered around the city. For example, on December 6, 1804, a day he describes as cloudy and cold, Sugita saw patients in Honmachi in Nihonbashi, Honjo, and Asakusa. The next day, he traveled to Ōtsuka Village and from there to Yoshiwara, a distance of roughly eight kilometers. After taking December 8 off to attend a social event, Sugita returned to work the next day, visiting a patient near his home in Hamamatsu-chō, before journeying to Kanda to see patients in Ogawa-chō and Surugadai, about five kilometers away.[47] To traverse the city, Sugita often used boats and sedan chairs but sometimes he simply walked from one destination to another.[48]

Sugita was by no means an ordinary doctor, and it is unlikely that all Edo's physicians were similarly in demand. Indeed, there is evidence of considerable fluidity in the medical marketplace. A comparison of the 1819 and 1825 editions of *Edo kinsei ika jinmeiroku* reveals that about 20 percent of the doctors listed in the first edition were no longer included in the second and had been replaced by a similar number of new names. The high concentration of doctors in Edo likely meant that not every doctor was successful in attracting patients, and a significant number seemed to have either moved on to other pursuits or relocated to an area with less competition. In this competitive environment, the physician directories also functioned to advertise the services of the doctors listed. This was particularly the case for the 1820 edition, which offered doctors the option of including additional information, presumably for a fee. Of the 1,503 doctors listed in the directory, 126 chose to insert additional information to advertise their services. These additions took a variety of forms. Some simply noted that the doctor lived within a daimyo estate, presumably a mark of distinction; others introduced the proprietary medicines they sold, the books they had written, or the history of their medical lineage, all ways of establishing their expertise.[49]

A more subtle form of advertisement is seen in the medical specialties that the doctors provided for their listings in the directories, information that was highlighted by listing it at the top of each entry. Of the doctors listed in the directories, 80 percent listed just a single area of expertise, most often *naika* or *honka*. Both terms refer to the orthodox form of Sino-Japanese medicine, which relied primarily on the use of medicinal compounds as treatment. However, some doctors listed multiple specialties, as many as five in a few cases. The most common specialties included *geka* or "external medicine,"

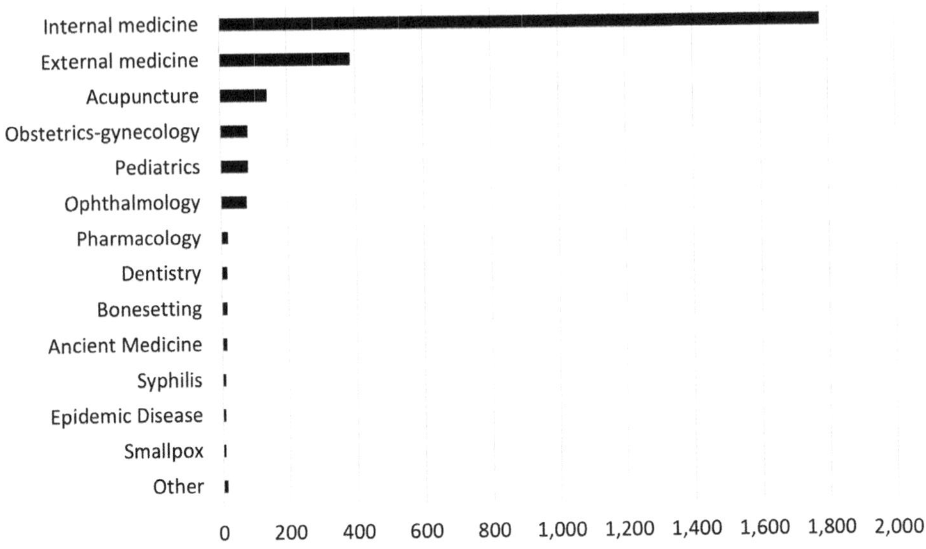

Figure 1.2. Number of medical specialties that appear in physician directories, 1819–1825. Data are from Takei and Inaba, *Edo kinsei ika jinmeiroku* (1819), Shiratsuchi, *Ika Jinmeiroku* (1820), and Takei and Inaba, *Edo kinsei jinmei roku* (2nd ed., 1825).

acupuncture, obstetrics and gynecology (OB-GYN), and ophthalmology, although bonesetting and dentistry were also represented. A minority of doctors claimed expertise in relation to specific ailments (listed under "other" in fig. 1.2), among them, syphilis, smallpox, edema, lung disease, and even "epidemic disease" (*ekibyō*). Interestingly, although medical histories of this era often draw attention to the tensions between different "schools"—"Dutch medicine" (*ranpō*) versus "ancient medicine" (*kohō*) versus "latter-day medicine" (*gōseihō*)—few doctors mentioned such affiliations. Only four doctors claimed to be practitioners of Dutch medicine, while another thirteen self-identified as practitioners of "ancient medicine." It thus seems likely that such designations meant little to prospective patients.

The services of an elite doctor like Sugita—or any doctor—would have been beyond the reach of many Edo residents, who instead turned to self-treatment using commercially available medicines. Although physicians, at least in theory, prepared medicinal compounds individually for a specific patient, adjusting a standard formula to suit the patient's constitution and specific cluster of symptoms, many mass-produced "prepared medicines" were advertised in broadsheets, handbills, and "efficacy pamphlets." It was not unusual for prepared medicines to be sold in single doses at a low cost, a practice that made them accessible even to the poor, while also facilitating a "try it and see" approach on the part of patients. However, prepared medicines were not necessarily the first resort for treating common ailments, they were also used in concert with the medicines prescribed and prepared by an attending doctor. In this period, many patients adopted a pluralistic approach to treatment, sometimes seeking out the care of multiple doctors, simultaneously or in succession, while also dosing themselves with prepared medicines they purchased or received as sickbed gifts.[50]

Residents of Edo had ready access to medicines from one of the many pharmacies in the city. The shopping guide *Edo kaimono hitori annai* (A Guide to Shopping in Edo on One's Own, 1824) lists 278 businesses dealing in raw and prepared medicines. Published in the form of a small portable volume (20 × 12 centimeters.), this work was a directory listing Edo's merchants, organized by categories of goods and services.[51] Fifty-five of the medicine shops listed in the guide were wholesalers, but the rest were retail pharmacies of one type or another. Many pharmacies (*kusuriya, yakushūya*) not only sold raw drugs and prepared medicinal compounds at the request of a doctor or patient but also manufactured and sold their own prepared medicines. According to the guide, twenty-nine pharmacies were involved in manufacturing proprietary medicines. Other pharmacies acted as the agents (*toritsugijo*) or distributors (*hiromejo*) for medicine manufacturers located outside of the city.

The *Edo kaimono hitori annai* reveals that Edo pharmacies distributed medicines produced by more than thirty manufacturers located in cities like Kyoto and Osaka, as well as those produced in more rural areas such as Ōmi, Ise, and Yamato. Almost 10 percent of the city's pharmacies (twenty-six shops) specialized in the sale of moxa, dried mugwort leaves that were burned on specific points of the body. "Moxibustion," as the use of moxa is termed, could be performed by a doctor but it was also a popular form of self-treatment. In addition to pharmacies, a variety of retailers (described as "other" in plate 7) sold prepared medicines. These included shops that specialized in sugar, sake, tooth powder, and incense, near Nihonbashi, where many wholesalers and some retail pharmacies and manufacturers were clustered. But beyond this area, retail pharmacies were scattered around the city. Business owners favored locations adjacent to the major highways that not only linked the city to the rest of Japan but also were used for travel around the city. Popular temples also became magnets for medicine merchants. One of these was Sensōji, a popular Buddhist temple in Asakusa that was known for its many amusements. Six pharmacies were located on or near temple grounds . But one did not need to journey to a pharmacy to buy a prepared medicine. Medicine peddlers (such as the person pictured in plate 8) plied their wares on the city's streets and at gathering places like temple grounds, where they performed tricks and displayed exotic oddities to capture the attention of audiences, who were then plied with exaggerated claims of efficacy. Although many prepared medicines drew upon orthodox formulas, manufacturers often claimed that their products were based on a "secret family recipe" or a "secret transmission" from some illustrious person of the distant past, presumably to heighten their appeal.

Another crucial part of Edo's medical marketplace was the many temples and shrines in and near the city that promised relief for common illnesses and other physical complaints to those who prayed, purchased amulets and votive talismans, and engaged in various forms of religious rites. The medical historian Tatsukawa Shōji has identified fifty-eight religious institutions in Edo and its outskirts that claimed the ability to help those suffering from poor health. Although a few asserted that they could relieve "all diseases," most were associated with one or more specific ailments. These included gynecological and obstetric issues like pregnancy and childbirth as well as eye problems, hemorrhoids, coughs, cancer, headaches, smallpox, and skin conditions. The rites they practiced varied. For example, Shiba Shinmeigū (now known as Shiba Daishingu), a branch of the famous Ise Shrine, was associated with the healing of eye diseases. Those who came in search of relief were offered access to the shrine's miraculous water, which was said to have healing properties when used to wash the eyes. In contrast, the Shingon temple Tōsenji, located in a village in the Katsushika District of Musashino (now Edogawa Ward), claimed to be able to cure cancerous growths by means of its fire ritual known as *goma-kitō*. Participants wrote their wish to be cured on little pieces of paper that were attached to small wooden sticks. The priest presiding over the ritual then tossed these into a purifying fire.

We can get a sense of how patients navigated the medical marketplace from the diaries kept by some families in this period as they nursed a family member through an illness. One such diary was kept by the family members of the popular author Takizawa Bakin as they dealt with the illness of Tarō, the grandson and heir of the family, who fell ill at the age of twenty.[52] His mother Michi nursed him through this illness and carefully recorded the family's efforts to return him to health. Between May 1848 and his death in June 1849, a period of thirteen months, Tarō was treated by at least eleven doctors, received regular moxibustion treatments at the hands of a specialist, and was dosed with a variety of prepared medicines purchased by Michi or provided by neighbors and friends. In addition to these medicalized treatments, the family pursued a variety of faith-based options. Michi and her daughter Sachi, Tarō's sister, visited a local temple, while friends brought amulets and, in one instance, introduced an exorcist. As his condition worsened, his mother became convinced that the family cat, taken in as a kitten about the time Tarō had fallen ill, was responsible for his illness, so she gave the cat away in a final desperate attempt to save her son.[53]

It is not surprising that the turn to faith-based and ritual practices was particularly pronounced in times of epidemic disease. Smallpox and measles, two of the most common infectious diseases in this period, were associated with malevolent deities, and efforts to control them took the form of both household-based and community-wide practices. Because the smallpox deity supposedly disliked the color red and dogs, children were sometimes dressed in red clothing and print images of red dogs were posted in entryways of houses to ward off the deity and the disease. Other rituals sought to appease the deity in question: some families set up temporary altars with an image of the deity and offered it sake and other delicacies; some families offered written apologies (*owabi sho*) to the deity, appealing to it to spare their relatives. Practices at the community level took the form of expulsion rituals (*hōsō yoke*, *hōsō nagashi*) that sought to drive the deity from the neighborhood.[54] These efforts did not mean, however, that smallpox and measles were not objects of medical care as well. Collections of formularies, treatises on therapies, and books offering advice to parents circulated in great number, attesting again to the pluralistic approach embraced by many.

The small number of "public" institutions and the booming medical marketplace meant that medical care in Edo at the time was both highly commercialized and highly stratified. Those of means could choose from among a variety of doctors, including even those who served the political elite of the day, and they also had access to an array of medicinal products, if for a price. Things were very different for the city's poor, many of whom would have lacked the funds to avail themselves of the goods and services on offer. The aid provided by the official medical facilities was always thin, and it would grow more frayed in the mid-nineteenth century as lack of funding, growing political tensions, and institutional change began to reshape medical care in the city.

Medical Edo in Transition

The fate of the Yōjōsho provides evidence of the fragility of the medical safety net available to Edo residents. Patient numbers at the clinic declined dramatically in the 1820s and 1830s, as conditions within the facility deteriorated. In some months, the Yōjōsho was only at half capacity. Driving the decline of the institution was a lack of funding. At the time of its founding, the town magistrates had provided 700 ryō of gold (a standard coin was about 37.5 grams) each year to support the institution and in 1732 they had increased their annual support to 800 ryō but that sum remained the same for the next hundred years, even as inflation eroded its value.[55] Lack of funds led to the disrepair of the buildings, although some renovations were made over the years, including the replacement of the thatched roof with tile in 1812.[56] The straitened circumstances of the clinic also contributed to the emergence of a new culture of corruption and graft. The poorly paid staff and administrators began to siphon off funds for their own use, as well as to extort kickbacks from patients, who were, as we have seen, among Edo's poorest residents.[57]

A report from 1832 suggests how bad conditions had become. In the building that housed the most seriously ill patients, the smell was so foul that "when people who are not even sick go to this place, they begin to feel ill." Another report, this one from 1836, noted that patients suffered greatly from the cold in winter and from heat and humidity in the summer and concluded that the building was not suitable for housing the sick. Eventually, the facility was rebuilt but with four rather than five wards, reflecting both the declining number of patients and financial constraints.[58] In 1843, in an attempt to improve the quality of care, oversight of the medical staff and patient care was turned over to fifteen town doctors.[59] The Yōjōsho would continue to function for another twenty years, but its impact on the health of the city's residents, always slight, was further diminished.

Growing political and ideological tensions also began to have an impact on the medical culture of the city. As ships from Europe, the US, and Russia appeared in Japanese waters, and news of the British victory in the Opium War with Qing China reached Japan, a rise in anti-foreign sentiment was bolstered by a nativist movement that celebrated Japan's "divine" nature. Some within the shogunate sought to exploit the moment to further their own interests. In 1839 one of the shogunate's official astronomers submitted a petition asking for greater scrutiny of the translation of Western astronomical works, which he characterized as heterodox and dangerous. Three years later, the shogunate responded by ordering the dissolution of the guild of book publishers in Edo, which had been entrusted with censoring publications according to shogunal restrictions. Instead of relying on self-policing by the guild, the shogunate made the town magistrates responsible for the screening of translations of

Western books.[60] In response, the magistrates entrusted the review of works on medicine to the heads of the Medical Institute, Taki Motokata and Tsujimoto Sūan. Both men were hostile to Dutch medicine, and they used their new role to try to crack down on its growing influence among doctors, if not patients.[61]

Their first opportunity came in 1843, when Mitsukuri Genpo (1799–1863), a physician, Dutch-learning scholar, and prolific translator, submitted the manuscript for a work he called *Taisei meii ikō* (Compendium of Articles by Renowned Western Doctors). Sometimes described as Japan's first medical journal, *Taisei mei ikō* was first published in 1836. This volume and those that followed offered readers access to articles by a variety of European authors.[62] Mitsukuri was a well-regarded figure in Edo, and in the 1850s he would be employed by the shogunate as a translator. Nonetheless, when he submitted the latest issue of his journal to the Medical Institute for inspection, the entirety of the work was banned, a decision that prompted the magistrate Torii Yōzō to inquire about the justification for this decision.

The response of the Medical Institute's leaders—that the popularity of Dutch medicine threatened the viability of Sino-Japanese medicine—made it clear that they were unlikely to approve the publication of any translation of a Western medical text. As we saw above, in the 1820s being identified as a practitioner of Dutch medicine did not seem to have been regarded as a selling point by most Edo doctors. Two decades later that had changed—at least in the eyes of Taki and Tsujimoto. Torii Yōzō pushed back, asserting that the important work of medicine was to preserve human life and that surely there were aspects of Dutch medicine worthy of consideration. In the end, however, Taki and Tsujimoto prevailed. Emboldened perhaps by this success, they successfully pressured the shogunate for new controls on the teaching and practice of Dutch medicine. In April 1849, the shogunate issued a ban on Dutch medicine in all its territories, and the Medical Institute was authorized to approve or reject the publication of all medical works.[63]

It was amid the Medical Institute's ascendancy that a transformative Western medical technology was introduced in Japan. Information about Edward Jenner's cowpox vaccination reached Japan as early as 1812, but it was not until mid-1849 that scabs containing cowpox matter were successfully transferred to Japan from the Dutch colony of Batavia. Vaccination of children quickly got underway, encouraged by a network of Dutch medicine physicians and supported by the daimyo of many domains. Within a few months, cowpox matter arrived in Edo, through the offices of Nabeshima Naomasa, the lord of Saga

Domain. Itō Genboku, a Dutch medicine physician employed by Nabeshima, used it to vaccinate Nabeshima's children and those of his vassals. He also shared the vaccine with fellow domanial physicians in Edo, who began to vaccinate the children of the domains they served as well as their private patients. What is noteworthy here is the lack of involvement of the shogunate, which played no role in the transfer of the vaccine to Edo or its use within the city.[64]

Ann Jannetta argues that this inaction indicated tacit approval rather than hostility on the part of the shogunate, but whatever the explanation, the early modern state played no direct role in what has been described by some as the origin of public health in Japan.[65] It was not until 1857 that the shogunate finally indicated approval for vaccination when a smallpox outbreak threatened the population of Ezo, as the island of Hokkaido was then known. In response, Edo's town magistrates recruited physicians in the city who could perform vaccinations and dispatched them to Ezo to vaccinate the children of the Indigenous residents of the island, known as Ainu.[66] By this time, the political situation in Japan had changed dramatically and so too had the shogunate's stance toward Western forms of knowledge, including medicine. After the arrival of Commodore Matthew Perry's fleet in 1853 and the "opening" of Japan to trade and foreign residents, many within and outside the shogunate came to believe that Western knowledge was key to national defense. In 1856 it created its own translation bureau, the Institute for the Examination of Barbarian Books (*Bansho Torishirabesho*); in 1857 it established a new medical school in Nagasaki under J. L. C. Pompe van Meedervort, a Dutch physician, as part of its new Naval Training Institute. The following year the ban on Dutch medicine came to an end, and two prominent Dutch medicine doctors, Itō Genboku and Totsuka Seikai, were hired to serve in the shogunal palace.

No doubt aware of the changing fortunes of Dutch medicine, some of Edo's most famous physicians organized to press for the creation of a clinic to facilitate the vaccination of city residents. Early in 1858, Mitsukuri Genpo, Itō Genboku, and Totsuka Seikai, among others, composed a petition to the town magistrates asking permission to establish such a facility. The shogunate ultimately agreed to this request, although it committed no funds. Instead, the vaccination clinic was financed by donations from Dutch medicine physicians in the city who jointly contributed more than 580 ryō to the project. These funds were used to establish the clinic on the site of the Kanda residence of a shogunal official named Kawaji Toshiakira, who had supported the petition effort. Unfortunately, only six months after its opening in June 1858, the clinic was destroyed by fire.

The loss of the vaccination clinic came during perhaps the most severe medical crisis in the city's history, one that revealed the devastating epidemiological consequences of the "opening" of the country. In July 1858 an American naval ship, the *Mississippi*, arrived in Nagasaki from China with infected sailors onboard.[67] This was in fact the second time cholera had been introduced in Japan. In 1822, in the midst of the first global cholera epidemic, the disease was transmitted to Japan, either from the Korean peninsula via the island of Tsushima or from the Dutch colony of Batavia via Nagasaki. Over the course of October and November the disease spread throughout Western Honshu, before stopping short of Edo.[68] Cholera is caused by *Vibrio cholerae*, a bacterium that originated in the warm waters of the Ganges Delta, and it cannot survive long in waters colder than about ten degrees Celsius. As a result, cholera epidemics often end with the onset of cold weather, and this seems to be what happened in Japan in 1822.[69] In 1858, however, the disease was introduced in July giving it ample time to spread during the warm months of summer, and within a month it had reached Edo.

The city's officials responded as best they could, distributing broadsheets that urged people to bind their abdomens with cotton or linen cloth, dress appropriately to ward off dampness, and avoid eating fruit, advice gleaned from European sources. The broadsheets also suggested possible treatments, such as drinking tea laced with *shōchū*, a distilled liquor, and sugar. This may have had some efficacy: heat and alcohol killed *V. cholerae* and the ingestion of fluids may have helped combat the dehydration that resulted from diarrhea and vomiting, the primary symptoms of cholera.[70] Meanwhile, the populace responded to the outbreak as they did to other more familiar forms of epidemic disease: they attached amulets to their doorways and charms to their persons and conducted rituals to appease the "epidemic deity" (*ekigami*) believed to be responsible for the disease. Contemporary accounts of the epidemic in Edo describe how crematoria in the city and local temple graveyards were overwhelmed by the unprecedented number of deaths.[71] By the end of the epidemic, it is estimated that between 40,000 and 200,000 people had died in the city.[72]

Even as the city was wracked by cholera, the proponents of vaccination regrouped to raise money to rebuild the clinic. A new site was chosen in Izumibashi-dōri in Shitaya, on a plot of land rented from two Tokugawa vassals. This was located not far from the home of Itō Genboku, who had transformed his residence into an ad hoc vaccination clinic after the Otamagaike clinic was destroyed.[73] Although the new clinic opened as a private institution in October 1860, within a few months the shogunate "bureaucratized" it, providing funding and official support. Ōtsuki Shunsai, a medical official of the shogunate, was made head of the clinic, and he developed an ambitious plan to transform it into an educational institution that would teach Western medical knowledge. In a petition submitted to the shogunate, he asked permission to conduct dissections at the clinic, arguing that this was the "foundation of Western medicine." All doctors, he wrote, required anatomical knowledge, and should have the opportunity to attend two or three dissections per year, and physicians in service to the shogunate would benefit from this training. The shogunate eventually approved this plan, and the clinic was officially renamed the Western Medicine Institute (Seiyō Igakujo).[74]

The shogunate's support for the vaccination clinic and the new medical school suggests a growing interest in medicine and the health of the populace, but the solidification of this stance was cut short by the events of the 1860s. In 1862, under pressure from the daimyo, who complained about the cost of maintaining their Edo residences while incurring the new expenses associated with national defense, the government announced that it was abandoning many of the requirements of the alternate attendance system, which had required daimyo and their retainers to reside in Edo every other year. In the wake of this change, many daimyo and their retainers left the city, reducing the population of Edo by half over the course of just a few years. The exodus of its warrior residents proved ruinous to the city. Areas given over to samurai residence were left unoccupied but for squatters who took refuge in the abandoned mansions and barracks that gradually fell into disrepair. The city's economy, largely fueled by consumer demand, soon collapsed. Merchants who had provided the daimyo households with food and goods were particularly hard-hit, as were the large number of people who had been employed as servants and part-time retainers in warrior households.[75]

The end of alternate attendance affected the medicine marketplace as well. As noted above, more than half of Edo's doctors were in the employ of one of the domains, and many accompanied their employers when they left Edo for their home domains. There are no contemporary statistics on the loss of doctors, but those compiled in the Meiji era tell us something about the situation. The earliest information available is from 1878 and reveals that Tokyo Prefecture, which included not only the city itself but also six adjacent rural districts, had a total of 1,878 doctors. Of these, 592 had passed or attempted the recently instituted licensing exam, which tested their knowledge of Western medicine. These were likely products of the new medical schools of the Meiji era. The remaining 1,296 were so-called previous practitioners—that is, doctors trained in the Tokugawa period who continued to practice.[76] Even allowing for deaths, retirements, and moves, this is significantly less than the number of doctors in Edo before 1862 and likely reflects the long-term impact of the loss of domanial doctors.

In the final years of the shogunate, conditions in the city continued to decline. As the historian Henry Smith has observed, "no city in Japan was so profoundly affected by the collapse of the Tokugawa regime as its political capital."[77] Partisan violence, crime, and poverty beset the city, and amid the confusion, the Yōjōsho and the vaccination clinic ceased to function. In January 1868, the Boshin War—the civil conflict fought between Tokugawa loyalists and pro-imperial forces—began, and in early July 1868 the conflict reached the city. The war itself prompted the establishment of new medical institutions as field hospitals began to be established to care for the wounded. William Willis, a doctor attached to the British mission, was an adviser to the anti-Tokugawa forces, and in that capacity played an important role in the establishment and running of these military hospitals, the first of which was in Kyoto.

As the conflict moved to the northeast, a military hospital was established in Yokohama to accommodate Willis's need to continue caring for members of the British community there. He was assisted by another British physician, Joseph Siddall, and by locally recruited Japanese physicians. Few Japanese doctors had any experience treating the bullet wounds that combatants suffered, but both Siddall and Willis found them a quick study and credited them with saving many patients from amputation. According to Siddall, "In the course of some three months, [they] learned the use of splints, and were able to apply them, and to bandage in a manner that would have been no discredit to a London hospital."[78]

As the fighting got underway in Edo, a hospital was established there using the Shitaya mansion of Tōdō Takayuki, a shogunal vassal who famously abandoned the Tokugawa cause in the aftermath of the Battle of Toba-Fushimi and then volunteered the use of his home to the pro-imperial forces.[79] The British doctors, again assisted by local doctors, found the large tatami rooms unsuitable for hospital care, so they brought in beds and mattresses from Yokohama. They noted, however, that the Japanese women recruited as nurses had no experience with such furnishings and required instruction in how to change sheets and manage the personal hygiene of bedbound patients.[80] With many patients requiring long convalescences, the hospital continued to function after the conflict had moved northward, and it began to offer care to civilian patients as well, thus assuming some of the functions of the now defunct Yōjōsho.

The Healthscape in Transition

This chapter has explored the healthscape of Edo as it evolved over the course of the early modern period. Unlike the new government that would replace it, the Tokugawa shogunate was only minimally concerned with the health of subjects, including those who resided in the city that was its seat of power. It provided only limited funding to the Yōjōsho and the Medical Institute, and, by design, these institutions provided medical care to only a small number of city residents. But this did not mean that Edo residents lacked access to medical care. As we have seen, the city was home to many physicians, including some of the most elite physicians of the day, and its residents were also able to turn to self-treatment via the booming market in prepared medicines. When doctors and medicinal products failed to improve a patient's condition, religious institutions offered renewed hope via the rituals of healing and pacification they offered and the amulets and talismans they sold.

The final decades of Tokugawa rule ushered in a new period in the city's medical culture that was characterized by both confusion and innovation. As the changing fortunes of Dutch medicine reveal, the shogunate's stance toward medicine was shaped by the vagaries of partisan conflicts. Even so, as old institutions like the Yōjōsho fell into disarray, others arose, such as the vaccination clinic, the Institute for Western Medicine, and the military hospital. The establishment of these facilities did not reflect the formulation of an explicit policy on the part of the city's government: rather, they were ad hoc responses to the exigent circumstances of the day. Contributing to the sense of crisis that befell the city was the mid-century arrival of cholera, an unknown and terrifying disease that brought unprecedented loss of life in Edo. Four years later, the end of alternate attendance and the dramatic loss of population (including many of the city's doctors) was yet another blow. In chapter 2, we examine the new government's interest in medical matters, the formulation of its medical policy, and the attempt to make the city into a testing ground for medical modernization.

2

The Medical Policy of 1874

Public Health, State-Building, and Tokyo

On January 3, 1868, the teenage emperor Meiji announced that political power would be restored to the imperial institution, marking the first step in Japan's transformation into a modern nation-state. The civil war with pro-Tokugawa forces would continue for another year and a half but amid the conflict, the leaders of the new government began a process of state-building that would last for several decades, culminating with the promulgation of a new constitution in 1889. As the new era began, medicine was soon identified as a target for reform. In February 1868, only a month after the emperor's announcement, Takashina Tsunenori, physician to the imperial household, submitted a memorandum to the new government in which he asserted, "The way of medicine too is a responsibility of government and is the best expression of benevolence." Noting that "in foreign countries, matters related to human life are profoundly valued and so in every country medical schools, hospitals, and asylums are established in order to provide relief to all people who suffer from disease," Takashina urged the emperor to follow this example by embracing Western medicine and establishing hospitals and other institutions that would "provide free care to widows, orphans, the poor, homeless, travelers and others experiencing hardship."[1]

This memorandum is remarkable not only for its criticism of the existing medical culture but also for its elevation of medicine to an object of imperial concern and a fundamental responsibility of government. Departing from the shogunate's limited involvement in medical matters, Takashina and others aligned with the new government asserted their concern for the health of the populace and the idea that the state must assume responsibility for ensuring it. As a result, the Meiji government (as the new regime came to be known) quickly announced its intention to embrace Western medicine, ordered the prefectures to vaccinate their residents against smallpox, and required manufacturers of prepared medicines to submit their products for inspection to ensure their efficacy. "New" medical institutions were quickly established as well, albeit simply by rebranding medical facilities established in the final years of Tokugawa rule. The Western Medicine Institute became the government-supported Medical School in 1869 and part of the Eastern College of the University (later University of Tokyo) in 1870, while the military hospital established during the civil war was designated as its affiliated hospital.

This chapter traces the government's efforts to reform the practice of medicine and establish a public health system and examines its decision to make Tokyo, just declared the capital of the new state in September 1868, a testing ground for reforms. Significantly, the Japanese government was not alone in making the promotion of health an important element of state-building in this era. As advances in biology and technology made disease control seem more possible than ever before, officials around the world realized that the safeguarding of health offered a means to forge a new relationship with the populace. The case of Latin America is revealing. Over the course of the late nineteenth and early twentieth centuries, postcolonial governments in Mexico, Ecuador, Argentina, and Brazil made "health public," in the words of Gilberto Hochman, by expanding state authority to address it, a process that required individuals and groups to collaborate with the state by, for example, accepting restrictions to their personal liberty or property rights for the good of the abstract national community.[2]

Similarly, in her work on the Yucatan in the period from 1847 to the 1920s, Heather McCrea, notes that public health policy became a potent "social instrument" of the Mexican government as it attempted, albeit with only limited success, to incorporate the peninsula and its Mayan population into the state. She noted that public health initiatives, such as the requirement for smallpox vaccination, allowed the state to "penetrate ever more deeply into the private lives of populations," creating a "Mexican presence" in a population that had long been ignored.[3] As these works suggest, medical reforms and the establishment of public health policy involved a complicated process of negotiation, subordination, and mobilization between the state and the people that often resulted in new social and political tensions. At the heart of the issue was the fact that while the reforms promised benefits to the people, in practice they were often experienced as oppressive rather than beneficial, or even simply benign.

In Japan, at least initially, interest in medical reform was not inspired by concerns about the extension of state power, or concern about population in the Foucauldian sense of the term. That is, the government did not yet seem to have linked the health of its citizens to the wealth and power of the state. Rather, the new government sought to demonstrate its "benevolent and compassionate intent" toward the people, still influenced by the idea of benevolent governance that had served to legitimate the Tokugawa shogunate. Takashina's concern about providing free medical care to those viewed as vulnerable ("widows, orphans, and the poor") and therefore worthy of aid is particularly revealing of this intent. But that would change as the reform efforts got underway and a new calculation of the value of a health citizenry emerged.

The Medical Policy of 1874

Discussion of medical reforms began even as the bureaucratic structure of the new state was evolving. By 1869, the government consisted of the Dajōkan or Council of State and a system of eight ministries, the Home Ministry, Foreign Affairs, Army, Navy, Imperial Household, Justice, Public Works, and Education. Power lay in the hands of twenty or so individuals, most of whom were samurai leaders of the military overthrow of the shogunate. They made up the Council of State and moved in and out of the various ministries often at a rapid pace. This "oligarchy," as it has been termed, initially governed via fiat, issuing and at times retracting edicts and decrees at a dizzying rate, a process that was aided by the new prestige of the emperor in whose name they acted. In short order, the government created a system of prefectures from the patchwork of domanial holdings, dissolved the long-standing status distinctions, established a new system of land tenure and taxation, and created a national army and navy.

In 1872 a governmental agency was created to deal specifically with medical matters. This was the Medical Section (Imuka), which was established within the Ministry of Education, reflecting concern for creating a new system of medical education. The following year the "section" was elevated when it was renamed as the Medical Bureau (Imukyoku). In 1875 the Medical Bureau was renamed the Hygiene Bureau and became a part of the Home Ministry.[4] Sagara Chian, a former samurai of Saga Domain (now Saga Prefecture), was already serving as the head of the Eastern College when he was appointed to lead the Medical Bureau in 1873. Like several other medical luminaries of the early Meiji period, Sagara was educated in Dutch learning, in his case under Satō Taizen, the founder of Juntendō, one of the most famous Dutch-learning academies of the day. From there, he went on to study at Nagasaki in the shogunate-supported medical school attached to the Naval Training Institute. This institution, while short-lived, would prove important to the process of medical reform as many of its former students became important figures in medical and public health administration.

As the head of the Eastern College, Sagara had successfully advocated for the adoption of the German "model" of medical training, which gave greater weight to educating medical researchers than clinicians. This stance angered some powerful governmental figures who favored the clinically oriented British system. Perhaps because of this, Sagara served in the Medical Bureau for only three months before he was dismissed.[5] Despite his brief tenure, however, Sagara left his mark on the process of medical reform: he drafted an ambitious plan for medical modernization that he called "An Abbreviated Medical Policy" (*Isei ryakusoku*). His inspiration seems to have been a series of medical reforms undertaken in the Netherlands in 1865 to address the credentialing of medical professionals and establish regulations for the pharmaceutical industry. He probably learned of these reforms from Anthonius Bauduin, a Dutch military doctor who had been an instructor at the Nagasaki Medical Training Center before joining the faculty of the Eastern College after the establishment of the new government.[6] Bauduin was but one of the thousands of foreign experts employed by the Meiji government in this period, which included many who worked at the government's medical school.

After Sagara's dismissal, Nagayo Sensai was selected to lead the Medical Bureau. Born the son of a physician of Sino-Japanese medicine who served the lord of Omura Domain (now Nagasaki Prefecture), Nagayo's education mirrored that of Sagara: he had studied at the Tekijuku, a Dutch learning academy in Osaka, and continued his studies at the shogunate's Nagasaki medical school.[7] After the overthrow of the shogunate, he remained in Nagasaki as director of the medical school's hospital before eventually joining the new government and relocating to Tokyo. In 1871 Nagayo was appointed a member of the Iwakura Mission, a diplomatic effort to revise the so-called unequal treaties signed with foreign governments in the 1850s and 1860s. Over the course of almost two years, the mission visited the US, Britain, and nine European countries. While senior members of the group were responsible for meeting with heads of state, Nagayo and other young officials were tasked with investigating the policies, practices, and institutions of the countries they visited. Nagayo's assignment was to gather information on medical matters, including medical education and physician licensing systems, evidence of the government's interest in reforming medical care.[8]

Nagayo was likely chosen for this task because he had obtained the most modern medical education available in Japan in the mid-nineteenth century. Even so, he would later write in his 1902 memoir that as he traveled across the US from San Francisco to Washington, DC, and on to London and Paris, he encountered a new, unfamiliar vocabulary of terms like "sanitation" and "health" that gave him pause. In Berlin he discovered the concept that would shape his later work, *Gesundheitspflege* (literally, "health care" but often translated as "hygiene"). Nagayo encountered this term at a critical moment. Until the early nineteenth century, "hygiene" referred primarily to personal cleanliness, although it was also tied to ideas about moral virtue. But the sanitary movement and the rise of germ theory had transformed hygiene from an individual concern into a public one, associated closely with the prevention of infectious disease.[9] In his memoir, Nagayo recalled his encounter with the idea of government management of the health of the citizenry: "At first I just understood it literally and did not pay much attention to it, but as my investigation progressed, I realized that it meant more than just health care [*kenkō hogo*]. As my questions multiplied, I began to probe [its meaning], and I discovered that it referred to the special administrative system that has responsibility for caring for the health of all the citizens of a country."[10]

Nagayo's confusion about now commonplace terms like "health" and "hygiene" was perhaps understandable. *Kenkō*, now the ordinary term for health in Japanese, was a neologism that had been coined only in the mid-nineteenth century as a translation for the Dutch *gezondheid* (German: *Gesundheit*).[11] In explaining its meaning in 1849, the Dutch learning scholar Ogata Kōan referenced the body in anatomical, physiological, and mechanistic terms: "'Health' describes a person when the body and all its organs are correctly formed and without defect, when blood and *ki* flow smoothly without obstruction, and when its workings are always in good order."[12] Notably, Ogata and others who adopted *kenkō* rejected terms then widely in use such as *sōken* (robust), *kyōken* (strong), *kenzen* (sound), *jōbu* (strong), and *sukoyaka* (vigorous). Presumably, these narrower terms did not capture the concern for anatomical correctness and bodily processes conveyed by *kenkō*. However, in translating *Gesundheitspflege*, Nagayo rejected compounds that would have incorporated this term. In his estimation direct translations such as *hoken* (preservation of health) or *kenkō hogo* (health care) would be "too frank and uninteresting." Instead, he chose the characters *eisei* (protecting life) from the Chinese classic *Zhuangzi*. He would later admit that this translation was "somewhat" imperfect, but he argued that *eisei* was "written with elegant characters" and was, moreover, pleasing to the ears. Later scholars would propose the alternative meaning of "policing life," in recognition of the invasive turn that Japanese public health efforts would soon take.[13]

As director of the Medical Bureau, Nagayo was positioned to act on his new understanding of *Gesundheitspflege / eisei*, and he ordered prefectural authorities to survey the state of medicine in their localities, soliciting information on doctors and their training, medical education, and pharmacies. Nagayo likely wanted to use this information to develop his own plan for reform, but it also reflected his view that the administration of public health should be a local matter. This position too emerged during his time on the Iwakura Mission, where he had observed the Anglo-American approach to public health, which eschewed national policies in favor of local initiatives. According to Nagayo, medicine and public health "intervene directly in the lives of people and their activities, and since customs and sentiments are different in each region, we should not impose restrictions uniformly."[14] However, when the Council of State ordered Nagayo to submit a plan for medical reform only weeks after he had taken up his new position, he quickly revised Sagara's plan for a highly centralized process of reform and submitted it for consideration.[15]

Consisting of seventy-six articles, the Medical Policy, as it was termed, was an ambitious plan to dismantle the existing medical culture to establish a new one that would be regulated by the state and serve its interests. It opened by declaring that government had a responsibility "to protect the health of the people, treat epidemic disease, and advance the study [of medicine]." The first topic addressed was the creation of a new bureaucratic structure to oversee medical matters at both the local and national levels. The Medical Bureau was to have authority over the country's medical professionals, hospitals, and other institutions, including medical schools, except for those under the army and navy. Beneath it, the country was to be divided into seven districts, each under a Hygiene Bureau (*eiseikyoku*; Sagara had termed these "health bureaus"). These were to "oversee everything related to medical affairs" with the cooperation of local officials in each district.[16]

To facilitate the relationship between local officials and the new Hygiene Bureaus, local administrations had to include "medical officials" (*imu kakari*), who would report to the Ministry of Education and the Medical Bureau, while at the grassroots level, the implementation of health policy would be placed in the hands of "medical supervisors" (*imu torishimari*), who were to be appointed from among local doctors, pharmacy owners, and veterinarians. They were charged with gathering information about their local communities and submitting it to their respective local Hygiene Bureaus. This included data on the number of doctors and other medical professionals, incidences of infectious disease, and information on adverse local factors affecting the health of residents (2:36–37).

The next section of the policy addressed medical education. Noting that at the time only two ostensibly modern medical schools were in existence (in Tokyo and Nagasaki), the Medical Policy called for the establishment of a government-funded modern medical school in each of the eight university districts established by the 1872 Educational Policy, another ambitious reform plan issued by the Ministry of Education. The new schools were to offer three-year preparatory courses, followed by five years of medical training. Students who graduated from the new elementary schools were to be admitted to the medical schools by examination. The preparatory course would instruct students in foundational subjects, including German, mathematics, and the sciences, with medical training taking place in the five-year course. Graduates would then have the option of pursuing further training in surgery, internal medicine, anatomy, and other specialized fields. In addition, a new government-funded hospital was to be attached to each medical school. These "national hospitals" (*kanritsu byōin*) would not only function as teaching hospitals but also provide broad access to modern medical care by offering free services to the poor (2:37–39).

The concern for making modern medical care widely accessible is also evident in the next section of the policy, which dealt with hospitals. Those seeking to establish public, private, or charitable institutions, including asylums and lock hospitals (that is, hospitals for syphilis patients) were required to make an application to the Ministry of Education via their local Hygiene Bureaus. This required submitting information about the credentials of the prospective medical staff, the available funding for the institution, and basic data about the proposed institution, such as the number of beds and whether a pharmacist would be on staff. Hospitals attached to private or prefectural medical schools were to be partially funded by local taxes, in exchange for which they were to offer reduced or free care to the poor. Hospitals were also integrated into the new public health system: their directors were required to submit detailed records about patient numbers, deaths, and causes of death to their respective local Hygiene Bureaus (2:39–40).

The Medical Policy also addressed the credentialing of medical professionals, including doctors, midwives, and pharmacists. Here Sagara and Nagayo attempted to negotiate a complex situation. The limited number of modern medical schools meant that it would be some years before training in Western medicine would be widely available. Meanwhile, what was to be done with the estimated thirty thousand doctors already in practice, albeit with differing forms and depths of medical education? To resolve this issue, the Medical Policy envisioned a transitional period in which a three-tier system of licensing would be instituted. Graduates of the new university medical schools would be licensed automatically, while those who obtained their education through a private school or an apprenticeship would have to take an examination that covered at least two medical specialties. Meanwhile, by submitting evidence of their medical education and a history of efficacious treatments, those already in practice could apply for a temporary license that would be valid for ten years. This was intended to provide these physicians with time to acquire the skills and knowledge needed to pass the licensing exam. Reflecting the assumption that younger doctors could make the transition more rapidly, the Medical Policy held that practicing physicians under the age of thirty should attempt the exam every three years. The rules for licensing midwives were similar: those already in practice could apply for a temporary license upon providing evidence of their expertise, while new aspiring midwives would have to take an examination (2:39–40).

The Medical Policy made no mention of the need to license other kinds of practitioners, such as acupuncturists and those who performed moxibustion, probably because these experiential skills did not lend themselves to testing and were outside the parameters of Western medicine. But it also did not call for banning them. Instead, the Medical Policy sought to delimit these forms of practice by requiring their practitioners to work under the supervision of a licensed doctor of internal medicine or surgery and forbidding them to provide medications. In addition, clearly aware that unqualified physicians could potentially continue to practice, Sagara and Nagayo designed a system to weed out bad doctors: if a complaint was made that a doctor had falsified credentials or neglected or injured their patients, the local Hygiene Bureau and local officials were to work with the medical supervisors to investigate the case. If the complaint was substantiated, local authorities could then ban the doctor from practicing (2:39–40).

Although the Medical Policy thus imagined a transitional period in which Sino-Japanese doctors would continue to practice, it also sought to fundamentally alter the economic basis of their work. In the early modern period, physicians typically derived their income by charging patients for the medicinal compounds they provided, although they also received seasonal gifts in-kind and cash from their patients during the Obon festival in late summer and at the New Year holiday (2:39–40). In contrast, the Medical Policy sought to institute a fee for services policy, in part because of the widespread belief that many doctors overcharged for medicines or substituted cheaper botanicals for expensive ones to maximize their profits. The Medical Policy aimed to ban doctors from providing medications directly: instead, they were to give the patient a prescription to be filled independently at a pharmacy. In the future, physicians were to charge standardized fees for their services, and these were to be disclosed to patients before any treatment was performed. In addition, the local Hygiene Bureaus were to investigate physician fees and work with local officials to ensure that they were reasonable for the specific locality (2:39–40).

The provisions of the Medical Policy clearly aimed to give the new medical administrative system it envisioned significant authority over private physicians. Not only was the local Hygiene Bureau to control their fees and their right to practice, but physicians seeking to relocate would be required to get permission from their local medical supervisor as well as the ward, town, or village head. In addition to these new constraints, private physicians were to be charged with performing new duties on behalf of the state. For example, whenever a patient died in their care, they were to notify the local medical supervisor within three days of the cause of death and the progression of the deceased's illness. There were similar requirements for instances of miscarriage, stillbirth, and live births. Furthermore, private physicians were to play a role in the control of infectious diseases, specifically cholera, smallpox, and measles. If a local physician became aware of an outbreak, he was to immediately inform the medical supervisors or local officials, who would then report it to the Medical Bureau in Tokyo (2:41–42). The concern for gathering data at the local level seen here and throughout the Medical Policy is significant. Reflecting the new concept of "population," Sagara and Nagayo sought to use the authority of the new state to gather what was now understood to be vital information for governance.

The final section of the Medical Policy was aimed at transforming the booming pharmaceutical industry that had been a central part of early modern medical culture. It called for the establishment of a drug testing center in Tokyo, with branches elsewhere in the country, that would examine proprietary medicines, although the new goal was no longer to determine their effectiveness but to identify those that were harmful. Like other medical professionals, pharmacy owners were to be licensed either by examination or by having graduated from a modern school of pharmacy. In addition, the Medical Policy required pharmacists to prepare drugs according to orthodox formulas and forbade altering them in any way. Producers of prepared medicines were required to include a complete list of ingredients and the cost of the product on the package or wrapper. The latter provision was designed to standardize medication prices by making it difficult for medicine peddlers and others to inflate prices. Medicine peddlers and retailers were the target of other provisions as well: they were required to be employed by a licensed pharmacist and were forbidden to pressure consumers to purchase medicines (2:42–44).

As this summary suggests, the Medical Policy envisioned a complete restructuring of the largely unregulated system of health care then in place. Until this time, a physician's "credentials" were established primarily by forging a teacher–student relationship with a well-known doctor or an established medical lineage. Of course, a reputation for good results mattered as well, both for ordinary doctors and would-be scholar-physicians, although the latter could also establish a name through their publications. Only in the early nineteenth century did some domains go beyond these ad hoc measures by attempting to develop policies for weeding out unskilled and dangerous practitioners. One such domain was Kishū (now Wakayama Prefecture). In 1812, as a first step toward exercising oversight of doctors, the domain issued an edict stating that those who wanted to study medicine should do so under either a domanial doctor or a private physician who was at least the third-generation successor within a medical lineage. After the completion of their training, would-be doctors were required to take an exam administered by the domanial medical school, and only those who passed were allowed to practice medicine within the domain.[17]

Kishū was not alone in adopting such measures. Other domains began requiring doctors practicing in their villages and towns to submit proof of their training, and some created local associations of reputable established physicians empowered to investigate cases of malpractice and to exclude poorly trained or itinerant doctors.[18] However, no similar regulations were enacted in Edo, perhaps because the competition among the large number of doctors in the city worked to eliminate those who were unskilled. This patchwork of local efforts was very different from the credentialing procedure envisioned in the Medical Policy. Now, a particular form of medical education (that is, university medical schools) was privileged, as was a specific body of medical knowledge. The intent was to eliminate those who could not prove their mastery of the latter. Similarly, the Medical Policy also aimed to create a system of strict controls over the heretofore unregulated manufacture and sale of prepared medicines. It called for a new transparency about their contents, origin, and pricing and sought to insert a new medical professional—the credentialed pharmacist—into the manufacturing process. If the early modern medical market was characterized by heterogeneity, lack of regulation, and the primacy of consumer choice, the Medical Policy sought to create one that was strictly regulated and highly centralized.

Tokyo as a Testing Ground

Although the Council of State had commissioned a reform plan and seemingly compelled Nagayo to quickly produce one, it was a full nine months before there was a response. When it came, it significantly scaled down the scope of the reforms. The Council of State ordered that the plan be implemented piecemeal and only in the three largest cities in the country, Tokyo, Osaka, and Kyoto. In its communication with officials in these three cities, the Ministry of Education explained this approach, stating that, "because of traditional practices, it would be difficult to implement [the Medical Policy] all at once."[19] By this time, the government was already confronting significant opposition not only from ordinary citizens but also from within the oligarchy itself. For example, Etō Shinpei, the former justice minister and onetime member of the Council of State, led a rebellion of erstwhile samurai against the new government in 1874. The members of the Council of State apparently feared that the medical reforms would result in more confusion and turmoil. As a result, the local governments of the three cities were instructed to "choose the policies that were most urgent at present" and implement them gradually while paying close attention to the results.[20]

The decision to make these cities the initial focus of reform was, arguably, a reasonable one. Not only were Tokyo, Kyoto, and Osaka the three largest population centers in the country and thus useful for monitoring the public's response, but they were also already centers of medical education and home to significant numbers of physicians, among whom were those who had at least some training in Western medicine. But the situation in Tokyo belied the assumption that the city was equipped to serve as a testing ground for medical reform. In the aftermath of the fall of the shogunate, the new capital was, in the words of Takashi Fujitani, a "dying city."[21] Population had fallen to 500,000, and the mansions and barracks that had once housed Tokugawa and domanial vassals had been abandoned and left to ruin, attracting both squatters and vandals. The social fabric of the city was frayed as well. According to the short-lived *Tokyo Prefectural Newspaper* (*Tōkyō-fu nisshi*), in 1868 three out of five Tokyo residents were living in poverty, and two of those three were suffering from extreme poverty. In that single year, almost 300 corpses and 160 abandoned children were found on the city's streets.[22] Natives of the city were joined by refugees, both villagers and samurai, from areas affected by economic dislocations and the ongoing civil conflict, and many gathered in what would become the city's new slums.

Initially help was hard to come by. The town magistrates' office had dissolved with the defeat of the Tokugawa shogunate, but a new system of city governance took form slowly. In the interim, some commoner-led organizations continued to function. One of these was the Machikaisho, an organization established in 1792 by order of the shogunate. Headed by prominent townspeople, it was tasked with collecting mandatory "donations" from the city's landlords and householders to provide relief for the poor population. Fortunately for the city's struggling residents, the Machikaisho remained in place until 1872, and it drew upon its financial reserves to provide food and housing for the swelling numbers of those living in poverty.[23] At the other end of the social spectrum was the beggar fraternity of Asakusa, which not only continued to manage the *tame* but also took on the management of new hostels established in 1869–1870 with Machikaisho funds to house the city's homeless people on abandoned daimyo estates in Mita and Takanawa in what would later become Shiba Ward and in Kōjimachi, close to the Edo castle.[24] Similarly, the *machi* headmen (*nanushi*) and *ienushi* continued to manage matters at the neighborhood level, and in some instances they organized their own relief efforts.[25]

The reliance on early modern institutions was not to endure for long. Over the course of a decade, the central government undertook a series of reforms that aimed to fundamentally reshape governance in the city. As a result, the prefectural administration had far less autonomy than other local governments and took orders directly from the Council of State until 1885. The position of the prefectural governor is revealing of this relationship. In the three and a half years between October 1868, when Tokyo Prefecture was formed, and June 1872, each of four governors served for only a matter of months. Two of the governors, Karasumaru Mitsue and Mibu Motoosa, were members of the Kyoto nobility who had aligned themselves with the anti-Tokugawa forces. Although they had no knowledge of the city or urban administration, they were rewarded for their support with this newly created position. Continuity came with the appointment of the fifth governor, Ōkubo Ichio, who was appointed in 1872 and served for four years.[26] Born in Edo as the son of a Tokugawa vassal, Ōkubo presumably knew the city well, and he would prove to be an efficient administrator. However, it was not until 1878, when the prefecture's elected assembly met for the first time, that the prefectural government began to gradually establish some degree of autonomy.

The early governors presided over a spatial entity that was itself evolving. The original Tokyo Prefecture (Tōkei-fu, as it was then known) consisted only of the parts of the city inside the so-called vermillion line. Dating from 1818, the vermillion line designated "Great Edo" (Ō-Edo) and clarified which parts of the city were under the control of the town magistrates. It included most of what are now Chiyoda Ward, Chūō Ward, Minato Ward, Bunkyō Ward, and Taitō Ward. But within months a hundred more villages that had been part of Musashi Prefecture were transferred to the prefecture. In 1869 the areas of warrior residence and temples and shrines were incorporated as well. For a brief period in 1870, at the order of the Council of States, three districts in Nemuro on the island of Hokkaido came under the authority of the Tokyo prefectural government, an initiative intended to facilitate the relocation of Tokyo's poor population to this region.

The attempt to relocate the city's poor people to Hokkaido is remarkable given the significant amount of unoccupied land and number of dwellings within the city. As noted in the chapter 1, the end of the alternate attendance system had reduced the warrior population of the city significantly, and the forced relocation of remaining Tokugawa vassals after the end of the shogunate further contributed to depopulation. It is estimated that about 11 million tsubo (3,636 hectares or 36 square kilometers) of land, much of it in the elevated areas of the city west of the Imperial Palace (formerly Edo Castle), lay unoccupied but for squatters. In 1871 these lands formally came under the control of the new state. However, the status divide that had organized the city for centuries, resulting in the densely populated commoner neighborhoods of the low-lying areas, went unaddressed. Instead, it was decided to use the remaining unoccupied former warrior lands for agriculture, specifically for the cultivation of mulberry and tea. But as the population rebounded, reaching almost 900,000 in 1882 and more than 2 million by 1897, this plan was abandoned and land began to be sold off to private buyers, who redeveloped it as rental, retail, and residential properties.[27]

Still, population distribution remained skewed. The wards of the eastern part of the city continued to be far more densely populated than those of the western city. Figure 2.1 shows population density by ward in 1883. Fifteen

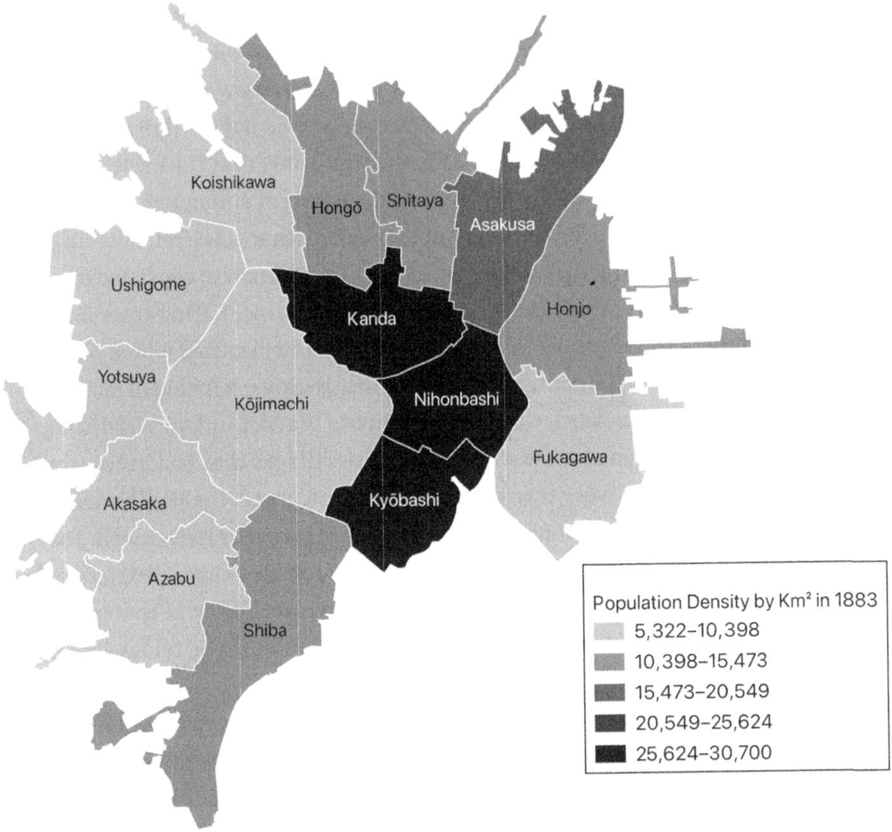

Figure 2.1. Population density in Tokyo, 1884. Data from Tōkyō-fu, *Tōkyō-fu tōkeisho, Meiji 16-nen–17-nen*, 22–23.

years after the fall of the shogunate, the former commoner areas of the city in wards such as Nihonbashi, Kyōbashi, and Kanda still had three to five times the population density of the areas of the city formerly reserved for warrior residence. Figure 2.2 shows population distribution in 1920. A half century after the fall of the shogunate, several of the eastern wards still had double the population density of wards east of the imperial palace.

The city's administrative structure evolved, too, as the new government grappled with how to gain control of both urban space and its residents. This required dismantling what remained of the Edo period administration system, specifically the local commoner elites who had participated in governance to this point. In 1869 the city was reorganized into a new system of fifty wards (*ku*), a move that allowed for the dismissal of the machi headmen, who

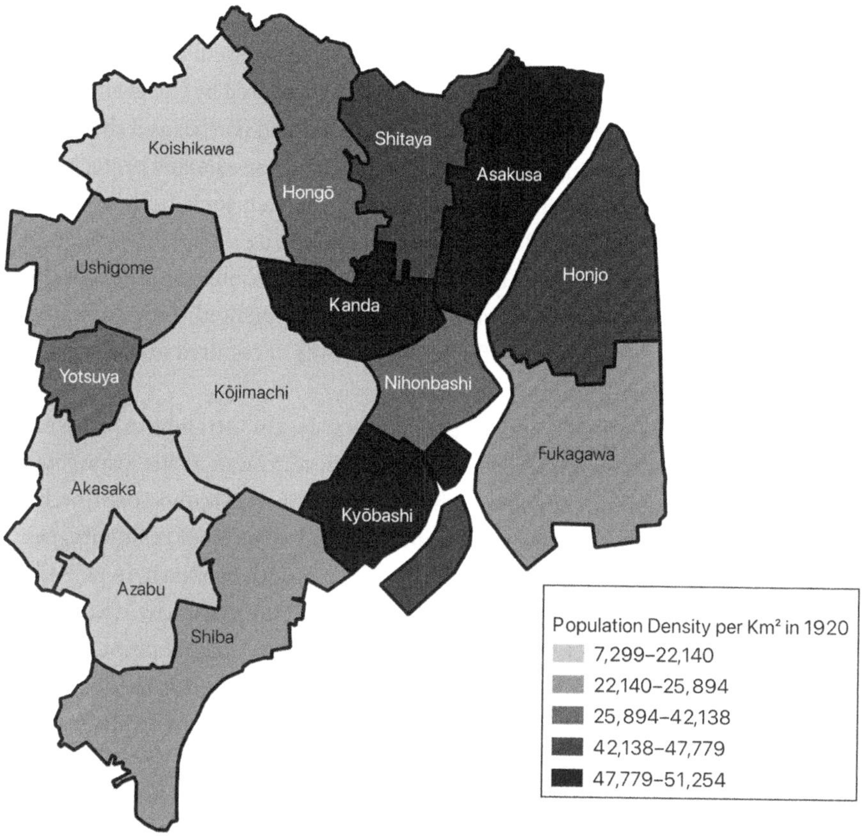

Figure 2.2. Population density in Tokyo, 1920. Data from Tōkyō-fu, *Tōkyō-fu tōkeisho, Taishō 10-nen*, 79.

had played an important role in managing the early modern city. They were replaced with allies of the new government, who were charged with a variety of novel responsibilities, from reforming "bad customs" to educating the populace about their new role as imperial subjects.[28] Once the new officials were in place, the unpopular and unwieldly system of fifty wards was abandoned, as a national plan to create new administrative units emerged in 1872. It called for the entire country to be divided into a system of "large wards" (*daiku*) and "small wards" (*shōku*) with the aim of dissolving existing village, town, and neighborhood communities and creating new rational ones that would be free of existing loyalties and relations of power.[29]

In Tokyo, there were other aims as well. The new wards incorporated the formally autonomous daimyo lands, bringing them under the control of the prefectural government. The new administrative units also made it possible to dismantle the surviving remnants of the Edo-era system of governance, the *ienushi*. They were replaced by new officials appointed by the prefectural governor: the large wards were headed by a ward head (*kuchō*) and the small wards by "heads of households" (*kochō*). The role of these salaried prefectural employees was to oversee the enlisting of those in their jurisdictions in the new household registries and to assist in implementing a local tax system to support the prefectural government. The plan was an ambitious one, but the large ward/small ward system was never fully implemented, and as a result, far from rationalizing the subprefecture-level units, it resulted in a confusing medley of old and new wards.[30]

Like the early establishment of the fifty wards, this attempt to erase existing communities engendered considerable resentment at the grassroots level—and at a moment of growing popular unrest. As Ōkubo Toshimichi, a powerful figure in the new government, noted, "For local residents, the wards and villages are independent units."[31] Faced with backlash, in 1878 the Council of State issued the "District, Ward, Town, and Village Law" to restore traditional administrative units around the country. At this point, Tokyo Prefecture was reorganized into a new system of fifteen wards in the urban area and six districts (*gun*) in the rural areas that would remain in place until 1932. Both the wards and the machi within them were officially identified using familiar historical place names.[32] In 1889 the de facto division between the urban wards and rural districts in Tokyo Prefecture was formalized when the fifteen wards became Tokyo City (Tōkyō-shi). Little else changed, however, since the prefectural governor simultaneously functioned as the mayor of the city. It was only in 1898 that the posts of mayor and governor were separated, and the city acquired a separate administration, including a municipal assembly.

Creating a Public Health Administration

The removal of the lowest level of officials in the city and the disestablishment of the old commoner elites complicated the process of medical reform. In 1869 the prefectural government consisted of five bureaus (*kyoku*) devoted to general affairs, law and crime, infrastructure, industry, and taxes, evidence of the priorities of the time. Despite Nagayo's stance that public health should be the responsibility of local government, no unit within the administration was specifically tasked with medical matters. Instead, public health initially fell under the authority of the general affairs bureau.

Complicating matters further was the establishment of the Tokyo Metropolitan Police (TMP) in 1874. The architect and first head of the TMP was Kawaji Toshiyoshi, a young samurai from Satsuma who had joined the new government. In 1872 the Ministry of Justice appointed him to an eight-person commission sent to Europe to examine their police forces. Upon his return, inspired by his observations of the Paris Police Prefecture, Kawaji wrote a report advocating for the creation of a special police force for the capital. He argued, based on the Parisian model, that social order in the capital was a matter of national concern and the police should have authority over a broad range of responsibilities that included the regulation of prostitution, theaters, and other forms of "entertainment," supervision of restaurants and lodgings, policing of public morals, and most importantly for our purposes, control over public health.[33] Kawaji's argument proved persuasive and in January 1874 the Home Ministry established the TMP, although it was not until 1876 that it was explicitly ordered to assume control over public health matters in Tokyo. We will look more closely at the struggles that ensued between the TMP and the prefectural government in chapters 4–6, but it is important to note the significance of the TMP's new role at this juncture.

The establishment of the TMP notwithstanding, prefectural authorities continued to make efforts to address health within in the city, and after a few years, multiple systems of local officials had been established with overlapping responsibilities. In 1877 the prefecture created a system of doctor-officials who combined the roles of the "medical officials" and "medical superintendents" outlined in the Medical Policy. Known as "ward doctors" (*ku'i*), these were physicians in private practice who were hired as part-time prefectural employees. It is unclear how much they were paid initially, but in 1895, the salary was forty-eight yen per year, a generous salary at a time when textile workers made about thirty-six yen annually, working ten to twelve hours per day.[34] Although advertisements for ward doctors appeared regularly in the newspapers, suggesting an open hiring process, a critic of the system would later claim that aspiring ward doctors often paid current office holders a hefty fee to write them a recommendation or otherwise help them attain this desirable and lucrative position.[35]

The responsibilities of the ward doctors evolved over the course of the first decade of their existence. Initially, their main responsibility was to facilitate access to medical care for the poor population living in their wards, evidence that the prefecture took seriously the Medical Policy's concern about creating access to medical care. Under the new system, a poor resident who needed to see a doctor was to go to the ward office and make a request for care. He or she was then issued a "charitable care ticket" (*seryōken*), which authorized the ward doctor to treat the patient without fees for examinations and medicines.[36] According to the historian Kitahara Itoko, the inspiration for this new policy was the system of charitable care in place in Washington, DC, and Boston. While traveling in the US in 1876, Nagayo had encountered the use of this public-private partnership to extend medical care to those in need.[37]

Initially, the number of people who sought care under the provisions was relatively small. In the first month after the new system was established, June 1877, only seventy-two people were granted a charitable care ticket. But efforts to publicize the program quickly got underway. For example, the *Pocket Guide to Tokyo* (*Kaichū Tōkyō annai*), a guide to the city that offered information on everything from leisure facilities to how to report a lost child, explained the system of charitable care tickets, and listed the names and addresses of all the ward doctors. The newspapers too played a role.[38] The *Yomiuri*, for example, related how a family of five was on the verge of starvation after the household head became ill. The agent for their landlord, taking note of their desperation, went to the ward office to apply for charitable care tickets, an act that won him high praise from the *Yomiuri* journalist.[39] By the second half of 1879, an average of 448 people per month were receiving medical care, and it was reported that in some months as many as 1,500 people were being treated by ward doctors under the charity scheme.[40] Gradually, the duties of the ward doctors expanded. They were made responsible for providing smallpox vaccinations to residents, issuing death certificates, reporting suspicious deaths and injuries to the police, and, during cholera outbreaks, identifying and reporting cases of infection.[41]

The creation of the ward doctors was a Tokyo initiative, but in 1879 the Home Ministry ordered all local governments, including Tokyo, to establish both a Hygiene Department (*Eiseika*) with responsibility for overseeing public health policy and a system of elected "hygiene officers" (*eisei iin*). As a result, the Tokyo prefectural government established an administrative unit dedicated to public health, a development that left the role of the TMP undefined, and the election of hygiene officers began. The number of officers per ward was based on population size and varied from three to seven per ward. Elections were held at the ward level and both candidates and voters were required to be over twenty, male, and to have the given ward as their registered domicile (*honseki*) within the household registry system, stipulations that limited the pool of aspiring hygiene officers to long-term ward residents.[42] As a result of these restrictions, most hygiene officers were landowners (*jinushi*), landlords (*yanushi*), or local merchants.[43] In other words, they were stable and relatively prosperous residents of the city.

Their social status within the ward may have aided the new hygiene officers in the performance of their duties since they were given considerable authority over both people and property. Monitoring the physical environment was one of their assigned tasks. They were required to regularly surveil their wards and take note of hygiene-related problems with roads, waterways, drains, drainage ponds, toilets, hospitals, schools, theaters, rental houses, markets, cemeteries, and crematoria listed as sites of particular concern. Any issues they discovered were to be reported to the ward head (*kuchō*) for investigation and action. In addition, the hygiene officers were required to compile information on the medical infrastructure of their wards, including the number of hospitals, pharmacies, doctors, veterinarians, and midwives, and they were asked to identify impoverished members of the community who needed medical care. Another responsibility was tracking the demographics of the ward. The hygiene officers were charged with recording marriages, live and still births, and deaths. Finally, the control of infectious disease was part of their portfolio. In addition to identifying unvaccinated people and ensuring they were vaccinated for smallpox, the hygiene officers were to report on cases of infectious disease among both humans and animals and to carry out the necessary disinfection when an outbreak occurred.[44]

As this summary suggests, there was considerable overlap with the duties of the ward doctors, although hygiene officers were not required to be doctors and thus were not involved in providing medical care themselves. Both ward doctors and hygiene officers were tasked with helping poor residents access medical care until 1881, when for reasons that are unclear, this responsibility was removed from the ward doctors.[45] But much of the redundancy remained in place. For example, both ward doctors and hygiene officers were responsible for ensuring that Tokyo residents were vaccinated against smallpox and for controlling infectious disease.

The situation became even more complex when in 1881 some of the ward doctors received new dual appointments as "reserve quarantine doctors" (*jōbi ken'eki i*), a position that put these prefectural appointees under the direction of the TMP during outbreaks of epidemic disease. As the name suggests, the "quarantine doctors" were primarily involved in determining whether patients should be transferred to a quarantine hospital, a topic that we will examine in chapter 6. To that end, they were to examine the sick and determine whether they were suffering from cholera or another acute infectious disease.

If the patient was infected, the quarantine doctor then had to decide whether the patient could be adequately cared for in the home or required transfer to a quarantine hospital.[46] During severe outbreaks, the reserve quarantine doctors were supplemented by "temporary quarantine doctors" (*rinji ken'eki i*) who were apparently recruited from physicians who lived in the ward.[47] Neither the temporary nor the reserve quarantine doctors seem to have received a regular salary but they were rewarded with "bonuses" (*irōkin*) paid by the TMP to compensate them for their efforts.[48]

With the creation of the hygiene officers and the quarantine doctors, the work of the ward doctors narrowed significantly. Nonetheless, the position continued to exist until 1895 when a dispute broke out between the ward doctors and the Tokyo City Assembly. The assembly, made up of sixty elected representatives, was established in 1889, with the founding of Tokyo City. The immediate issue was petty: the doctors asked the city to supply them with microscopes, an expensive piece of equipment. At first the prefecture agreed to this request, but it failed to follow through, prompting a protest on the part of the ward doctors. In response, one member of the assembly, Aoki Kinshichi, who was on the finance committee, publicly rebuked the doctors, suggesting that they were overpaid for their limited duties and that their selection process was flawed. He charged that ward doctors were chosen based on their connections rather than their skills and that some resorted to bribes to foster the necessary ties. But Aoki went further: he also claimed that some doctors sought the position not out of a desire to serve the public but for prestige and money. In his words, "As soon as someone becomes a ward doctor, he becomes very busy with visitors arriving incessantly." Aoki's remarks were reported in the press, and the ward doctors responded by asking for a public apology and threatening to resign if one was not forthcoming. Apparently, others assembly members agreed with Aoki's comments, and in August 1895, their resignations were accepted, and the ward doctor system came to an end.[49]

Tokyo City's government then tried to create a new system of citywide medical officials under its direction. In September 1895, the assembly announced the new position of "city doctor" (*shi'i*), although it was more than a year before the details of the post were defined. In October 1896, it was announced that in addition to a "chief city doctor" (*shi'i chō*), there were to be twenty city doctors below him: two in Kanda, Nihonbashi, Asakusa, Shiba, and Kyōbashi, the most densely populated wards, and one in each of the remaining ten wards. Unlike the ward doctors, this was to be a full-time position and correspondingly came with a more substantial salary. The chief city doctor was to receive an annual salary of three hundred yen and the rank-and-file city doctors, two hundred yen.[50]

Like the ward doctors they replaced, the city doctors were charged with assisting in the prevention of infectious diseases and in the care of those infected during outbreaks. Similarly, they were to be responsible for developing strategies to disseminate the smallpox vaccinations and to ensure that the poor people in the city were vaccinated. But there were new responsibilities as well. By this time, there was considerable criticism about the ineffectiveness of the elected hygiene officers, with one city official commenting that "hygiene officer" was little more than an honorary title.[51] The city doctors were to be responsible for sanitary measures, including ensuring that drinking water was safe, public toilets cleaned, and wastewater properly removed. But some of their new duties were decidedly more intrusive. The city doctors were charged with examining stillborn and miscarried fetuses delivered by poor women in the city.[52] This policy clearly related to the criminalization of abortion and infanticide and the widespread assumption that these were crimes of poverty. Both acts were criminalized in 1873, with stiffer penalties defined in the 1880 criminal code and later in the 1907 code that replaced it.[53] City doctors were to play a role in policing reproduction by determining whether a miscarried fetus was the result of an abortion or if a supposed stillbirth masked a case of infanticide. Similarly, the city doctors were charged with diagnosing men who failed the medical examinations that were part of the conscription process, presumably to ensure that they were not malingering, and overseeing their treatment. In addition, they were to play a role in the system of charitable medical care: the city doctors were to examine the circumstances of applicants to determine if they were actually in need.[54]

The heterogeneous set of responsibilities assigned to the city doctors reflected local and national concerns as well as medical and extra-medical ones. Their new duties reveal the city government's new, less generous approach toward impoverished residents. The coupon system of the late 1870s had allowed city residents considerable agency. Poor people needing medical attention could apply directly for aid and if approved were allowed to seek care from a doctor of their choice. In contrast, at this juncture the health of the poor population was subject to new scrutiny. This reflected the discourse on poverty that emerged at the turn of the century, which distinguished between the worthy and unworthy poor. Those who were deemed unable to work—the very young and old as well as people with disabilities or illness—were viewed as legitimate recipients of public aid, while those judged to be capable of supporting themselves were not.[55] Another consideration was the turn from "protecting health" to "policing health" as the underlying principle of public health policy. This will be explored further in chapters 4-6, but it is important to note that in 1898 the Hygiene Bureaus within local governments around the country were transferred from the civil administrations to police control. As a result, as in Tokyo, public health came under police authority.[56]

The implementation of the city doctor system was delayed for almost six months, and its final form differed from that of the original proposal. For one thing, the plan for this to be a full-time position was dropped, as was the proposed salary of two hundred yen. Like the ward doctors they replaced, city doctors would be part-time officials with an annual salary of sixty yen. A newspaper article of February 1897 offered two explanations for this change. First, the job of city doctor was described as a "meritorious position," implying that those so employed should not be interested in a high salary. Second, the low salary would help engender public confidence in the city doctors, presumably because of their willingness to undertake this work for low pay, which was viewed as evidence of their good character. No changes were made to the list of duties, but the number of city doctors was increased from twenty to thirty-six.[57]

The hiring process for city doctors also proved contentious. The ward doctors had been hired by the prefectural government, but as noted above, rumors circulated that the process was compromised by the payment of bribes and other improprieties. As a result, the Tokyo Physicians Association (Tōkyō Ikai) proposed that it should be made responsible for the selection of the city doctors. This organization has its origins in an 1882 Hygiene Bureau directive that ordered the formation of "private physician unions" (*kaigyōi kumiai*). The Tokyo organization was established in 1886 and by 1887 it had 1,592 members, drawn from the fifteen wards and rural districts.[58] According to Ikai Shūhei, the 1882 order was intended to make it easier for the Hygiene Bureau to exercise authority over private physicians, but conversely, this organization also allowed physicians to collectively respond to initiatives from the local and central governments and sometimes to resist them.[59]

In 1897, when the hiring of city doctors became an issue, the association was headed by Hasegawa Tai, a prominent physician, official, and politician. Like Sagara Chian, he began his medical training in the Juntendō and went on to study in the shogunate's medical school in Nagasaki. Beginning in the 1870s, he quickly moved through a series of official positions in Tokyo, serving as director of both the prefectural hospital and the prefectural asylum. In 1890 Hasegawa entered politics, serving three terms in the House of

Representatives. In 1899 he became the head of the Hygiene Bureau within the Home Ministry. Thus, he argued from a position of considerable authority that his organization was best situated to assess the training and skills of candidates for city doctor positions. Not everyone agreed. The ward heads objected to turning the hiring of officials over to a professional organization. In the end, it was decided that the city would be responsible for hiring the city doctors, but all viable candidates would be drawn from the association's members.[60]

The two-decade struggle to create a public health administration reveals some of the tensions surrounding the process of medical modernization in this period. Despite the initial view that public health was a matter for local government, the central government's Hygiene Bureau and the Tokyo Metropolitan Police—both under the authority of the Home Ministry—complicated efforts in Tokyo to craft an effective system of local officials with authority over the physical environment and residents of the city. This resulted in overlapping systems of officials and a good deal of redundancy. Further complicating the situation were the interests and motives of the doctors and local elites who served as ward doctors, hygiene officers, quarantine officers, and city doctors during this period. The public discourse surrounding these officials suggested that they were to be selfless public servants who aspired only to improve the health of the city's residents. But the situation was more complicated, and personal ambitions for prestige, power, and financial gain all came into play. As a result, rather than an effective, rational, and nimble system of knowledgeable officials, the public health administration was shaped by contradictions and conflicting realms of authority that made it unclear who was ultimately responsible for managing the city's material environment and residents.

From Policy to Practice

The Medical Policy of 1874 was an ambitious plan to disestablish the early modern medical marketplace to create a new medical and public health system that would improve the health of all citizens, with special provisions made to ensure medical care for the poor population. Sagara and Nagayo, the authors of the policy, believed that education and licensing were key aspects of the plan, as was the appointment of new local officials who would mediate the relationship between local communities and the Home Ministry's Hygiene Bureau. Tokyo, unsurprisingly given its status as the capital and largest city, was one of the cities chosen to initially implement the Medical Policy, but at the time, the city itself and its government were in a state of disorder: still recovering from the fall of the shogunate and the destruction and economic turmoil it brought, Tokyo suffered from frequent changes of leadership and an evolving administrative structure. Amid the confusion, fundamental questions remained.

Was public health a local or national concern? Was it a matter of "protecting" or "policing" the public? Should it be in the hands of the civil administration or the police? The ambitious goals of the Medical Policy came to be shaped by a series of compromises, the result of competing priorities, popular resistance, and economic constraints, with the result that health care within the city assumed a form very different from that envisioned in the Medical Policy.

3

Creating the Infrastructure of Medical Modernization

Doctors and Hospitals in Tokyo

In 1910 Nagao Setsuzō, a physician, journalist, and sharp critic of the modern medical marketplace, wrote a brief report in the *Asahi shinbun* in which he commented on the recent popularity of hospitals in Tokyo: "There are many people who want to enter a hospital even though their illnesses could easily be treated at home. This is not because the hospitals pressure them; they themselves want to be hospitalized."[1] The popularity of hospital-based care by the turn of the century is striking given that before the 1870s medical care outside the home was both rare and associated with poverty and marginal status. This chapter explores the formation and proliferation of hospitals in Tokyo and the new medical professionals who staffed them. The Medical Policy of 1874 had addressed the role of hospitals at length, and as medical modernization got underway, they quickly became the most ubiquitous and visible of the new medical institutions within the city's evolving healthscape. Although the central government's priority was the establishment of teaching hospitals, which were to train modern doctors, prefectural authorities were initially more interested in creating a public hospital that would offer care to a broad range of city residents. In 1873 the Tokyo Prefectural Hospital was established with this in mind. It would function for only eight years before being dissolved, and in the following decades, private "for profit" hospitals became the norm.

Implicated in the proliferation of private hospitals were the physicians who founded, administered, and worked in them. One aim of the Medical Policy was to gradually replace practitioners of Sino-Japanese medicine with those trained in "Western medicine" through the establishment of new medical schools and a licensing system. To achieve this, practitioners of Sino-Japanese medicine were issued temporary licenses but were encouraged to take the licensing exam as soon as possible. The result was a multitiered system of physicians with different forms of training and credentials, who competed for paying patients. Many of them opposed the new policy of subsidized medical care for the poor population, which they argued was an illegitimate use of local taxes that threatened their livelihoods. The need to cultivate a paying clientele also led doctors to establish their clinics and hospitals in more prosperous neighborhood, with the result that poor and working-class areas of the city were poorly served.

Discovering the Hospital

In 1870 Tokyo had a single hospital, the military field hospital, still housed in a former daimyo mansion but now renamed as the hospital of the Eastern College, as the government medical school was then known. Forty years later, there were more than a hundred hospitals in Tokyo, all but ten of which were privately owned (see plate 9). What accounts for the rapid proliferation of hospitals, particularly private hospitals, in the city? And how can we explain the spatial order they assumed?

A point of origin for the modern hospital in Japan was the Nagasaki Yōjōsho, the first purpose-built medical facility in Japan that reflected European conceptions of hospital design. It was established in 1860 as part of the shogunate-funded Medical Training Center in Nagasaki, where the first generation of the modern medical elite studied under European instructors. Pompe von Meedervort, the Dutch physician in charge of the Nagasaki medical school and instrumental in its construction, stressed the need for his students to receive clinical training. Unlike the Edo Yōjōsho, which was modeled on typical commoner housing in the city, the Nagasaki hospital was an entirely novel structure. Its design reflected Florence Nightingale's 1858 work *Notes on Hospitals*, now regarded as a foundational work for modern hospital architecture. In her book, Nightingale stressed the need for ventilation to ensure good air flow, large windows to allow in sunlight, and small wards of twenty or so patients to reduce noise, improve care, and promote cleanliness. For these reasons, she favored the so-called pavilion-style hospital consisting of multiple long, narrow buildings with windows on both sides connected by covered walkways. Influential too was a Dutch architectural manual on civil and military architecture that Pompe apparently brought to Japan, which included a design for a pavilion-style hospital.[2]

The Nagasaki hospital was an H-shaped structure consisting of two two-story pavilions joined by a central corridor. The pavilions each measured about 45 meters × 32 meters, featured large glass windows, and had a capacity of 124 patients who were accommodated in eight fifteen-bed wards and four private rooms.[3] Although smaller in scale than contemporary European hospitals, many of which could house hundreds of patients, it was a modern space that reflected contemporary ideas about hygiene and care. The architectural historian Jeanne Kisacky has argued that architects who designed hospitals in the mid-nineteenth century "overwhelmingly privileged the building's therapeutic potential over its ability to facilitate medical treatment." In her words, the hospital in this era was intended to be "an orderly, sunlit, well-aired place in which the urban poor could be returned to health (and moral behavior)."[4] This may have been the intent, but a stay in the Nagasaki hospital must have been an unnerving experience for its Japanese patients, not only because of the novelty of institution-based medical care but also because Pompe insisted that they sleep in beds and be served Western-style food.[5]

The Nagasaki hospital introduced the idea of institutionally based medical care to the samurai students at the medical school, but many Japanese likely encountered the idea of the hospital by other means. In 1866 Fukuzawa Yukichi, who would later become one of the most famous public intellectuals of the day, published the first three volumes of the influential work *Conditions in the West* (*Seiyō jijō*), a bestseller by the standards of the day. It is estimated that more than a quarter million copies of the work were sold.[6] Fukuzawa had traveled to the US and Europe as part of two official Japanese diplomatic missions in the early 1860s, and upon his return to Japan he sought to introduce the public to the political, economic, and social institutions he had observed while overseas.

Hospitals were among the facilities that caught his attention. In London, Fukuzawa had toured St. George's Hospital, King's Cross Hospital, and St. Mary's Hospital. All were of recent origin: King's Cross was established in 1840 in an area surrounded by slums, while St. George's was founded in 1733 but was rebuilt in the mid-nineteenth century. The building Fukuzawa toured was completed in 1844. St. Mary's, established in 1851, was the last of London's great charitable hospitals to be founded. All three of these London hospitals were housed in neoclassical buildings, featuring multiple floors, a central staircase, and corridors that provided access to wards and private rooms on two sides of the building.[7] So, too, was, the famous Charité hospital in Berlin, which Fukuzawa also visited. In Paris, however, he toured the Hôpital Lariboisière. Built in the new pavilion style, it was completed less than a decade before Fukuzawa's tour, in 1853.[8]

Fukuzawa thus had the opportunity to visit some of the largest and most modern hospitals in Europe. In *Conditions in the West*, he described them as an important feature of urban life in all major European cities, noting that they made health care available to a wide swath of urban residents. The very poor paid nothing, while others who had some income paid according to their means. This, he explained, was possible because hospitals were either supported by the government or funded by donations from the wealthy. For his readers, who were likely unfamiliar with private philanthropy, Fukuzawa explained that in Europe, people made donations to hospitals as the Japanese did to temples and shrines. He also described the organization of the hospitals: they had multiple doctors on staff, thirty or more, and men and women were accommodated in different wards and cared for by nursing staff of the same gender, with one nurse responsible for ten patients.[9]

Fukuzawa, an astute observer, was correct in his assessment about the prominent place of hospitals in nineteenth-century European and US cities. As cities had grown in size and complexity, absorbing immigrants from both the countryside and abroad, concerns arose about the deleterious effects of urban life along with a newly recognized need to provide health care for poor and working class urban residents. In Paris, New York, and London, public and charitable hospitals became the object of civic pride and government support as the idea of the "hospital" began to evolve. No longer were they to be warehouses for people who were elderly, indigent, and dying. Instead, modern hospitals should be light, airy spaces staffed by skilled, caring professionals, where "citizen-patients" would be returned to health, and the next generation of skilled physicians and nurses trained.[10] It was this optimistic vision of the hospital that impressed Fukuzawa and perhaps his readers as well.

A Hospital for the Nation

This rosy picture of hospitals notwithstanding, Tokyo's first hospital of the modern era had little to do with the institutions that Fukuzawa had toured or the first generation of modern doctors had experienced in Nagasaki. With the establishment of the new government in 1868, the military hospital in

Shitaya was renamed the Daibyōin (Great Hospital), and the Western Medical Institute was placed under the direction of its staff. This was the first step in the process of building a modern medical school and a teaching hospital but frequent changes in both administration and naming followed. Early in 1869, the hospital and medical school were given equal status and renamed the Medical School and Hospital (*Igakkō-ken-byōin*). Later that year, the name was changed again, and the school became the Eastern College (Daigaku Tōkō). In 1870, Sagara Chian, the future head of the Medicine Bureau, and Iwasa Jun, the emperor's treating physician, were appointed to oversee the project of institutionalizing Western medicine. Like Sagara, Iwasa had been trained at the Medical Training Center in Nagasaki. While Dutch was the language of instruction, many of the books used at the Nagasaki school were translations from German, and both Sagara and Iwasa were aware of the achievements of German physicians and scientists. Impressed by the results of German medical training, they advocated successfully for the establishment of a research-focused medical school, and when the new school opened it was staffed by German military physicians.[11] Even as instruction got underway, name changes continued. In 1874, the school was renamed Tokyo Medical School. In 1877 the medical school, which had moved to Hongō the year before, became part of the new University of Tokyo.

Little is known about the functioning of the hospital during this time, but Leopold Müller, one of the German instructors at the medical school, later wrote that "the most basic hygienic requirements" for a hospital were "neglected." According to Müller, garbage was disposed of carelessly in courtyards, bedding went unaired, and the air itself was befouled by the smoke of the many charcoal braziers that were used both for cooking and heat. He also took note of the crowded conditions. In addition to its patients, the hospital housed their family members as well. They prepared meals, laundered clothing, and provided basic nursing care to their relatives.

Japanese officials were apparently aware of the poor conditions in the hospital. Müller noted that they wanted to build "a huge European monumental building with the newest of ventilation, heating, and facilities for disinfection" within what is now Ueno Park.[12] Given that the prefecture's Poorhouse and the Public Asylum were in the park at this time, the intention was apparently to make it a campus for medical and social welfare facilities. Although the architect of the planned hospital is unknown, his design is striking.[13] The plan shows an elaborate building with seventeen separate pavilions connected to walkways in the shape of a triangle, providing for light and air to enter the

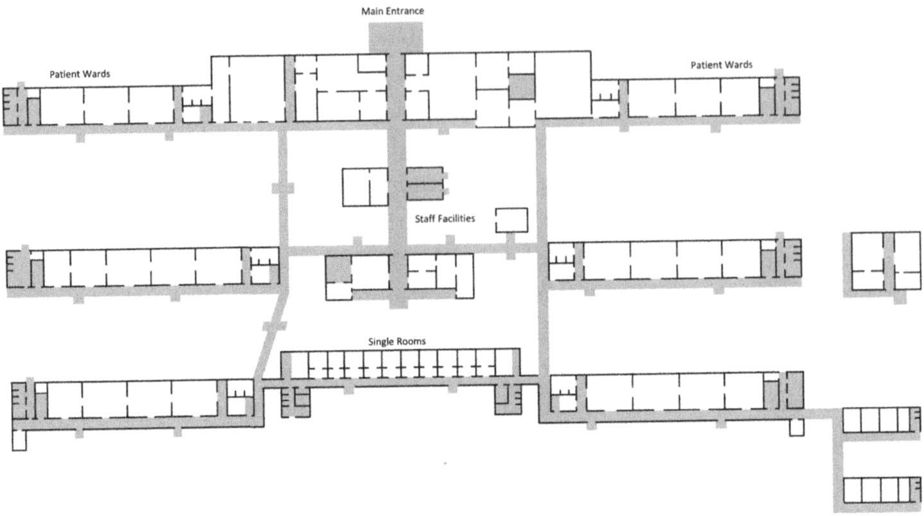

Figure 3.1. University of Tokyo No. 1 Hospital, constructed 1876–1877. Image by Hannah Tomio, based on Tōkyō Daigaku Igakubu, *Tōkyō Daigaku Igakubu ichiran Meiji 13-nen–14-nen*, 4.

building from three directions. Additional facilities such as lecture rooms, a pharmacy, a surgical theater, administrative offices, and a morgue were situated at the base of the triangle and in the central courtyard, while student dormitories were clustered around it, signaling the hospital's intended role as a teaching institution.[14]

This ambitious plan was opposed by Müller and the other German instructors of the medical school who proposed building a simple structure that would be ready more quickly than the "monumental building" envisioned by some. In the end, a far simpler design was adopted (see fig. 3.1), and the building was completed in 1877. By the time construction got underway, there were new plans for the Ueno site, and instead the hospital was built on the new medical school campus in Hongō Motofuji-chō on the grounds of a former daimyo estate. Dubbed the No. 1 Hospital, it had 134 rooms and a total capacity of 348 patients, with the number of patients capped for each medical specialty. The internal medicine and surgical wards had a capacity for 91 patients and 88 patients respectively, while pediatrics could care for no more than seven.[15] The new hospital did not, however, entirely replace the original one. Instead, the latter was designated the No. 2 Hospital with a capacity to house 134 patients. Reflecting the difference in facilities, a stay in the No. 1 Hospital cost from 35 sen to 1 yen per day in 1881–1882, while the No. 2 Hospital cost 30–60 sen per day.[16] At the time, an elementary school teacher made about 5 yen a month, so even a brief hospital stay would have strained the finances of many Tokyo residents.[17] Moreover, these room charges did not include meals, medications, and physician fees, and given that hospital stays in this period tended to be lengthy, the cost of treatment at the hospital would have been beyond the reach of many.

There were, however, provisions for the treatment of poorer patients. According to the Medical Policy, every hospital that received government funding was to provide charitable care for poor people, and all medical schools (both public and private) were required to have a hospital attached. These two provisions were to ensure that medical students received clinical training while providing wider access to modern medical care. The dual aim of using hospitals to supply both medical training and charitable care resulted in something akin to a Faustian bargain, at least from the perspective of impoverished patients. According to the 1881–1882 catalog (*ichiran*) of the medical faculty, "This hospital is attached to the University of Tokyo Medical School, and patients will be admitted who are beneficial for purposes of scholarly study and the staff's educational lectures to students."[18] What this meant in practice was that the hospital could be selective about who would be admitted for care. A later guide to the hospital put it more bluntly: "Only charity patients whose symptoms are recognized as necessary for scholarly research will be admitted."[19]

Once admitted, nonpaying patients were subject to several requirements. They had to agree to accept the treatments offered as well as to an autopsy if they died while hospitalized. To enforce compliance with the treatment regime ordered, patients were required to sign a contract stating they would follow the directives of the teaching faculty under threat of financial penalty; this provision would have made it difficult for nonpaying patients to leave the hospital or refuse further treatment.[20] Because charity patients typically had few financial resources, the hospital required that a patient's guarantor (*hoshōnin*) also sign the contract, promising to pay the penalty if the patient could not.[21]

Despite these provisions for poor patients, most of those treated at the new hospitals were well off. Indeed, in 1876, a Bureau of Hygiene official commented, "The hospitals in our country are very different from those in Europe and America in that they are, generally, places that offer treatment to those above the middle class."[22] The initial step in being admitted for treatment required patients to queue up during clinic hours in the hope of being examined by one of the medical school's professors, but the number of patients seen each day was limited, and many were turned away. In 1890 Erwin Bälz, the famous German physician who counted the Meiji emperor among his patients, saw patients Monday, Wednesday, and Friday mornings, but no more than an eighteen per day. Other members of the faculty were less generous than Bälz. His colleague Julius Scriba, the head of the surgery department, saw patients only two days a week and no more than ten patients per day.[23]

Not everyone was forced to wait in hope of seeing a doctor: the well-connected were easily able to gain admittance to the university hospitals even if their symptoms were not "beneficial for the purpose of scholarly study." Bälz's diary for this period reveals that he saw a steady stream of elite and well-off patients, including family members of former daimyo, high-ranking military officers, members of the peerage, nobility, and diplomatic communities, and a high-ranking priest associated with Honganji Temple.[24] Given the popularity of the hospital among Tokyo's elite, administrators eventually established quotas for charity patients to ensure that the university's hospitals met their obligation to provide care for poor residents as well as wealthy and well-connected citizens. In 1876 only 40 patients were to be treated without cost each year, but by 1896, hospital regulations required care for 328 charity patients annually.[25]

A Hospital for the City

The university's hospital was never intended to serve as a general hospital for city residents. The prioritization of research and teaching and the burdensome restrictions placed on poorer patients meant that it had a limited impact on the health of Tokyo residents. But even before the role of the university hospital was fully defined, plans were underway for the founding of a different kind of institution. In the early 1870s, amid the organizational changes shaping the medical school and its hospital, the health of the city's residents concerned many. In 1872 Satō Naokata, then director of the medical school's hospital, petitioned the Imperial Household Ministry (the government agency in charge of matters related to the imperial family, including its finances) for permission—and money—to establish a public hospital that would provide modern medical care for the city's residents. The ministry agreed and offered a grant of 10,000 yen, in one of the first instances of the imperial family's growing involvement in public philanthropy.

Initially, Hatchōbori in Kyōbashi, one of the city's most densely populated areas, was the proposed site of the new public hospital, but the plan was soon abandoned, perhaps because the purchase of a suitable plot of land was too costly. At the time, land values in Kyōbashi were second only to those of neighboring Nihonbashi.[26] Eventually, the city acquired a plot of approximately 1.6

hectares (about 4 acres) in the area known as Atago in what was then the Second Ward and after 1878, Shiba Ward.[27] This part of the city bore little resemblance to Hatchōbori. Before the Restoration, it had been home to the estates of daimyo and other high-ranking vassals of the Shogun, as well as important religious institutions, including Zōjōji temple, where the mausoleums of several Tokugawa shoguns stand, and the Atago Shrine, founded by Ieyasu, the first Tokugawa shogun. After the Restoration, much of this land was confiscated by the new government and gradually repurposed.

But there was another aspect to Shiba. Situated close to Edo Bay, it stood on low-lying land, adjacent to the 250-meter-high hill that housed Atago Shrine and was subject to flooding during times of high tides and heavy rains. The hospital was also near Shin'ami-chō, which by the late 1870s was already known as one of Tokyo's largest slum districts. In the Edo period, this area had been home to various groups of entertainers, officially classified as outcasts.[28] However, in the period just before and after the fall of the shogunate, it began to attract new residents. Located near the Tōkaidō, the great highway that linked Edo to Kyoto, dislocated people who flowed into the city came to settle here. After the Restoration, the number of residents continued to grow. By 1890, an estimated 3,400 people lived in Shin'ami-chō, an area of less than 2 hectares.[29] Like many parts of the city at this moment of transition, Shiba was the site of a heterogeneous mix of people and institutions.

Initially known as the Prefectural Hospital and as the Atago Hospital, and later officially named the Tokyo Prefectural Hospital, the new institution was, from the outset, an ambitious endeavor. The building itself was about 3,200 square meters in area and was built at a cost of 9,227 yen, although unfortunately, no photos, sketches, or plans for the building seem to have survived.[30] At the time of its opening, the hospitals had a staff of seventeen doctors, including one "hired foreigner," an American physician named Albert Ashmead. Ashmead had been educated at the University of Pennsylvania and Jefferson Medical College in Philadelphia and had come to Japan at the invitation of Prince Kachō Hirotsune. When the prince fell ill while studying at the US Naval Academy, he was treated by Ashmead, an encounter that resulted in Ashmead's employment by the Japanese government. Iwasa Jun and Sasaki Tōyō (another graduate of the Nagasaki Medical Training Institute) were appointed director and associate director, respectively.[31]

All three men would be employed at the hospital for less than a year, although this was not particularly unusual at the time. Iwasa left to establish his own private hospital; Sasaki became director of the university's hospital; and

Ashmead returned to the US. Iwasa was replaced by Tsuboi Shinryō, formerly a physician in the shogunal household, who served as director of the hospital from 1874 to 1877. He was succeeded by Hasegawa Tai, by then an important figure in the Tokyo medical world. Two new foreign doctors also joined the staff. Tjarko W. Beukema was a Dutch physician, and C. J. Manning was a British surgeon who had trained at University College Hospital London.[32]

The hospital opened in May 1873 and initially had to work hard to attract patients. Advertisements for the hospital appeared frequently in the newspapers and often included references to the schedule of the clinics conducted by Manning and Beukema, presumably because readers would be interested in care at the hands of a foreign expert.[33] This, after all, was one of the attractions of the university's hospital. Treatment was available for both inpatients and outpatients, and, following Edo-period practice, outpatients were not charged for diagnostic examinations but only for the medicines they were prescribed.[34] The cost for inpatient care was also relatively low, at least compared to the university-affiliated hospitals. There were four types of rooms, with the most expensive costing 1 yen per day, and the least expensive, only 25 sen per day.[35]

Still, the location of the hospital, far from the more populated areas of the city, seems to have been a problem. In this period, public transportation was not yet available, and potential patients had to walk or take a rickshaw to the hospital. The rate for a rickshaw was standardized with a distance of 1 ri (approximately 4 kilometers) costing 6 sen 2 rin. Tokyo was still a relatively compact city at the time, but a trip from Asakusa or Honjo to the hospital would have been an expensive endeavor for many. For the convenience of patients, two branch clinics were established in 1876. The first, located at Bakurō-chō near Asakusa Bridge, opened in May; the second, in Fukagawa, opened in September. Both facilities were about 297 square meters (3,200 square feet) in area, considerably smaller than the main hospital.[36] Other branch clinics were planned for Shinjuku and Shinagawa, but these never materialized.[37]

Hospital staff also used the newspapers to publicize the hospital's efforts to educate the public about health and hygiene. For example, between March 24 and April 7, 1878, the *Yomiuri* newspaper published a twelve-part series on the care of infants and children. Topics addressed included the use of cow's milk and other substances as alternatives to breastmilk, treatments for common childhood ailments like colic as well as weaning and the introduction of solid foods.[38] The press also publicized the hospital's success in tackling difficult cases. Articles in 1878 and 1879 reported on successful amputations, removal of tumors, the use of tracheotomies in diphtheria cases, and even the birth of a child to a woman who had suffered multiple miscarriages. The public image of the hospital was thus that of a thoroughly modern medical facility, where miraculous treatments were available.

Despite these glowing press reports, evidence indicates that some residents of Tokyo were suspicious of the hospital. In January 1879, the *Yomiuri* published a letter from a woman named Masu, a resident of Ryōgoku Hisamatsu-chō, who had recently given birth at the hospital as part of a new program that offered poor women midwifery care at no cost. Masu wrote explicitly to dispel rumors about the hospital—that "living blood" was stolen, that patients were treated as "guinea pigs" for trainees, and that the poor were subject to abuse at the hands of the hospital staff. Instead, she described her experience in positive terms.[39] The relatively sophisticated language and style of the letter, however, suggests that it may have been penned by someone other than Masu to counter rumors that were circulating about the quality of the care on offer.

From the time of its establishment, the hospital played an important role in early public health initiatives in Tokyo. The campaign to control syphilis will be the topic of chapter 4, but it is worth noting at this point that when the examination of prostitutes for syphilis began in 1873, infected women were required to be transferred to the hospital for treatment, the cost of which was borne by owners of the brothels where they worked. Smallpox was another concern for city officials. Although vaccination had been available in Edo from 1858, the number of vaccinated city residents remained relatively small, and outbreaks of the disease were common. In 1876, the government passed the Smallpox Prevention Law, which mandated vaccination for infants under the age of one. Both the main hospital and the branch clinics offered smallpox vaccinations for a small fee, and when a smallpox epidemic broke out in 1876, vaccination was made available to the poor at no cost.[40] Similarly, when cholera broke out in 1877, the hospital created a quarantine unit for cholera patients and offered advice for how to avoid infection.[41] In that same year, the hospital became involved in the treatment of leprosy, forging a relationship with Gotō Masafumi, a doctor of Sino-Japanese medicine who had gained fame for the treatment he offered at his private leprosy hospital. Although Hasegawa was skeptical of the effectiveness of Gotō's "cure," he agreed to designate Gotō's facility in Kanda a "branch" of the prefectural hospital, an arrangement that made it possible for the hospital to pay for the care of impoverished sufferers of the disease. This arrangement, however, was short-lived. In 1879, concerned that Gotō's costly treatment brought only a temporary improvement in symptoms, Hasegawa severed ties with him.[42]

Training Modern Doctors

An important function of the public hospital was the training of medical professionals. The Medical Policy had outlined a procedure for the licensing of physicians, requiring those who wanted to take the credentialing exam to present proof of graduation from a medical school and of experience in two specialized fields. However, "for the time being," those already in practice could receive a "temporary license," with the caveat that they must take a licensing exam within ten years. Initially, localities determined the content of the exam, until a national medical exam began to be offered in 1878. In 1882 new standards were established for medical schools, which were divided into two ranks: those who graduated from the higher-rank schools (which included university medical schools) were granted licenses without an examination, and those who graduated from lower-ranked schools were required to pass a licensing exam.[43]

The earliest information on the number and credentials of doctors dates from 1882, and it reveals the progress of medical modernization less than a decade after it got underway. There were then 2,346 doctors in Tokyo (2.6 per 1,000 people) but only about 25 percent were fully licensed. Of the 75 percent practicing under a temporary license, 396 or almost 30 percent had attempted the exam but failed.[44] Another issue was the unequal distribution of doctors, licensed or not, around the city. In 1882 the ratio of physicians to population (see fig. 3.2) was greatest in the central and western wards of the city, while the two wards east of the Sumida River, Honjo and Fukagawa, had relatively few doctors, as did Koishikawa, then the most agricultural of Tokyo's wards.[45]

Increasing the number of doctors trained in Western medicine was a priority in this period, and medical schools took a variety of forms. As noted above, the Tokyo Medical School (from 1877 the Medical Faculty of the University of Tokyo) trained the medical elite, with particularly promising students sent to Europe for further training. On the other end of spectrum was Seisai Gakusha, a medical school founded by Hasegawa Tai. Unlike the research-oriented university-based medical schools, Seisai Gakusha focused on quickly preparing aspiring doctors and established doctors trained in Sino-Japanese medicine to pass the new licensing exam. Its low fees and open admission policy (women were accepted as students) made it extremely popular. Lectures were offered from 5:00 a.m. to 9:00 p.m., and, at least in theory, it was possible to pass the licensing exam after only one year of study. While it was disparaged as a "cram school" by some, including the army's surgeon general, Mori Rintarō, Hasegawa himself defended the school as the most expeditious way to train

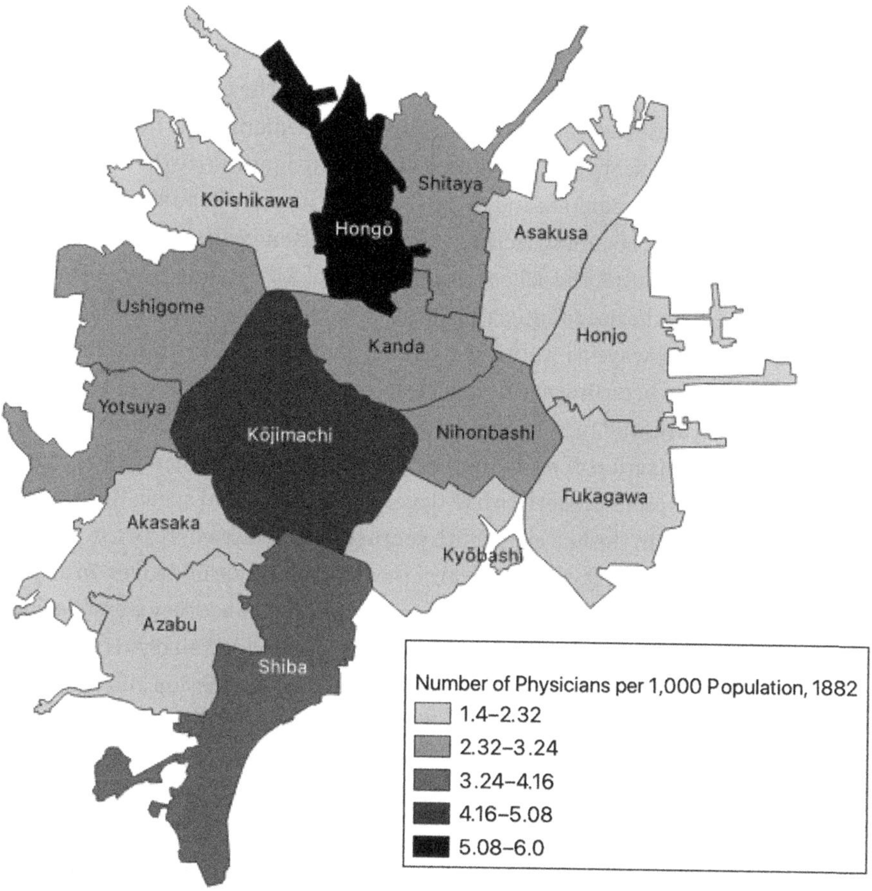

Figure 3.2. Number of doctors per 1,000 population, 1882. Data from Tōkyō-fu, ed., *Tōkyō-fu tōkeisho Meiji 15-nen*, "Eisei," 7.

doctors in Western medicine. In fact, the school's teachers included many notable doctors, among them faculty members of the Tokyo Medical School, who worked on a part-time basis. Initially, there were no provisions for clinical training but in 1886 a hospital was established adjacent to the school. Somon Hospital, as it was known, had two wards and twenty beds. It functioned as both a charity and teaching hospital: patients were only charged for the medicines they received, but in return had to agree to be subjects of clinical lectures and submit to examinations by Seisai students.[46]

The Tokyo Prefectural Medical School (1873–1878) occupied a middle ground between these two approaches to medical training by offering students both academic and clinical training. In the five years of its existence, 87 students had graduated, and another 93 were studying at the time of its closing. Another important pedagogical role of the prefectural hospital was the reeducation of doctors of Sino-Japanese medicine. The hospital staff offered extension school–style lectures designed to familiarize them with the tenets of Western medicine, and these seemed to be quite popular. According to newspaper reports, these lectures were often attended by well over a hundred doctors.[47] In 1878, the school reported that of 248 attendees, 171 had successfully passed the licensing exam. The hospital was involved in the licensing process in other ways as well. Until the unified national examination was established, the licensing exam was prepared and administered at the level of the prefecture, and in Tokyo the prefectural hospital assumed this role.[48]

The modernization of midwifery was another project undertaken by the prefectural hospital. Obstetrics had developed as a medical specialization in Japan beginning in the late eighteenth century, and as elsewhere in the world, male obstetricians were often critical of the skills of female midwives. In addition, midwives came under criticism on ethical grounds since they were known to perform abortions and aid in acts of neonatal infanticide.[49] In 1876 Hasegawa Tai petitioned the prefectural government to ask for permission and funds to start a midwifery school at the prefectural hospital. After the prefectural government approved this plan, announcements were made in the newspapers, soliciting thirty students for what would be Tokyo's first midwifery school.[50] Students were to be between the ages of twenty and thirty and had to be able to read and write. The course took eighteen months to complete, with classes meeting for two to three hours per day. Although there was no fee for the course, and textbooks and equipment were to be provided free of charge, initial applications were fewer than the intended class of thirty, and the application date was extended several times. The course finally got underway in October 1877.[51]

As a textbook for the students, the hospital sponsored the publication of a translation of *Lehrbuch der Hebammenkunst* (Textbook of Midwifery, 1860) by the German obstetrician Bernhard Schultze under the title *Sanbaron* (Treatise on Midwifery). Advertisements at the time describe this work as a "must read" for both midwives and women generally, and it became a standard textbook for midwifery students for several decades, with the fourth and final edition published in 1896.[52] To aid in the training of modern midwives, in 1878 the hospital opened an obstetrical unit and offered free obstetrical care to women who agreed to give birth in the hospital—something that would remain uncommon until the postwar era.[53] However, as discussed above, the efforts

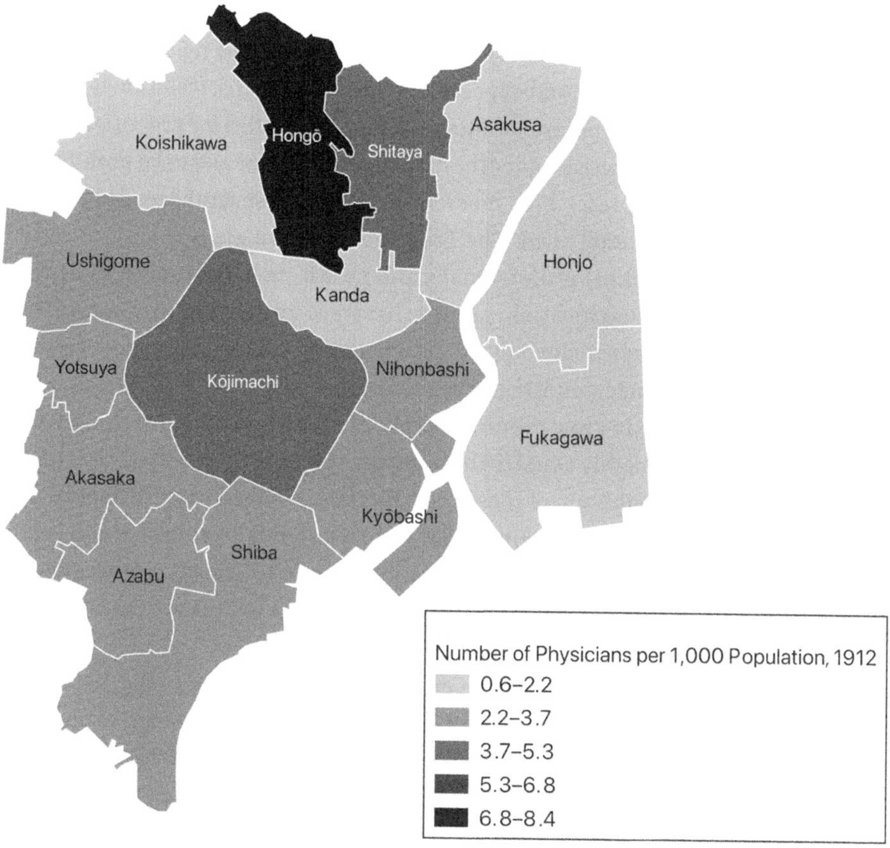

Figure 3.3. Number of doctors per 1,000 population, 1912. Data from Tōkyō-fu, ed., *Tōkyō-fu tōkei-sho Taishō gannen*, 267–78.

to recruit poor women to give birth in the hospital for training purposes was greeted by considerable suspicion on the part of some Tokyo residents.

With this varied landscape of medical education in place, the number of licensed doctors in the city increased steadily over the late nineteenth and early twentieth century. By 1912, there were 4,234 doctors in Tokyo, almost double the number three decades earlier, and all but 265 of these were fully licensed, evidence of the success of the government's gradualist approach. However, the increased number of doctors did not keep up with population growth: by 1912, physician density had fallen to 2.1 per 1,000 population.[54] Moreover, the uneven distribution of doctors around the city continued. Fukagawa and Honjo, by this time the center of Tokyo's industrial zone and home to many members of the new working class, continued to be underserved, even as doctors began to practice in less populated western wards of the city (see fig. 3.3).

Despite the growing number of credentialed physicians, traditional therapies continued to be popular. The Medical Policy had called for practitioners of these therapies to practice under the direction of a doctor and to be prohibited from preparing or prescribing medicines, but it was several decades before regulations were established. The Tokyo government already kept records on numbers of medical professionals, and now it included practitioners of acupuncture and moxibustion, groups that were growing in this period. In 1882, there were reportedly only 452 practitioners, a suspiciously low figure that may reflect undercounting, given that three years later it was 1,230. The number continued to grow over the next two and half decades, reaching 3,114 in 1906, a figure roughly equal to the number of doctors in the city at the time. However, the distribution of these practitioners was strikingly different. In Honjo and Fukagawa, for example, the number of moxibustionists and acupuncturists was almost double that of licensed doctors.[55] It may have been then that traditional practitioners established themselves in areas of the city that had few credentialed physicians.

The new availability of modern doctors then did not lead to the displacement of traditional practitioners. Rather, practitioners of massage, acupuncture, and moxibustion too became part of the modern medical marketplace, and like the city's doctors, they were shaped by it. These nonphysician practitioners created professional associations, advertised heavily in the newspapers, and began to explain their methods in biomedical terms. They also proclaimed the efficacy of their therapies for the diseases that were the targets of public health discourse, such as cholera and beriberi, aligning themselves with the new discourse of public health, and some even began integrating the use of electricity into their practice.[56]

Gradually, however, efforts to regulate these therapies got underway, perhaps because practitioners were making increasingly expansive claims of efficacy, or because of reports of serious complications following treatment.[57] In 1880 Tokyo Prefecture issued an edict forbidding acupuncturists, moxibustion practitioners, and massage therapists to prepare or provide medications to patients.[58] In 1885 the Hygiene Bureau in the Home Ministry ordered prefectural governments to require practitioners to submit their training history to prefectural authorities for review. In response, the Tokyo prefectural government followed a procedure like the one used for doctors: already established practitioners were issued temporary licenses, while new ones were required to take a licensing exam.[59] Initially, at least, the pass rate seems to have been quite high, because in 1907 the Tokyo government announced that a more rigorous exam would be developed.[60]

A final turning point came in 1911 when the Home Ministry issued new national regulations that required practitioners of acupuncture and moxibustion with less than four years of experience to take a new national licensing exam that tested their knowledge of anatomy, disinfection, theory, and practical skills. There were additional restrictions: acupuncturists and moxibustion practitioners were now forbidden to use electricity or do any procedure regarded as surgical in nature, and they were prohibited from treating those with mental illness or an infectious disease.[61] Faced with these new requirements, some acupuncturists and moxibustion therapists, willingly or not, abandoned their trade, and traditional therapies became an increasingly marginal part of the city's medical culture.

Caring for the Poor Population

From the time of its founding, the prefectural hospital made provisions for the care of people living in poverty, but in 1877 new policies were established to expand its role in relation to the "ward doctor" system discussed in chapter 2. Although the ward doctors continued to be authorized to treat minor illnesses and injuries themselves, patients who were seriously ill or in need of specialized care were now to be referred to the prefectural hospital, and even patients suffering from minor ailments had the option to request that their ward office issue a ticket for use at the hospital or one of its branches. Based on where they resided, charity patients were required to seek treatment at specific facilities. Residents in the Second and Third Wards were to go to the main hospital, residents of the First and Fifth Wards were to go to the Bakurō-chō Clinic, and those in the Sixth Ward to the Fukagawa Clinic. Residents of the Fourth Ward were sent to Juntendō Hospital, a private general hospital in Yushima.[62]

In a very real sense, the attempt to create a system of free or low-cost care to improve the health of Tokyo's poor was a victim of its own success. From the outset, those who developed the ticket system were aware of the potential for the cost of the program to spiral, and they put into place measures designed to control expenses and to ensure that a black market for tickets did not take form. Only a limited number of tickets were issued for any single month, the names of recipients were recorded, and tickets expired at the end of the month for which they were issued. Still, there were many unknowns: ward doctors prepared and supplied medicines to patients, and under the ticket system they could seek reimbursement for these expenses. Tokyo officials recognized the potential for abuse by the doctors who could prescribe expensive medications or charge exorbitant fees. To counter this, they originally planned to establish a Tokyo Prefectural Charity Pharmacy (Tokyo-fu seryō chōsetsu yakusho) to prepare and distribute medicines, but this was never accomplished.[63] As feared, the actual cost of the program grew, exceeding the budgeted amount by 60 percent in the period from June 1879 to July 1880. Tokyo officials responded by limiting the number of charity patients to 190 per month, less than half of those who had been seen in an average month in the previous year.[64]

The growing resentment of doctors in private practice was another looming problem. After he became director of the prefectural hospital, Hasegawa Tai sought to use the new system of ward doctors to improve the quality of medical care offered by the city's physicians. Four of the ward doctors were selected to organize a new General Practitioners Assembly (Kaigyōi shūkai) offering doctors edifying lectures on medicine, public health, and professional ethics. These meetings were held in the Prefectural Assembly Building, a locale that gave them an aura of authority.[65] Some Tokyo wards went even further and organized such assemblies at the ward level: in Ushigome, for example, doctors in the ward met on the third of each month beginning in February 1878 in a local school.[66] Ironically, this attempt to create a professional organization that would further the prefecture's goals instead inspired doctors to create a new, parallel organization with a very different goal: to dismantle the prefectural hospital and the ward doctor system. The Society to Protect the Rights of Tokyo's Independent Doctors, as it was called, was headed by physicians who, in fact, benefited from the charity ticket system, including Satō Naokata and Satō Susumu, both of whom served as directors of Juntendō, the private hospital that had been integrated into the charity care system.[67]

At its first meeting, the new organization put together a memorandum to the prefectural government that laid bare the deep resentment of many doctors toward the prefecture's involvement in medical care. The memorial asserted that the prefecture's proper role in medical matters should be limited to the control of infectious diseases and that all other medical matters should be left to "independent doctors." The prefectural hospital and the charity ticket system, it was argued, threatened the livelihood of Tokyo's doctors. The organization's members were also critical of the prefectural medical school. They argued that its students included many who resided outside the prefecture, and support for their education thus constituted an abuse of taxpaying prefectural residents. The memorial also made the point that the current system of charitable care required the poor to make their financial situation public, which some were unwilling to do.

To resolve these issues, the society called for the prefectural government to scale down its involvement in medical matters. The prefectural hospital, they asserted, should be turned into a "poverty hospital" (*hinbyōin*) that would serve the city's destitute, and private doctors should take responsibility for offering charitable medical care to members of their local communities, without the involvement of the government. This would save tax dollars, protect the livelihood of the city's doctors, and respect the dignity of the deserving poor.[68] It is worth noting that the Tokyo doctors were not alone in their opposition to governmental involvement in health care: elsewhere, too, private doctors organized against the establishment of prefectural hospitals and medical schools.[69]

The plan put forward by the society presented a radically different vision of an urban health care system, one organized simultaneously by old notions of voluntarism, self-regulation, and limited government and by new concepts of rights and professional advocacy. Unfortunately for supporters of the prefectural hospital, the organized opposition of the city's doctors came as the prefectural government was grappling with an acute public health issue, the cholera epidemic in 1880 that killed 1,700 people and sickened many more. In addition, during this period, the country was beset with rampant inflation that prompted the central government in 1881 to adopt a set of deflationary policies. These included cutting expenditures and raising taxes, policies that shifted responsibilities for public services downward to the local level. Even before the central government announced the retrenchment policies, Tokyo Prefecture took a first step toward defunding the charity ticket program: in 1880 it cut the budget for subsidized medical care by 25 percent.[70] The arguments advanced by the society—that public health should be the Tokyo government's central concern and that the other functions of the prefectural hospital could be shifted to the private sector—found a newly receptive audience in the prefectural assembly. In 1881, the ambitious experiment in publicly funded health care and medical education came to an end when the assembly voted to close the prefectural hospital and its branches and end the charity ticket system.

To be sure, not everyone was happy about this development, especially since the prefectural government's retreat from public medical care was complete. That is, there was to be no publicly funded charity hospital, an institution that even the Society to Protect the Rights of Tokyo's Independent Doctors had thought necessary, given the number of Tokyo residents who lived in poverty. One critic of this decision took action. Takaki Kanehiro (1849–1920), a naval physician, would later gain fame for his discovery that beriberi could be managed through dietary measures. Born into a samurai family in Satsuma, Takaki had begun his medical studies under a domanial physician. Still in his teens at the time of the Boshin War, he served as a medic for the anti-Tokugawa forces and later studied under the British physician William Willis, who in 1870 had found employment in a new medical school established in Kagoshima. Two years later Takaki joined the navy and in 1875, he was dispatched to London for further medical training, interning at St. Thomas' Hospital, one of the city's great charity hospitals. This was a significant departure from the government's later practice of dispatching promising students to German universities for medical training, and it clearly influenced Takaki's conception of social responsibility for the poor. Takaki spent five years at St. Thomas' and upon his return to Japan he devoted considerable energy into replicating the aspects of British medical culture he admired. He founded one of Japan's first medical societies, the Seiikai or Society for the Advancement of Medical Science, which published a medical journal in both English and Japanese.[71]

Takaki soon set about establishing a charity medical hospital on the British model that Fukuzawa had praised a decade and a half before. He started with fundraising, seeking donations from a wide range of public figures including Totsuka Bunkai, a prominent naval doctor; Tashiro Motonori, founder of the journal *Medical News* (*Iji shinbun*) and director of the army's medical school; Koyasu Takashi, founder of the *Yomiuri shinbun*, and Narushima Ryūhoku, publisher of the *Chōya shinbun*, as well as other journalists and businesspeople. Together they raised more than 100,000 yen in capital for the new hospital and identified more than 126 subscribers who agreed to support a privately financed charity hospital. They then approached the prefectural governor and requested permission to rent the now closed prefectural hospital and its furnishings and equipment.[72] The petition they submitted to the governor makes it clear that they were responding to the closing of the prefectural hospital. It opens with a description of the dilemma that the city's poor confronted: "They struggle day and night just for food and clothing and when on top of that they become ill, there is no way for them to get help even when they know that death could result. And so some die at the hands of Chinese medicine doctors while others end their lives having turned to patent medicines and prayers." The petition goes on to note that this pointless loss of life occurs "even in the imperial capital" where many poor people lived in crowded city neighborhoods. Recognizing their plight, early on the government had taken on the worthy task of providing medical care to the poor but regrettably had abandoned that effort. "Lamenting this," Takaki and his colleagues had decided that they must work to establish a hospital.[73]

The strong tone of reprimand was effective and the prefectural government both approved the founding of the new hospital and agreed to rent the buildings that had housed the former prefectural hospital to the new venture. According to its charter, the new hospital was to be funded by the interest on the capital Takaki and his compatriots had raised, together with voluntary subscriptions and money from fundraising activities. The Tokyo Voluntary Cooperative Hospital (Yūshi Kyōritsu Byōin) opened its doors in August 1882. In its first year it provided care for 186 inpatients and 349 outpatients, just a fraction of the number of patients who had been cared for in the prefectural hospital. In 1883 the hospital acquired some important patrons, which greatly improved its visibility and financial situation. These included Prince Arisugawa Taruhito, uncle of the Meiji emperor, who became its president, and a group of aristocratic women headed by Princess Arisugawa, who created a Woman's Aid Society to support the hospital by fundraising. In 1886 the Meiji empress became an official patron of the hospital, replacing Prince Arisugawa as president. The following year, at the suggestion of the empress it was said, the name of the hospital was changed to Tokyo Charity Hospital (Tōkyō Jikei Byōin).[74]

The name signaled an important change in the nature of the institution. While the term "voluntary cooperative" had brought attention to the community effort to support the poor, the term "jikei" (written with the characters that mean "benevolence" and "mercy") were strongly associated with the imperial institution. Takaki fully embraced this rebranding of the institution he had pioneered. In 1893 he submitted a report to the International Congress of Charities, Corrections, and Philanthropy that met in Chicago, which portrayed the hospital as part of a long tradition of imperial philanthropy that stretched back to the reign of Emperor Kinmei (509–571 CE). He suggests that the empress was deeply involved in every aspect of the hospital: she approved the members of the Aid Society, appointed the members of the medical board, and of course served as the hospital's president.[75]

But while the hospital provided good publicity for the imperial family, its impact on the health of Tokyo's residents was slight. Between 1886 and 1897, the hospital had on average fewer than 400 inpatients per year.[76] In his 1893 report to the Chicago congress, Takaki noted that at the time of his writing only about half the hospital's 120 beds were filled.[77] In actuality, the Charity Hospital functioned more successfully as an outpatient clinic. In the late 1880s, it was treating fewer than 200 outpatients per month, but that number increased substantially after 1890: between 1890 and 1898, the hospital saw, on average, almost 1,000 patients per month, likely consisting of people with minor and chronic ailments. The Charity Hospital was better equipped to deal with this population, since it was staffed entirely by volunteer doctors who donated their time on an occasional basis, making the treatment of difficult or acute cases more challenging. A letter of complaint published in *Yomiuri* in 1893 suggests that the hospital did indeed prefer to treat outpatients. It tells of an impoverished man who had fallen seriously ill. At the suggestion of the local police officer, he sought out treatment at the Charity Hospital but the journey to and from the hospital day after day proved difficult. He repeatedly asked to be hospitalized but was refused admittance with no explanation. Interestingly, two days later the paper issued a retraction describing the complaint as "baseless."[78] The facts of the case are unclear, but the apologetic tone of the retraction suggests that criticism of the Charity Hospital may have ruffled some powerful feathers.

The Tokyo Charity Hospital was not the only philanthropic medical institution founded in the aftermath of the dissolution of the prefectural hospital, nor was it unique in its connections to the imperial institution. In 1877 the civil conflict known as the Seinan War was raging in Kyushu, pitching the new conscript army against disaffected samurai, who were led by Saigō Takamori, formerly a member of the oligarchy that controlled the central government. In response, Sano Tsunetami (1822–1902), formerly the minister of war, established the Hakuaisha (Philanthropic Society) to care for the wounded. He was inspired by the activities of the International Red Cross, an organization he had learned of when he traveled to Paris as a member of the Japanese delegation to the Paris Exposition of 1867.[79] The International Red Cross had been founded only four years earlier by Henry Dunant, a young Swiss man who had been horrified when he witnessed the suffering of soldiers during the Battle of Solferino in 1859. From the beginning, Dunant had two aims, to create a relief organization for those involved in international conflicts and to create a legal basis to compel armies to provide care for all wounded.[80]

Initially, Sano's willingness to extend aid to enemy combatants—who in this case were former samurai fighting against the Imperial Army—evoked outrage among many both in Tokyo and on the battlefields of Kyushu, but he eventually found some powerful supporters, including Prince Arisugawa, Prince Komatsu Akihito, and Hashimoto Tsunatsune, surgeon general of the army from 1877 to 1886.[81] After the end of the conflict, Sano and his compatriots worked to institutionalize and expand their efforts. When Hashimoto traveled to Europe in 1883, he carried out a survey of the Red Cross's activities, organizational structure, and funding in various countries. After his return to Japan in 1885, he compiled a report for the government outlining the widening influence of the Red Cross movement. It proved convincing, and in 1886 the Japanese government signed the Geneva Convention, paving the way for the Hakuaisha to join the Red Cross Federation in 1887. From the beginning there were close ties between the new organization and the imperial household. Prince Komatsu became the first honorary president of the Japanese Red Cross, and the Meiji empress is credited with designing the organization's coat of arms.[82]

While these negotiations were ongoing, Hashimoto began advocating for the establishment of a hospital that would further the Hakuaisha's goals and public standing. In this instance too, he was influenced by developments in Europe, which had seen the founding of Red Cross hospitals in several countries. According to Hashimoto, such a facility would aid in training doctors and nurses who could be used in times of conflict, and it could provide care to wounded combatants if war broke out. With this vision of the hospital in mind, originally its focus was to be on surgical care, reflecting the type of injuries that might result from battle. Hashimoto approached the minister of the army with a request for a grant of property in central Tokyo where the new institution could be constructed, asserting that the hospital would serve national interests. In response, he was offered a plot of land in Iidabashi-chō in Kōjimachi, a part of the city that was both dotted with military installations and close to the imperial palace. There were other links with the military as well. At the time of its opening on November 18, 1886, all the doctors on staff were military doctors who volunteered their services to the hospital, although the application to the prefecture declared the hospital to be a private venture.[83] The imperial family also made a very public show of support for the new institution: the empress attended the opening ceremony, together with Prince Arisugawa and Prince Komatsu, and upon its conclusion she privately toured the new hospital in the company of Hashimoto.[84]

This support of the imperial household expanded after the hospital formally became the Japanese Red Cross Hospital in 1887. In 1888 it was decided to move the hospital outside the city proper to Shibuya Village to increase its capacity. The imperial household provided 80,000 yen to fund the purchase of land and construction, a generous gift that made it possible to build an impressive new pavilion-style hospital with 57 rooms of varying size and a capacity of 101 beds (see fig. 3.4). Designed by Katayama Tōkuma, one of the most famous architects of the day, it was almost ten times the size of the old hospital and incorporated a large Japanese garden in an interior courtyard. The support of the imperial family did not end with this initial gift. The Crown

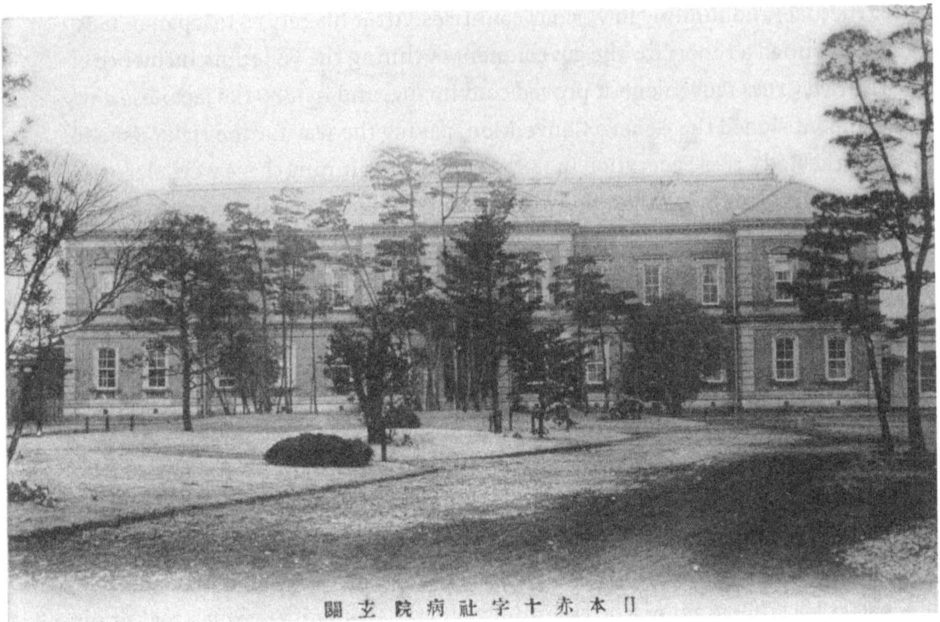

Figure 3.4. Postcard of the Japanese Red Cross Hospital in Shibuya. Author's collection.

Prince endowed an additional 500 yen to the hospital, and the empress pledged an annual donation of 5,000 yen for ten years.[85]

From the outset, the hospital accepted both charity and paying patients, although the rules for charity patients were arguably more restrictive than those in place at the university hospital. A patient wishing to receive free care was required to obtain a letter of introduction attesting to their poverty from a reliable person residing in the same ward or village. Those who obtained such a letter then faced additional hurdles: the hospital would treat no more than thirty outpatients per day on a charity basis and only sixteen charity patients could be hospitalized at any given time—and for no more than six days. Charity inpatients also had to provide the names of two guarantors to ensure their good behavior, and all patients were to remember that their care was provided through the benevolence of the imperial household. Even after death, patients were to show due deference to hospital. If their case was deemed interesting, doctors were authorized to conduct an autopsy without the prior consent of the patient or family members, although surviving family members would be compensated by a "condolence gift" of 2–5 yen.[86]

Paying patients had a very different experience of the hospital, which offered five different types of rooms, with fees ranging from 4.5 yen for a first-class room to 50 sen for the cheapest in 1901.[87] The price for a first-class room was three to four times more expensive than similar accommodations in private hospitals in the city at the time, making the Red Cross Hospital one of Tokyo's most costly hospitals. It quickly became the hospital of choice for many of the city's elites. In the late 1880s and 1890s, prominent patients included Ōki Takatō, the senior statesman and former head of the national assembly; Kurizuka Seigo, a prominent jurist; Saigō Kikujirō, the son of Saigō Takamori and a politician and diplomat in his own right; Sudō Rikuzō, a politician; and Itō Hirokuni, the adopted son of the oligarch Itō Hirobumi.[88]

Established in the wake of the demise of the prefectural hospital, the Tokyo Charity Hospital and Red Cross Hospital were framed as civic responses to the medical needs of the urban poor, although certainly the Red Cross Hospital had additional aims. Even so, the care they offered was clearly inadequate for the needs of the city. Both institutions were shaped by ideological imperatives that had little to do with concern for social welfare. They were a powerful means to publicize the benevolence of the imperial institution and the generosity of Tokyo's social and political elite. For this goal to be served, it was not necessary to attempt to provide care on a mass scale, which had been the original goal of the charity ticket system. Instead, a few of the deserving poor would suffice. The stringent requirements of the Red Cross Hospital for those seeking medical care at no cost—letters of introduction and guarantors—surely posed barriers for many, and they reveal how little interest this institution really had for the dignity and privacy of those it claimed to serve.

Private Hospitals and the Commodification of Medical Care

The closing of the prefectural hospital not only propelled medical philanthropy but also marked the beginning of another new development in Tokyo's medical modernization, the proliferation of private for-profit hospitals. To be sure, private hospitals had been a feature of city life as early as the 1870s. Matsumoto Ryōjun, another former student of the Nagasaki Medical Training Institute, is credited with founding the first private hospital in Tokyo. A Tokugawa loyalist who had fought on the losing side in the Boshin War, Matsumoto was briefly jailed in 1868–1869. Upon his release he quickly set about founding a Western-style hospital that he called Ranchū Hospital, using funds he borrowed from two European merchants from whom he had bought arms during the civil war. The new hospital was styled after the Nagasaki Yōjōsho's "H" construction and had a capacity of about seventy patients. Matsumoto also opened a private medical academy in Waseda, where his students assisted with patient care at the hospital. The model of the Nagasaki hospital prevailed in other ways as well: patients were served Western-style food and encouraged to drink milk. The success of the hospital and medical academy was cut short, however, when Matsumoto, now fully rehabilitated, was offered a position in the new government. In 1873 he became the surgeon general of the Japanese Army. His hospital did not close immediately, however, instead being briefly converted into a temporary military hospital.[89]

By 1878, the first year for which there are records, the city had seven private hospitals. Five of these were relatively small institutions devoted to specific ailments: leprosy (2), psychiatric care (2), and beriberi (1). Despite their embrace of the term "hospital," these institutions were established by doctors of Sino-Japanese medicine and offered long-term treatment for chronic ailments to a small number of patients. The Tōda Beriberi Hospital, founded by Tōda Chōan, for example, housed a total of only 47 patients in 1878, and in the same year the Shūsai Hospital in Kanda, which specialized in treating leprosy, cared for only 50. The two private "general hospitals," in contrast, were far larger institutions. Juntendō Hospital treated almost 6,000 patients in that year, some of whom were charity patients whose care was funded by the prefecture. The other, Kōseidō Hospital in Nihonbashi, was founded by Iwasa Jun, the first director of the prefectural hospital, not long after he resigned from that position. Almost 10,000 patients were treated here in 1878, and the hospital continued to prosper over the next two decades, prompting the establishment of two branch hospitals, one in Kōjimachi in 1883 and the other in Senju in 1896.[90]

Figure 3.5 indicates the relatively slow growth in the number of private hospitals until 1894, when it rose sharply and began an upward trend that would continue for more than a decade. We know a good deal about hospitals around the turn of the century because of the many guidebooks that were published in this period. Some of these were general guidebooks to Tokyo that included information on hospitals, but there were also two specialized guides to medical care, *Medical Matters in Tokyo* (*Tōkyō iji tsūran*, 1901) and *A Guide to Health Care in Tokyo* (*Saikin chōsa Tōkyō iryō annai*, 1911).[91] While not comprehensive—*A Guide to Health Care in Tokyo* describes 68 of the 104 hospitals in the 15 wards—these works supplied detailed information on the city's hospitals, addressing matters such as the credentials of the staff, facilities, and fees. *A Guide to Health Care in Tokyo*, which seems to have imagined a reader who resided outside of Tokyo who came to the city in search of medical care, offered information about how to get there, hire a rickshaw, what to bring, hospital

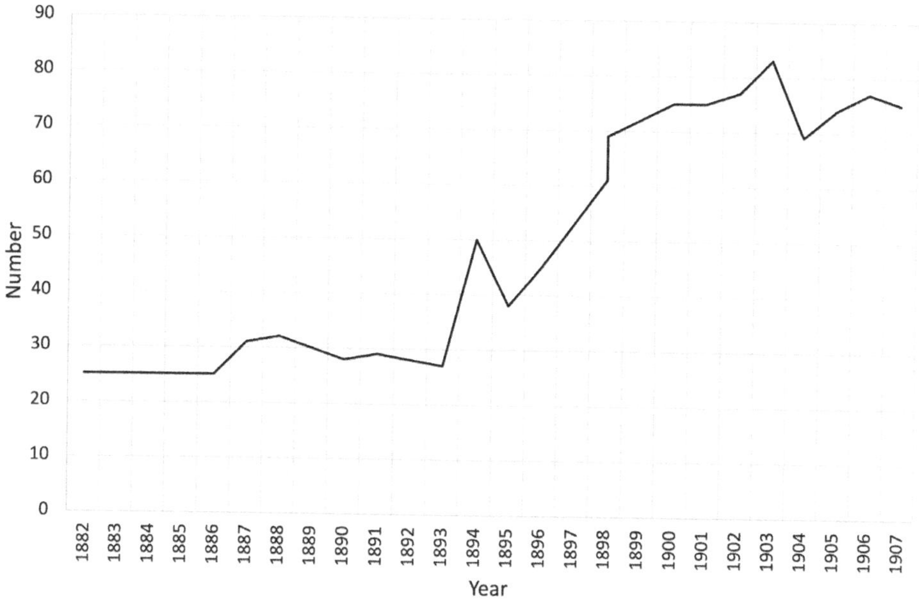

Figure 3.5. Number of private hospitals in Tokyo by year. Data from Tōkyō-fu, *Tōkyō-fu tōkeisho, Meiji 15-nen–43-nen.*

procedures and rules, and notably, information about the cost of medical care. The author advised that private hospitals charged for the initial examination and that hospitalization typically entailed many expenses in addition to the basic daily fee. He advised that a monthlong stay in a third-class room would cost about 70 yen.[92] This would have been a substantial expense for many. In 1900 the monthly salary of an elementary school teacher in Tokyo was 10–12 yen. Skilled artisans (tailors, plasterers, tatami makers, etc.) earned 12–15 yen a month, and day laborers made less than 10 yen, even when fully employed.[93]

In fact, the estimated fee of 70 yen was on the low side. Tokyo had 43 general hospitals in 1901, and their fees varied greatly. One of the largest and most expensive hospitals in Tokyo was Juntendō. It was established in 1873, but its origins date back to 1838 when Satō Taizen, a famous physician of "Dutch Medicine" established an academy in Edo. Satō's adopted son Takanaka went on to study medicine with Pompe van Meedervort in Nagasaki, and as a result he was acquainted with Hasegawa and other prominent physicians in Tokyo. The hospital, a splendid Western-style building, had 150 patient rooms and a capacity of 274 patients, who were cared for by 19 physicians. The cost of rooms differed dramatically based on their size and amenities: special-class rooms had a fee of 2.7 to 6.5 yen per day; first-class rooms, 1.2–1.5 yen; and third-class shared rooms were charged at a rate of 1.2 yen. Patients of means could also choose from a menu of extra services. The hospital provided private nursing for a fee of 40 sen to 1 yen per day, based on the nurse's qualifications and experience. A special medicinal bath, which supposedly replicated hot spring waters, long favored as a treatment for dermatological and gynecological disorders, was available at a cost of 20 sen per day, as was massage for a fee of 15 sen.[94] If one took advantage of these various offerings, a stay in Juntendō would easily have cost more than 200 yen per month.

Of course, less expensive hospitals were also available. Kanda Hospital had only 8 rooms and capacity for 17 patients. It charged 1.5 yen for a first-class room, 1 yen for a second-class room, and 80 sen for a third-class room, making it one of the least expensive hospitals in the city.[95] Most hospitals were somewhere between these two extremes, with a room charge of 1–2.5 yen. But as *A Guide to Health Care in Tokyo* noted, medical expenses could quickly add up. The fee for an initial consultation could be between 50 sen and 5 yen, and even greater if the patients chose to have the doctor visit them at home. In the latter case, the patient was not only charged a fee that was at least double the cost of a clinic visit but also was expected to pay for the doctor's round-trip travel by rickshaw. Once hospitalized, patients were charged for special foods such as milk and eggs, as well as for medicines, ice, bandages, laundry services, special treatments, and heating in the winter. Those who wished to have a family member or acquaintance stay with them were charged a daily fee, with an additional cost for their meals. And those who were hospitalized with an infectious disease were also charged a special disinfection fee. In some cases, it seems that hospitals advertising low daily fees tacked on additional costs, thereby making them more expensive than hospitals with higher daily fees.

The less expensive hospitals did not necessarily provide a lower level of medical care. By the turn of the century, the directors of private hospitals, even small facilities with modest fees, were often products of the new medical schools. Okamoto Kenji, the director of Kanda Hospital and apparently its only full-time physician, was a graduate of the University of Tokyo Medical School. Similarly, Torii Haruhiro, the director of Meiji Hospital, another relatively low-cost hospital, was not only a graduate of University of Tokyo Medical School, from which he received a doctorate in medicine, he had also spent five years in Europe where he "visited" universities in Berlin, Bonn, and Vienna (124–25, 142–43). This, in fact, was the profile of many hospital directors, for whom the experience of studying abroad was a mark of distinction. Nor did medical costs necessarily reflect the scale of the institution. Kyōundō Hospital in Kanda and Kōseidō Hospital in Asakusa were large institutions for the time with sixty-two and fifty rooms, respectively, but their fees were about average (110–11, 159–60).

Hospital directors surely recognized that many Tokyo residents simply could not afford the high cost of hospitalization, and a small number of institutions advertised that they provided charitable care. Sanyūdō Hospital, a general hospital with a capacity of ninety patients in Kanda, offered to waive the initial examination fee of 1 yen for students and the poor, a policy that was unlikely to have made a huge difference to those in desperate circumstances. Far more generous was the policy of Kyōundō Hospital. It offered to treat fifteen patients each year at no charge, with the provisions that charity patients must have resided in Kanda for at least two years and must make their application through their local police station (which presumably would confirm that they were indeed impoverished). Other hospitals offered little more than empty promises. Kusuda Hospital in Nihonbashi advertised that it would treat a "limited number" of patients at a reduced cost (94–95, 110–11, 151–53). As these provisions suggest, the claim made by the city's doctors in 1881—that medical care could be provided to the poor without the prefecture's involvement—proved to be false.

Specialty hospitals, which offered treatment for specific illnesses, were an important part of the medical landscape in this period. Until the turn of the century, on average 40 percent of private hospitals were devoted to a single disease, condition, or medical specialty. That said, new specializations emerged over time even as the hospitals dedicated to the treatment of leprosy, syphilis, and beriberi continued to operate. Ophthalmological hospitals appeared in the mid-1880s; obstetrical hospitals, in the early 1890s; and a hospital specializing in respiratory ailments, including tuberculosis, in 1893. In 1901, of seventy-eight private hospitals in the city listed in *Medical Matters in Tokyo*, thirty-four were specialty hospitals. Nine of these were obstetrical or lying-in hospitals, making this the most popular type of specialty hospital.

Like general hospitals, specialty hospitals varied greatly in size, facilities, personnel, and fees, and this was certainly true of Tokyo's obstetrical hospitals. For example, the Tokyo Obstetrics and Gynecology Hospital in Kanda had fifty rooms with a capacity for fifty-seven patients and offered its patients a choice of Western- or Japanese-style rooms. Its director Hamada Gentatsu had graduated from the University of Tokyo Department of Medicine and went on to serve as director of Kumamoto Medical School before traveling to Europe to study obstetrics at the University of Strasbourg as a government-funded student. He returned to become a professor of obstetrics at the University of Tokyo Medical School in 1888 before resigning in 1899 to devote himself full-time to the private obstetrical hospital. The Tokyo Obstetrics and Gynecology Hospital had a staff of five doctors and six nurses and offered patients a menu of added amenities. The private special-class room cost 5 yen per day, a fee that included a private nurse and 180 milliliters of milk twice a day. A third-class room, shared with another patient, cost 1.5 yen a day, but for that price patients had no private nurse and no milk (101–2).

In contrast, the Mizuhara Hospital, also in Kanda, had only two doctors on staff, including its director Mizuhara Susumu, and one midwife. Housed in a Japanese-style building, it offered only two classes of tatami rooms, one costing 1.2 yen per day and the other 90 sen per day. In keeping with the modest scale of his hospital, Mizuhara's training differed significantly from that of Hamada. His formal training was at the University of Tokyo Medical School's preparatory course, and he passed the licensing exam in 1886. Three years later, he founded a midwifery school in Tokyo that held classes at night, allowing women who had other employment to study after working hours. The school attracted many women in their forties, some of whom were likely practicing midwives who wanted to pass the licensing exam. In 1893 Mizuhara returned to the university to take a specialized training course in obstetrics and two years later he founded his hospital.[96]

Given their high fees, one might think that hospitals were guaranteed to be profitable, but in fact running a hospital was a risky undertaking, especially as the number of hospitals increased, making competition for patients stiff. Hospital directors worked hard to gain a competitive advantage. Many advertised heavily in the newspapers, sometimes offering treatments for ailments that were then the object of collective anxiety. We will look more carefully at this phenomenon in chapter 4, which examines the popularity of the syphilis treatments offered by a wide range of hospitals and clinics, including those that specialized in dermatology, obstetrics and gynecology, and urology. Other popular specialties included ophthalmology and gastroenterology.

Location was another way to gain an advantage over competitors. Plate 9 reveals that by 1912, both general and specialty hospitals were clustered in specific areas, with many of the city's hospitals located in just three wards: Kanda (21), Kyōbashi (13), and Nihonbashi (12). This is perhaps not surprising, given that these were three of the most densely populated wards, but there were other reasons as well. As we saw in chapter 1, Kanda had been home to many of the Edo-era medical facilities, including the Igakukan, the vaccination clinic, and the Institute for Western Medicine, with the military hospital in neighboring Shitaya. The association of Kanda with medicine may have continued into the modern era, but there were also more pragmatic reasons for establishing a private hospital there. For one thing, Kanda was well situated to attract patients who had unsuccessfully sought care at one of the Unversity of Tokyo's hospitals, located in Hongō and Shitaya. In addition, the university's medical school was in Hongō, and private hospitals often hired junior members of the medical faculty on a part-time basis. Finally, as the case of Hamada Gentatsu discussed above suggests, it was common for professors on the medical faculty to serve as directors of private hospitals, sometimes lending their names to these institutions even if their day-to-day involvement was limited.

As public transportation developed in the city, initially in the form of horse-drawn trollies in 1880, proximity to stations became another factor in the location of hospitals, and this trend continued after electrification began in 1903. Indeed, a guide to using the streetcars published in 1910 included a list of hospitals and helpfully noted the closest station to each.[97] By 1912 many hospitals were located adjacent to or near subway lines (see plate 9). Travel by streetcar certainly made economic sense: a ride by rickshaw from Shinbashi station to Kanda cost between 20 and 28 sen, four or five times as much as the same journey by streetcar [98]

It would not have been possible for the very ill or those with infectious diseases to travel by public transportation, so the clustering of hospitals in the city center created issues of access for many of the city's residents, particularly those who lived on the city's periphery or in the wards east of the Sumida River. Fukagawa is a notable example: not only was it poorly served by public transportation, but it also had only a single hospital for some years. The situation was similar in Azabu and Yotsuya, then undergoing transformation into residential neighborhoods. In general, as one moved away from the city center, hospital-based care became more difficult to access.

But even a prime location did not guarantee success. A significant number of hospitals located in Kanda, Kyōbashi, and Nihonbashi closed in the period between 1901 and 1912. Hospitals in other locations were even more likely to be short-lived. This was the case for Honjo and Fukagawa, two wards that had a relatively small number of private practice doctors and few hospitals. In 1901 these two wards had a total of nine hospitals, but five of these had closed by 1911. Four of the five had been established in 1897–1899 and were thus in operation for at most fifteen years. Except for a single maternity hospital, these were small-scale general hospitals that employed only one to three physicians. The hospital guidebooks do not mention the academic background of the directors of these hospitals, suggesting that they were credentialed through the licensing system. Poor and working-class people in these wards thus had limited options for high-quality medical care locally.

The Hospital as a Modern Experience

The material form of the "hospital" evolved over the course of the Meiji period. While the founders of the earliest institutions had embraced aspects of the Western hospital, insisting that patients sleep on beds and eat Western-style foods, by the turn of the century many private hospitals were built in a more familiar domestic style of architecture (see fig. 3.6), like that of a traditional inn (or a brothel, as one author noted) and offered patients the homey comfort of tatami rooms. According to the 1901 *Medical Matters in Tokyo*, 40 percent of Tokyo's hospitals were built in the Western style, and 60 percent were described as "Japanese style" or "hybrid Western-Japanese style." In contrast, *A Guide to Health Care in Tokyo*, published ten years later, classified 60 percent of Tokyo's hospitals as "Western style." While Japanese-style hospitals offered patients the familiar comfort of a tatami room, the "hybrid" hospitals allowed patients to choose between a hospital bed or a tatami room. But the differing architectural styles did not necessarily align with the therapeutics available. Even Juntendō, housed in a monumental Western-style building, offered patients traditional therapies in the form of mineral baths and massages. And unlike European and British hospitals, which enforced strict visiting hours and put nursing in the hands of professionals, in Japanese hospitals, the long-standing practice of having family or friends care for the sick was another accommodation to patient preferences, although hospitals were quick to capitalize on this practice and charged 35–50 sen per day per person for the privilege of staying with a patient.

Of course, the experience of the hospital differed greatly depending on one's financial resources. While private hospitals offered a familiar and comfortable environment within which to regain one's health, charity and university hospitals imposed considerable restraints on both the dignity and liberty of the poorer patients for whom they cared. In 1903 Kondō Tsunejirō (1864–1904) offered a compelling critique of hospital care in his memoir, *Bed-bound for Three Years* (*Gyōga sannen*). A doctor himself, Kondō had trained at the University of Tokyo Medical School. He then became an army physician and

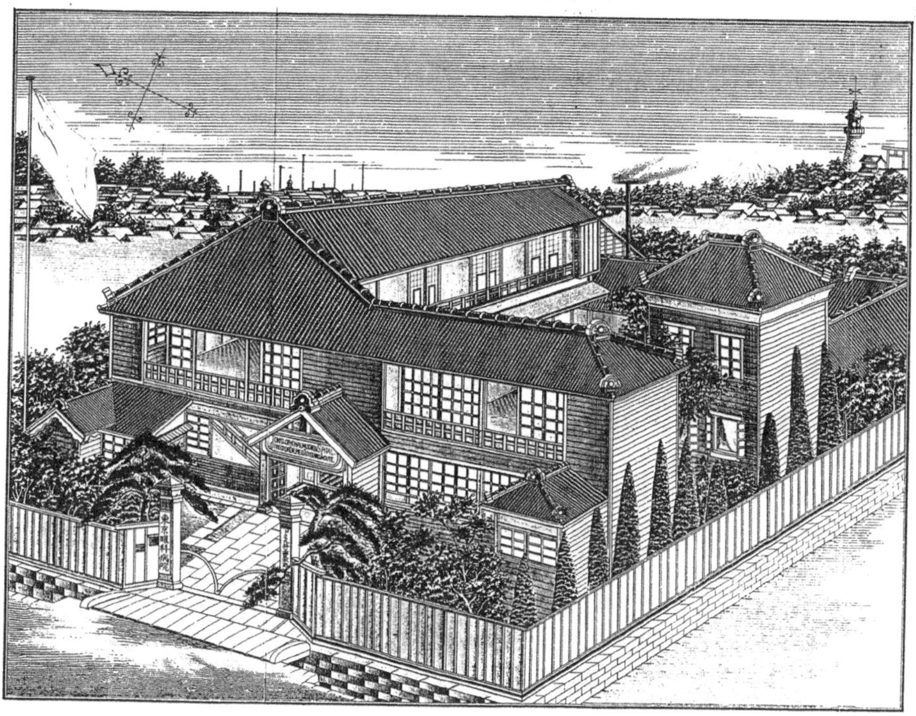

Figure 3.6. Tokyo Ophthalmology Hospital (Kōjimachi), ca. 1906, an example of a hospital housed in a traditional-style wooden building. *Tōkyō Ganka Byōin nenpō*: front matter.

served during the first Sino-Japanese War of 1895. After the war he traveled to Europe for further study, but upon his return he fell seriously ill with a chronic illness that caused his death at age forty-one. Over the course of his illness, Kondō stayed in both private and university hospitals, and found both lacking:

> As for private hospitals, they are just like brothels that are greedy for profit. The sick who should be pitied are viewed like brothel customers. They will not be set free until they have emptied their pockets. The assets of the average man, accumulated over ten years, will be completely exhausted if his wife enters the hospital for a single stay. . . . The attitude of the hospital director is just like that of the madam of such an establishment, while the attending doctors and other staff are like the accountants and bouncers, respectively, and the nurses are like prostitutes who have just started in the business.[99]

But if private hospitals made patients into customers, university or national hospitals were even worse, according to Kondō: "National hospitals are nothing more than prisons. The attitude of the hospital director and the revered and distinguished doctors beneath him are indeed intimidating. They view the sick person as a criminal: when the doctors make their rounds, they question him about his symptoms, just like a prosecutor interrogating a suspect."[100] Kondō's remarks, however, obfuscate the very real distinction between the two spaces he evokes metaphorically to describe the hospital experience. In the case of the brothel, one enters voluntarily seeking bodily pleasure, while one enters prison under duress, to be "disciplined and punished," in the words of Michel Foucault. Of course, Kondō's intent was to expose the commercial nature of the private hospital, but his choice of reference, particularly when considered in light of Nagao Setsuzō's observation about the popularity of hospitalization, even for relatively minor ailments, suggests that the metaphors of brothel and prison do not capture the full significance of the hospital for Tokyo residents at this time.

Another perspective is offered by the poet and journalist Ishikawa Takuboku. On February 4, 1911, Ishikawa entered the University of Tokyo Hospital as a charity patient. He was suffering from peritonitis, a complication of the tuberculosis that led to his death the following year at the age of twenty-six. An avid diarist, Ishikawa wrote, "From today, I will record the journal of my hospital life in red ink," apparently to convey the special nature of his hospital stay.[101] Writing in red on his first night in the hospital, he stated, "I feel as if I am already left behind by the rest of the world, and I am already longing for that second-floor apartment that until now seemed so noisy." These sentiments notwithstanding, during his five-week stay, Ishikawa wrote repeatedly of the simple pleasures of hospital life, its solitude and tranquility and the escape it offered from work and family. He noted more than once that he had become "lazy" (*namakemono*) in the hospital. Rather than writing poetry, he spent his time reading, playing shogi, and chatting with his ward mates about socialism and other matters. After being told by his doctor that he could do some work, Ishikawa noted that the effort to write "burned up" at least two weeks' worth of his hard-won sense of health and tranquility. For Ishikawa, then, the hospital was neither a brothel nor a prison; instead, it was a kind of refuge that offered a respite, albeit a brief one, from the frenetic and competitive world outside its walls.

Medical Capitalism and Tokyo's Healthscape

The establishment of hospitals had been an early goal of both national and local authorities in Tokyo. Hospitals would not only provide clinical training for the new medical professionals but also make it possible to extend "Western medicine" to the city's residents, transforming them into healthy citizens who could contribute to the nation. By the second decade of the twentieth century, it seemed that this aim had been achieved. Hospitals had become an important part of Tokyo's healthscape, visible to those who navigated the crowded streets of central Tokyo, on foot, in a rickshaw, or on a streetcar. But as we have seen, the formation of these hospitals did not necessarily follow the plan of the Medical Policy. Doctors of Sino-Japanese medicine founded many of the early private hospitals, and although the University of Tokyo Hospital did indeed become central to research and teaching, it also served the powerful and wealthy residents of the city. The prefectural hospital, on the other hand, quickly became an important node in the life of the city offering education, care, and training to many, but its very success contributed to its demise. Underfinanced, even as patient numbers grew, and opposed by many of the city's private doctors, it was abandoned after only eight years.

Similarly, the new system of medical education and licensing of physicians had mixed results. The number of licensed doctors grew steadily over the course of the period, but it lagged behind the growth of the city's population, and physicians were not evenly distributed around the city, leaving poorer working-class wards underserved. The situation was similar with other medical professionals. In 1883 Tokyo had only 74 licensed midwives, about 14 percent of the total.[102] By 1912, the number of midwives was 2,114 and all but 273 were licensed. But as was the case with doctors, the distribution of midwives around the city was profoundly uneven: the central ward of Kōjimachi had 2.6 midwives per 1,000 population, while in Fukagawa, the figure was .43.[103]

As for-profit private hospitals became the norm, the earlier concern to replicate the material form of European hospitals gave way to a new intention to appeal to paying patients. As a result, hospitals began to offer patients an array of familiar comforts for a price: one could stay in a tatami room, eat Japanese food, and be cared for by family members all within the space of these new institutions. What failed to emerge in the wake of the demise of the prefectural hospital and the charity ticket system was a viable means to provide medical care to the city's poor and working-class residents. For the city's elites, the Tokyo Charity Hospital and the Red Cross Hospital became important sites to perform philanthropy and thereby demonstrate their benevolence to the lower classes along with their concern about the national good, but they did little to improve health within the city. In a city of about two million people in 1912, the total number of hospital beds available to the poor at the Tokyo Charity Hospital, the Red Cross Hospital, and the University of Tokyo Hospital institutions numbered only a few hundred. As the experiences of Kondō Tsunejirō and Ishikawa Takuboku reveal, those who found themselves within these heterogeneous spaces struggled to understand the new experience of hospitalization and their place within new economies of care that valorized clinical training and profit over patients.

In the chapters that follow, we will explore how the infrastructure of medical modernization examined in this chapter and the public health administration discussed in chapter 2 were implicated in efforts to address three specific concerns that emerged at the intersection of medicine and public policy, syphilis (chapter 4), mental illness (chapter 5), and cholera (chapter 6). These case studies reveal how public health policy toward these ailments reshaped the built environment and spatial order of the city—and the lives of those within it.

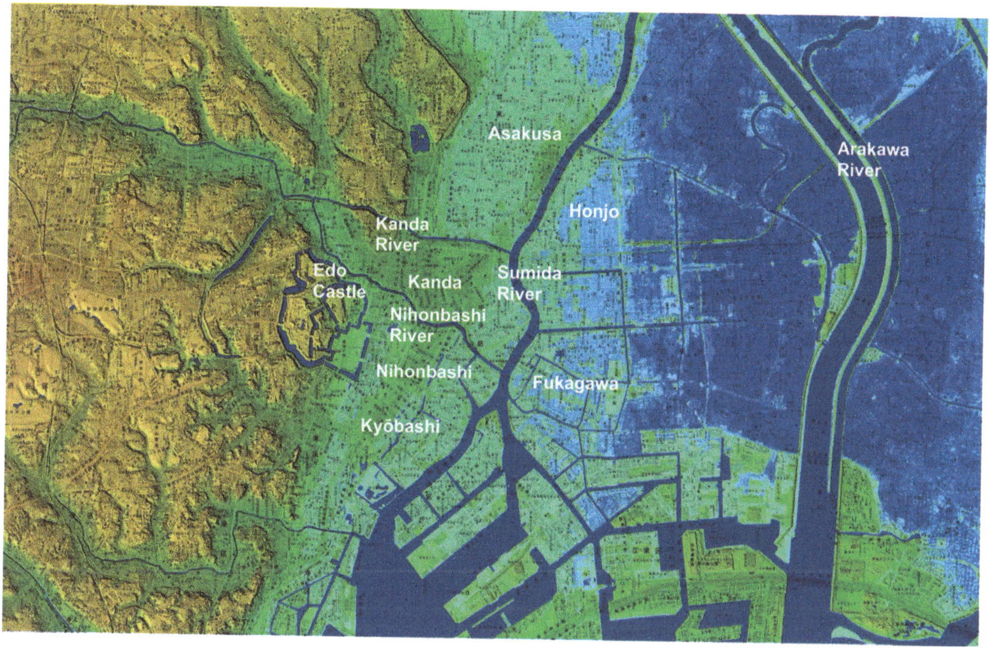

Plate 1. Elevation map of Tokyo today. Dark blue areas are less than 5 m. in elevation; medium blue, 5–10 m.; light blue, 10–50 m.; green areas, 50–100 m.; yellow areas, 100–500 m. From the Geospatial Information Authority of Japan, https://maps.gsi.go.jp.

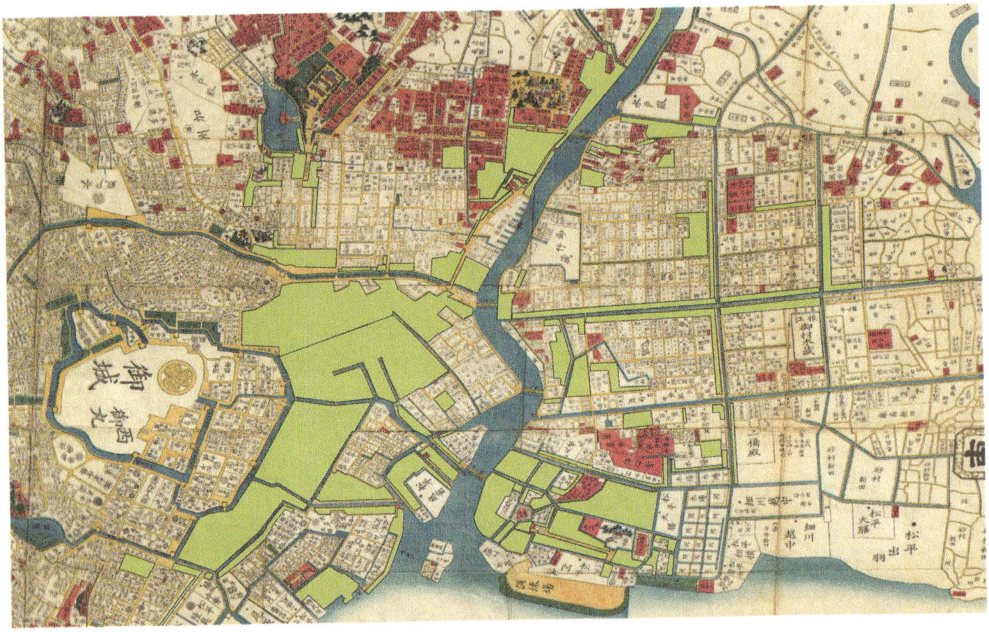

Plate 2. Major areas of commoner residence in the western part of Edo, ca. the mid-nineteenth century, are shown in green. Original red coloring represents sites of religious institutions. Other areas were reserved warrior residences, storehouses, and the like. The base map here and in plates 3, 5-7 is *Bunken Edo ōezu : kan* / Fusai Mori. Ansei 5 [1858] (Raster Image), Courtesy of the David Rumsey Map Collection, David Rumsey Map Center, Stanford University Libraries. https://purl.stanford.edu/bj558ct3072.

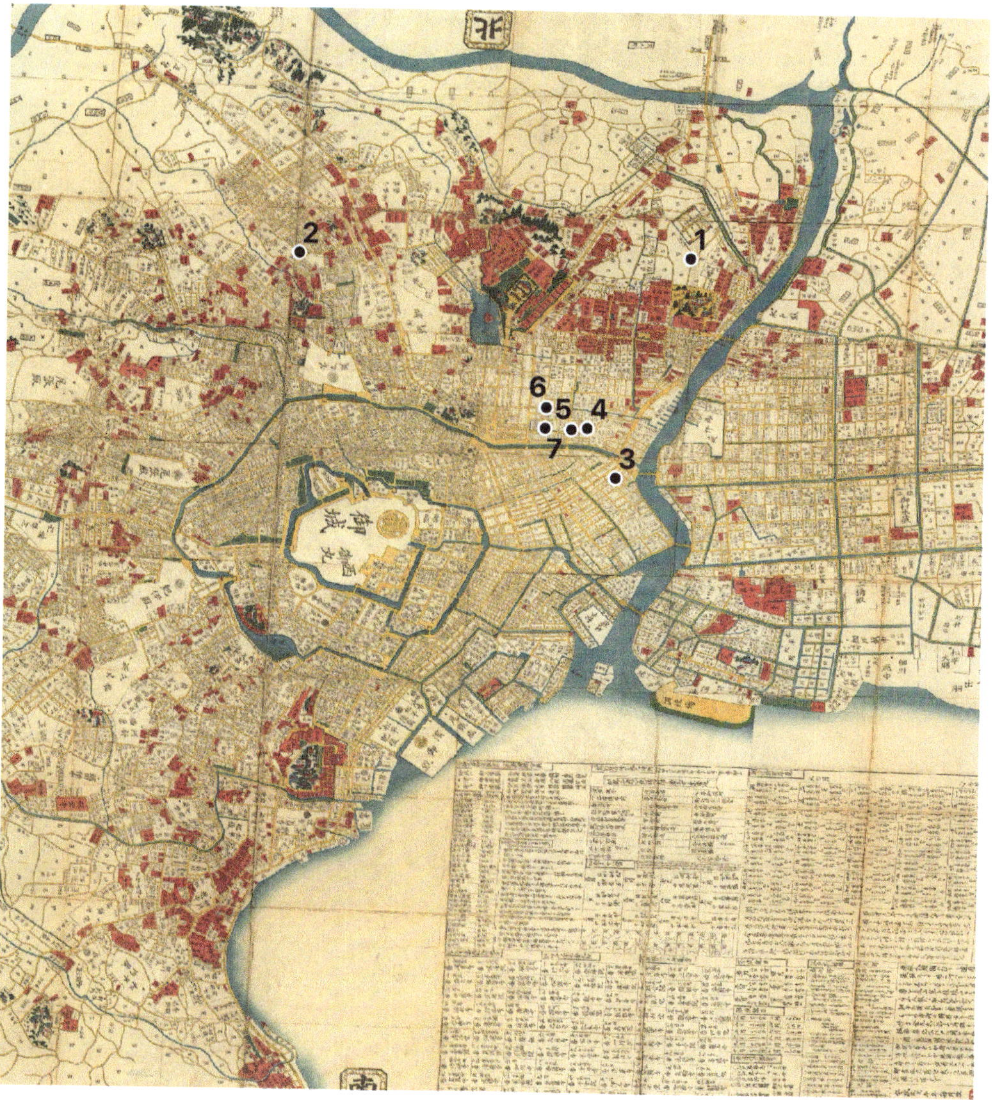

Plate 3. Medical facilities in Edo: (1) Tame, (2) Yōjōsho, (3) Otamagaike Vaccination Clinic (1858), (4) Igakukan (1765–1806), (5) Igakukan (1806–1869), (6) Vaccination Clinic/Institute of Western Medicine (1860–1869), and (7) military hospital (1868).

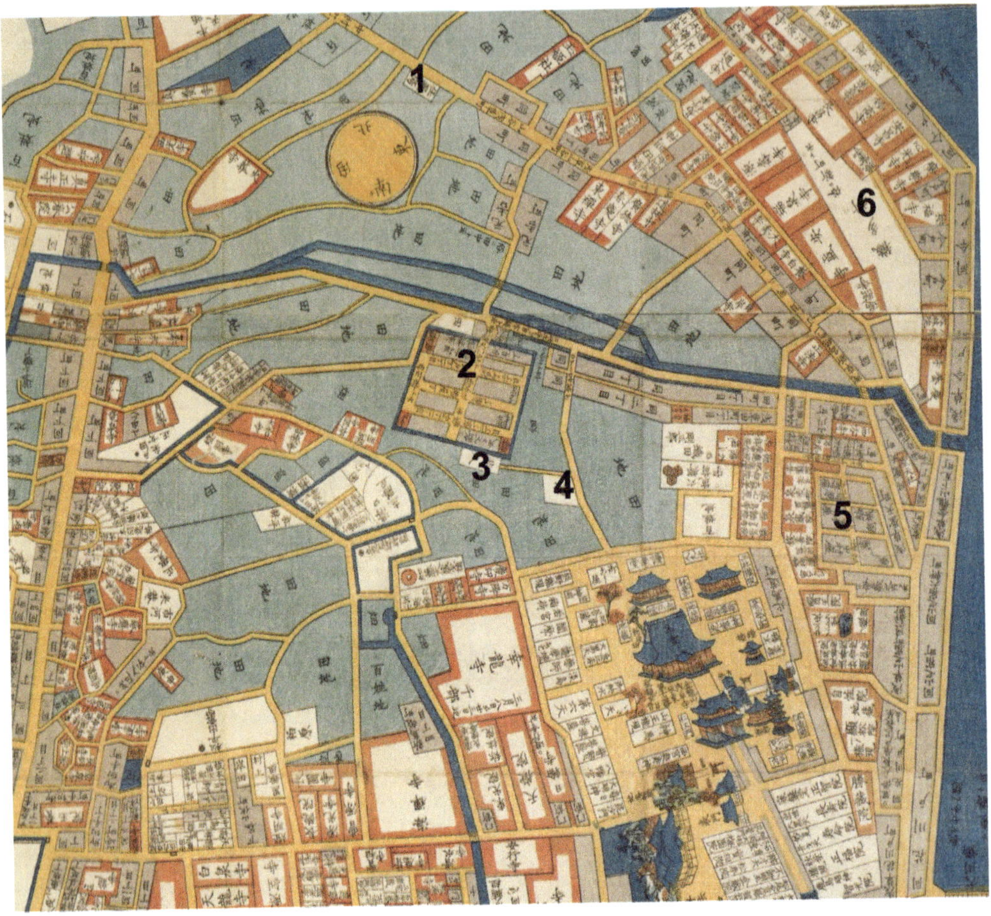

Plate 4. Environs of the Asakusa Tame: (1) Execution Grounds, (2) Yoshiwara, (3) Asakusa Outcast Hut, (4) Tame, (5) Theater District, and (6) Eta Village. Detail from Tomatsu Masanori, *Imado Minowa Asakusa ezu: kaisei shinkoku* (Edo: Owariya Seishichi, 1853). International Center for Japanese Studies (Nichibunken) Digital Map Collection, https://lapis.nichibun.ac.jp/chizu/map_detail.php?id=002149656. Used with permission.

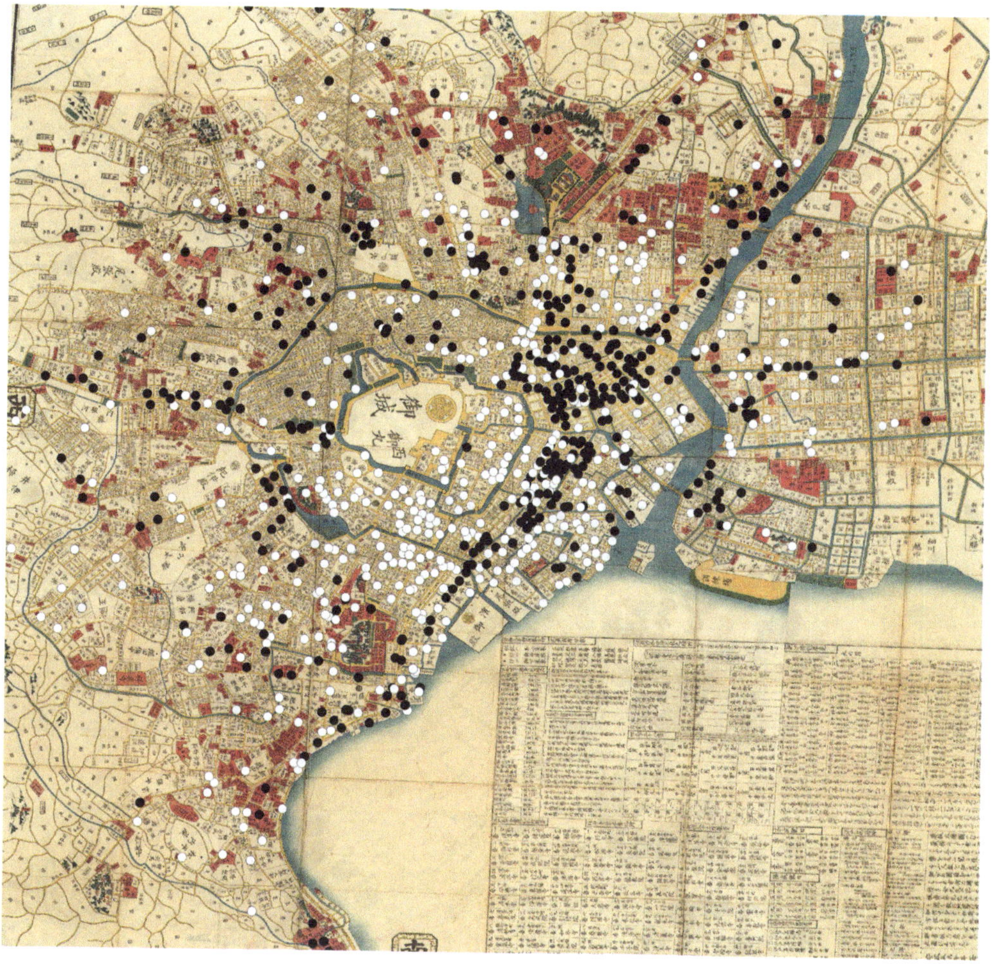

Plate 5. Distribution of doctors in Edo, ca. 1819–1825. Data are from Takei and Inaba, *Edo kinsei ika jinmeiroku* (1819), Shiratsuchi, *Ika jinmeiroku* (1820), and Takei and Inaba, *Edo kinsei ika jinmeiroku* (2nd ed., 1825). White dots show the location of domanial doctors, and black dots show the location of commoner or "town" doctors.

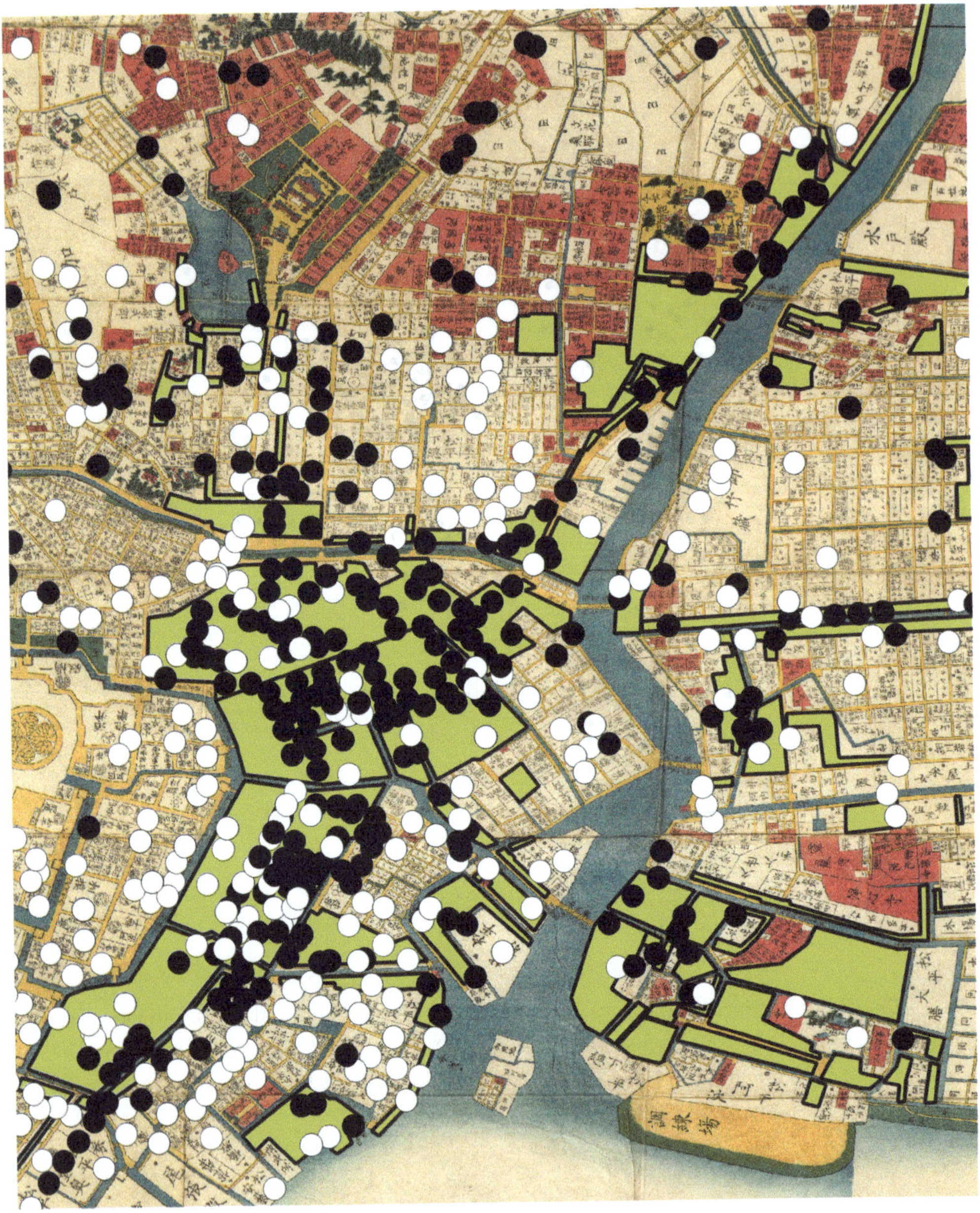

Plate 6. Detail of plate 5 showing the distribution of doctors in the commoner neighborhoods east of Edo Castle.

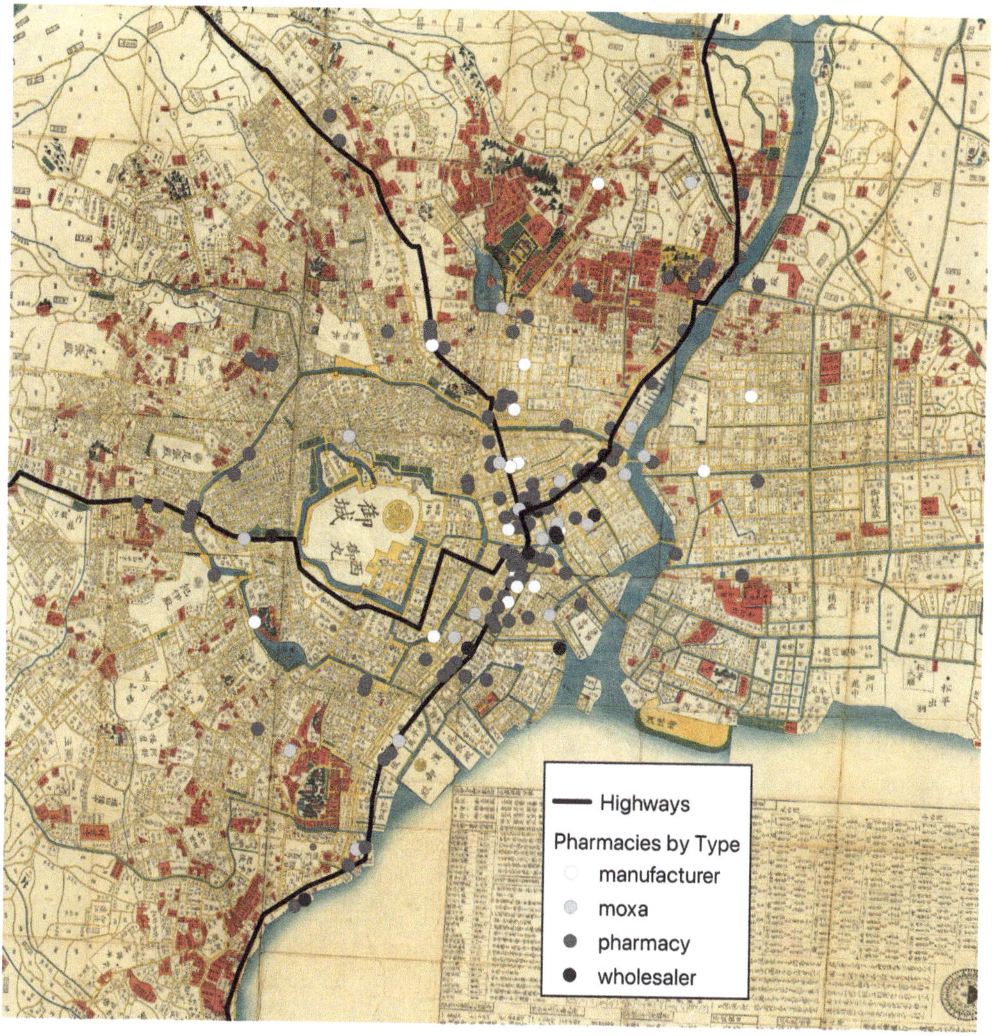

Plate 7. The medicine trade in Edo, ca. 1820s, data on the location of pharmacies are from Nakagawa and Katsushika, *Edo kaimono hitori annai*, vol. 2.

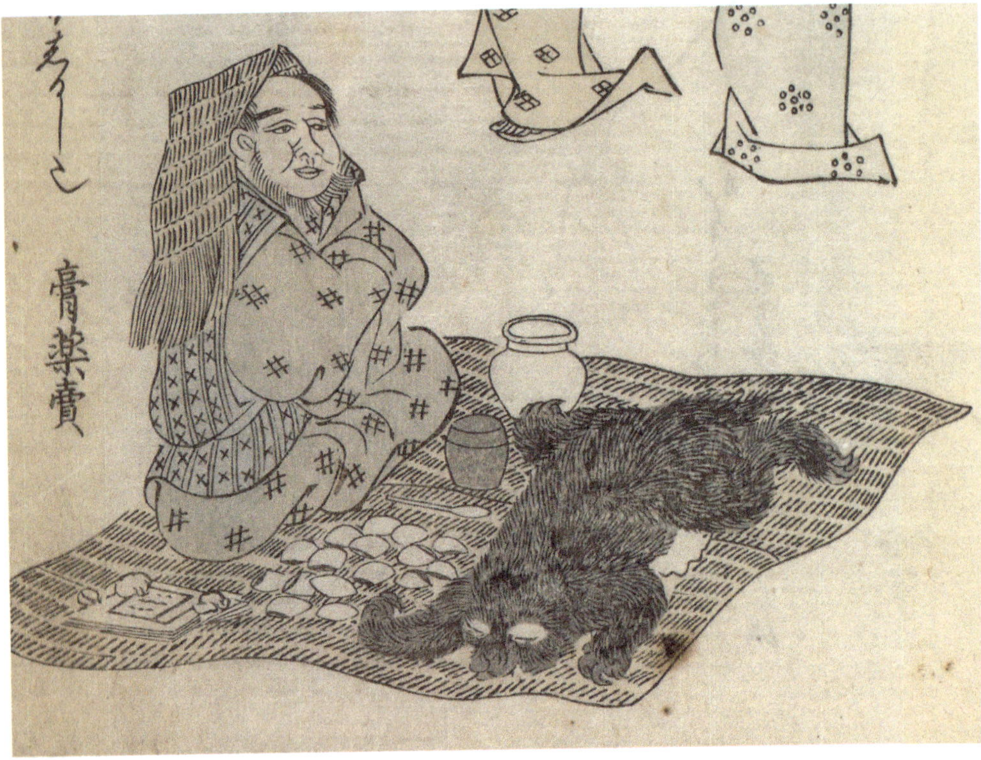

Plate 8. A medicine peddler selling a popular ointment that incorporated bear fat—hence the bear pelt on display. From Kitao Masayoshi, *Imayō shokunin zukushi uta-awase* (Edo: Shinsen'en Sagimaru, 1825). National Museum of Asian Art, Smithsonian Institution, Freer Study Collection, Purchase, The Gerhard Pulverer Collection—Charles Lang Freer Endowment and the Harold P. Stern Memorial fund in appreciation of Jeffrey P. Cunard and his exemplary service to the Museum as chair of the Board of Trustees (2003-2007), FSC-GR-780.345.

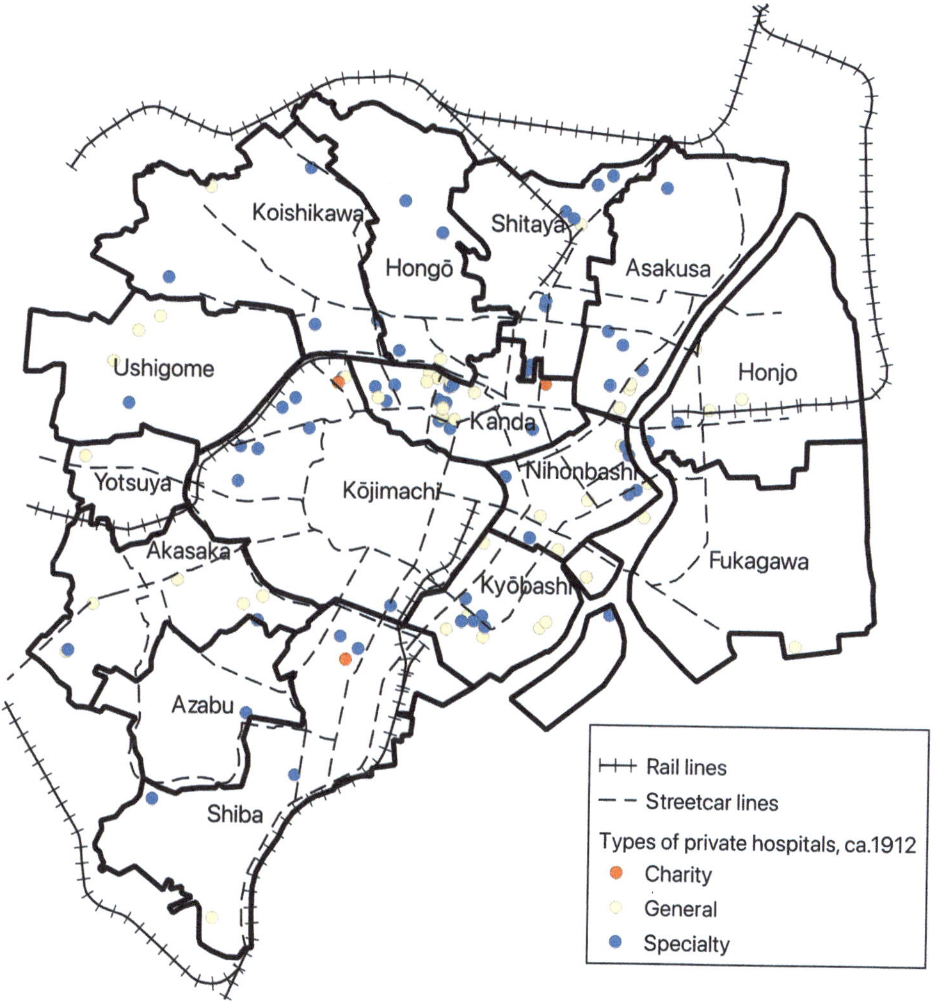

Plate 9. Private hospitals in Tokyo in 1912. Data from Tōkyō-fu, *Tōkyō-fu tōkeisho, Taishō gannen*, 56–60.

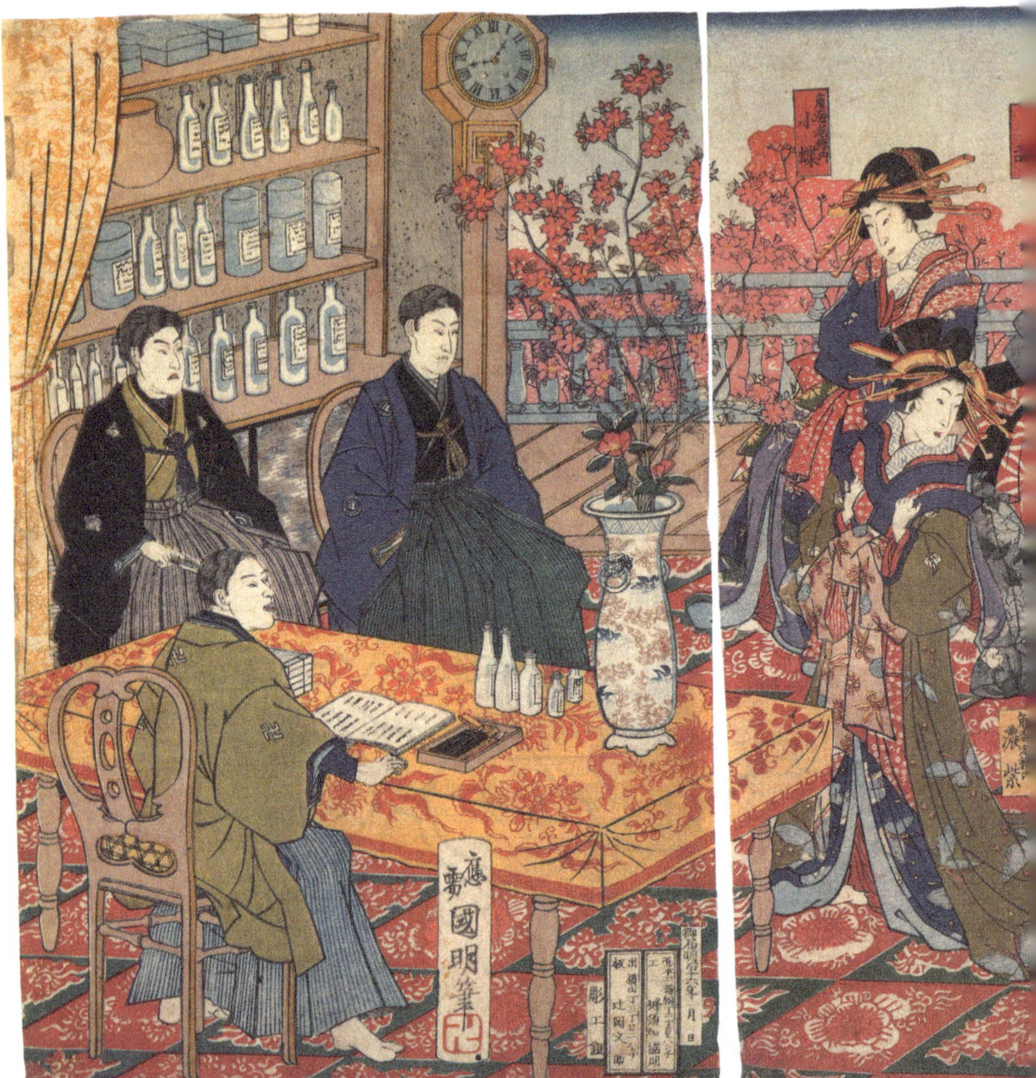

Plates 10, 11, and 12. Illustrations of examinations of prostitutes at the syphilis hospital of New Yoshiwara. Utagawa Kuniaki II, “Shin Yoshiwara shōgi baidoku byōin kensa no zu,” in Nakano Misao, *Nishikie igaku minzokushi* (Kanehara Shuppan, 1980), plate 4. Used with permission.

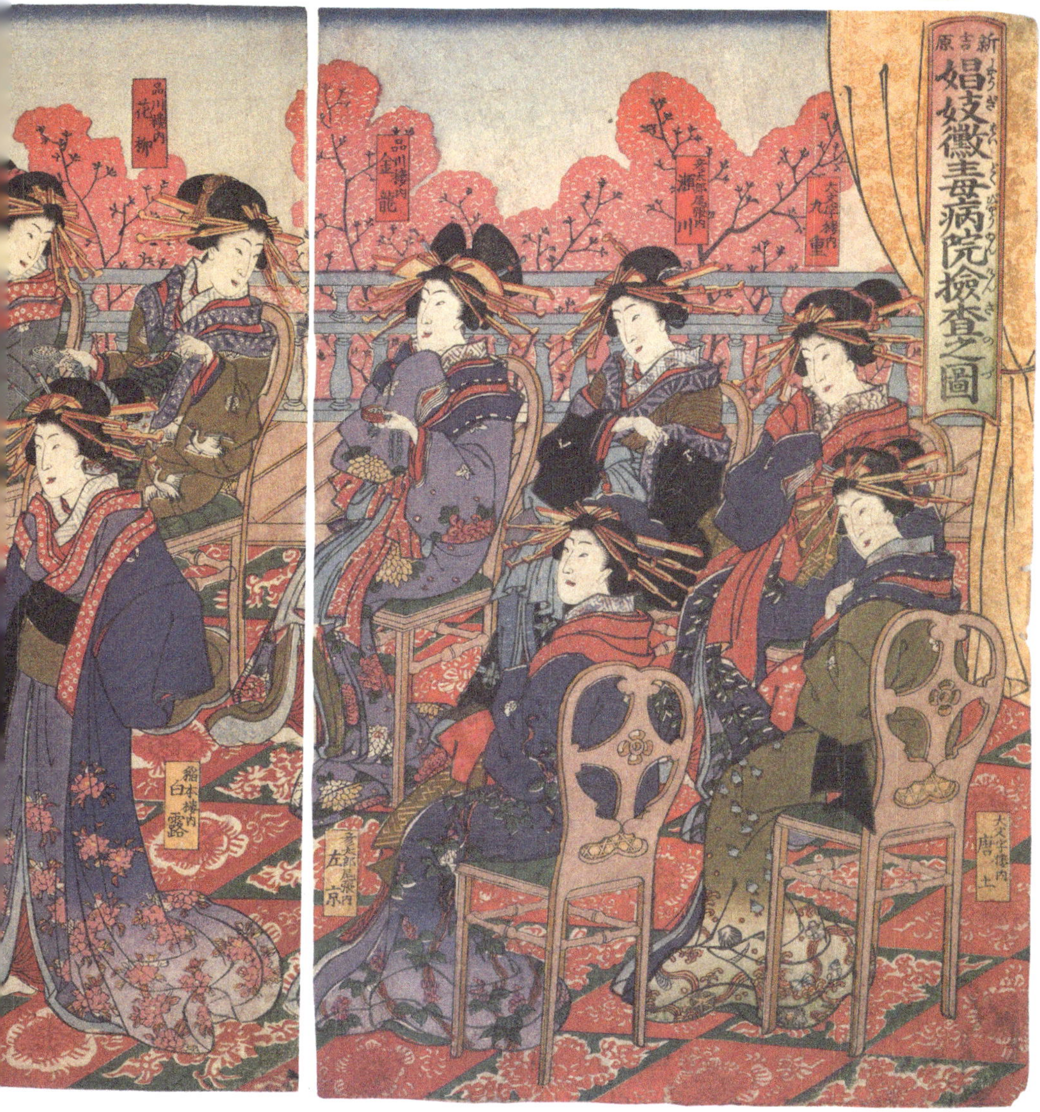

新吉原
娼妓黴毒病院撿査之圖
品川楼内 花柳
品川楼内 金龍
瀬川
大文字楼内 九重
稲本楼内 白露
左京
大文字楼内 唐土

4

Sex(ually Transmitted Diseases) and the City

Syphilis and the Healthscape

On November 15, 1909, a twenty-year-old woman named Nakajima Yoshi jumped from the Komatsuka Bridge in Mejirodai into the cold waters of the Kanda River below. Yoshi survived her suicide attempt due to the quick action of a passing fireman, who managed to pull her from the river. We know about her desperate act because of a brief article in the *Yomiuri shinbun* two days later. It explained that Yoshi, suffering from a serious case of syphilis, was in despair, fearing that she would never be able to marry and that her stepfather, who operated a shoe shop in nearby Waseda, would be unwilling to support her.[1] Nothing else is known about Yoshi, not how she became infected, nor the aftermath of her attempted suicide, but she was not the only Tokyo resident whose suicide was attributed to having contracted syphilis. Between 1875 and 1912, newspapers reported on more than twenty-five successful or attempted suicides by sufferers of the disease in Tokyo, poignant evidence of the devastating impact of this diagnosis at this time.

By the time Yoshi made her way to the Komatsuka Bridge, Tokyo authorities had been attempting to curb the spread of syphilis for four decades. In the 1870s, the prefectural government began requiring the examination of licensed prostitutes for signs of the disease, but as the Tokyo Metropolitan Police (TMP) assumed control over matters of public health, licensing, examinations, and treatment all became matters of police procedure. Meanwhile, the spread of the disease among the general population of the city was left unchecked—a situation that was soon addressed by the city's booming medical marketplace. An array of Tokyo's private physicians began claiming expertise in the treatment of syphilis and other sexually transmitted diseases, with the result that clinics and hospitals for those who were infected became a feature of the capital's healthscape. This chapter explores the emergence of this de facto public-private collaboration, its limitations, and its impact on the city and its residents.

Edo's Pox

Syphilis is a systemic infection caused by the bacterium *Treponema pallidum*, which was first identified in 1905 by two German researchers, Erich Hoffmann and Fritz Schaudinn.[2] Transmission of syphilis occurs primarily through sexual contact with an infected person or congenitally from an infected woman to her fetus. The disease progresses in stages. The most obvious symptom of the primary infection is the development of a lesion known as a chancre at the site of infection, typically on the genitals, in the perianal region, or in the mouth, about three weeks after intimate contact with an infected person. However, some of those infected either never develop the chancre or fail to notice it before it disappears within a few weeks. Visual symptoms are thus not a reliable means of diagnosis but no other way to identify the disease was available until 1906, when the bacteriologist August von Wassermann developed a test that identified antibodies of *T. pallidum* in the blood.

The secondary stage of the disease begins one to two months after the appearance of the chancre and is marked by a diverse set of dermatological symptoms, including a red raised rash over much of the body, wartlike pustules on the mucous membranes, and hair loss, as well as fever, fatigue, headache, and swelling of the lymph glands. Following this second stage, the disease becomes latent: the patient can be asymptomatic for many years, creating the mistaken perception that the disease has been cured. If untreated, approximately a third of patients will eventually develop tertiary syphilis, the most serious form of the disease. At this stage, some patients develop cardiovascular symptoms; others have neurological impairment after the disease invades the brain and central nervous system; and some fall victim to so-called bone syphilis.[3]

There is general agreement that syphilis arrived in Japan in the early sixteenth century, most likely via Chinese merchants, following the introduction of the disease to south China by European traders. By the late sixteenth century, cases of syphilis were common in Kyushu and Kyoto, prompting European missionaries then resident in Japan to comment on the Japanese lack of shame about the disease.[4] Over the course of the early modern period, the disease continued to spread, becoming a major focus of medical discourse. Between 1764 and 1866, at least thirty works devoted to syphilis were published, including several that were directed at ordinary readers, and case reports and discussions of diagnosis and treatment were common in general medical works as well.

As was common in Sino-Japanese medical discourse, syphilis was attributed to multiple causes, including "self-generation" (*jihatsu*), "fetal poison," and sexual contact with an infected person. However, by the late eighteenth century, sexual transmission was recognized as the primary means of infection, and syphilis was increasingly identified with prostitution and the urban brothel districts (*yūkaku* or "pleasure quarters"), where prostitution was permitted. Brothel quarters, which were typically segregated from the rest of the city by moats, walls, and gates, were a feature of Japanese cities in this era, and the culture of play associated with the quarters found expression in popular literature and art. As a result, syphilis acquired an ambivalent set of meanings. While some associated it with sexual immorality, others viewed it as evidence of worldly sophistication.[5]

Over the course of the early modern period, Edo became ground zero for Japan's syphilis epidemic, leading some to describe it as "Edo's pox" (*Edo no tōsō*), and giving rise to a popular aphorism that stated, "You are not an Edoite until you have drunk the water and caught syphilis."[6] In 1810, the physician Sugita Genpaku, whose work was discussed in chapter 1, wrote, "Of the more than a thousand patients I examine each year, seven to eight hundred are syphilitics."[7] While this may well have been an exaggeration, other evidence supports Sugita's claim about the prevalence of syphilis among Edo residents. The physical anthropologist Suzuki Takao examined human remains excavated from five Edo-period burial sites looking for evidence of tertiary syphilis. Based on the frequency that bone necrosis occurs among infected people and Edo's population, he hypothesized that close to 50 percent of the city's residents may have been infected with syphilis in the early nineteenth century.[8]

Some historians have suggested that the prevalence of syphilis was attributable to the sex imbalance in the city's population, the result of the large number of samurai retainers garrisoned in the city. Although the number of women increased over the eighteenth century, men still constituted almost 60 percent of the city's population in 1800. Another explanation is the evolution of the sex trade in the city. By the mid-nineteenth century, the reputation of

Yoshiwara, Edo's celebrated brothel district, had declined, and the women who worked there were increasingly viewed simply as prostitutes rather than as courtesans. In part, this reflected the increasing number of women offering sexual services in Yoshiwara, from about 2,000 in the 1720s to more than 3,700 in the mid-nineteenth century, and many of these women lacked the musical and other skills associated with courtesans.[9] Prostitution expanded outside of Yoshiwara as well. The city was home to a growing number of "private" or illicit prostitutes, who offered sexual services at restaurants and inns in the post-stations leading into the city and the recreational and entertainment districts that formed on or near the grounds of temples, shrines, and firebreaks.[10]

As illicit prostitution proliferated and the reputation of Yoshiwara declined, syphilis came to be closely identified with prostitution in overtly negative terms. For example, Honma Genchō, a domanial doctor from Mito, wrote in 1837 that not only was syphilis transmitted by prostitutes, but in fact the disease originated in their sexual organs. In his words, syphilis developed when "the viscous fluid within the vagina [of the prostitute] stagnates and then ferments to produce [the disease]."[11] But while many doctors advised that the best way to prevent syphilis was to avoid sex with prostitutes, others argued that the disease, at least in its early stages, was curable, and thus abstinence was unnecessary.[12]

Early modern doctors employed a variety of treatments, some of which would continue to be used until the development of Salvarsan, the first effective antimicrobial agent, in 1910. The use of mercury was introduced from Europe as early as the late sixteenth century, and it was used orally, as well as in the form of ointments applied to the skin and via fumigation with mercury vapor. In addition, in an interesting example of the multidirectional flow of medical knowledge in the early modern world, many treatments incorporated the dried root of the plant known in Japan as *sankirai* (*Smilax glabra*, also known as chinaroot). An herb used in Chinese medicine to remove toxic substances that supposedly cause skin eruptions from the body, *Smilax glabra* was introduced in Europe in the sixteenth century as a syphilis cure.[13] The ingestion of both mercury and *Smilax glabra* induced sweating, diarrhea, and increased urination and salivation, symptoms that were regarded as evidence that the "poison" responsible for syphilis was being flushed from the body.

Syphilis and the Treaty Ports

As in Japan, in Europe growing concern about the spread of syphilis prompted new scrutiny of prostitution in the nineteenth century. France established a system for licensing brothels in 1804 that required the women who worked in them to submit to twice weekly medical examinations, and this approach was widely emulated elsewhere. Amsterdam began requiring prostitutes to be examined for syphilis in 1806, and local officials in some states of the German confederacy adopted this practice in the early decades of the nineteenth century. In 1843 prostitutes in Russia were ordered to undergo regular medical exams. Although Britain did not follow suit until the Contagious Disease Acts were passed in 1864, the examination of prostitutes in British colonies had begun decades earlier. In India, as early as the eighteenth century, the British army established "lock hospitals," as syphilis hospitals were known in Britain, in areas where troops were stationed.[14]

In Japan, the policy of examining prostitutes for syphilis originated in the politically charged spaces of the treaty ports, the semicolonial spaces that were created in response to the "unequal treaties" signed by the Tokugawa shogunate with Western powers in the 1850s. Throughout the period of their existence, the Japanese treaty ports were populated largely by men, many of whom expected access to Japanese women for sexual services as a matter of course. In 1860 when a Russian naval ship called the *Posadnik* sailed into Nagasaki, its commander asked permission for his men to visit Maruyama, Nagasaki's brothel district. The city's magistrate quickly approved this request, but he was dismayed when the Russian commander then insisted—following Russian practice—that the women in the quarter be examined for syphilis. When the magistrate conveyed this request to the brothel owners of Maruyama, they refused.

The conflict was eventually resolved by creating an alternative brothel quarter for the Russian sailors. Poor women from outside the city were recruited to staff the new brothels, but they were required to submit to regular genital examinations. These were carried out by students of the shogunate's Medical Training Institute. One of those involved was Matsumoto Jun, the former Tokugawa vassal who later went on to establish Tokyo's first private hospital before becoming the first surgeon general of the army. Matsumoto participated in the syphilis exams, but he found the procedure distasteful and soon turned responsibility over to his junior colleagues. Even so, at some point after his return to Edo in 1862, Matsumoto began advocating for the examination of prostitutes in the city. According to Matsumoto himself, once back in Edo he was dismayed by the rise of licentious behavior on the part of city residents, something he attributed to the declining morals that had resulted from the opening of the country. As a result, syphilis was spreading like fire and "the failure to control the disease was worse than allowing arson.

Fire destroys property, but the spread of syphilis continues without limits from children to grandchildren. . . . It destroys the strength of the realm."[15]

Matsumoto quickly moved into a series of influential positions within the shogunate that allowed him to act on his new concern about syphilis. He became a medical official within the shogunate, then the head of the Western Medicine Institute, and by 1864 he was the treating physician of Shogun Tokugawa Iemochi. In the mid-1860s, he began campaigning for the implementation of syphilis examinations in Yoshiwara, approaching brothel owners and the town magistrates with this proposal. However, as in Nagasaki, brothel owners resisted efforts to compel women to submit to the exams. As a result, Matsumoto eventually abandoned the idea of introducing examinations in the existing brothel quarters and instead, based on his Nagasaki experience, formulated a new plan. He would create an alternative brothel district that required syphilis exams from the outset.[16]

Matsumoto's chance to put his plan into action came in 1866, after Yoshiwara was largely destroyed by a fire and its brothels were temporarily relocated to a location near the Nezu Gongen (now Nezu Shrine), one of the best-known sites of private prostitution (see fig. 4.1) Prompted by Matsumoto, Ishikawa Toshimasa, one of the town magistrates, sought the approval of the magistrate of temples and shrines (*jisha bugyō*), who had jurisdiction over Nezu, and the commander of the shogunate's army (*rikugun bugyō*) to conduct syphilis examinations in the temporary brothels. The involvement of the commander is noteworthy. Ishikawa argued that the establishment of this alternative brothel site and its syphilis clinic was necessary to protect the strength of the troops in this turbulent era of political unrest.[17] The argument that syphilis was endangering the military, a concern that would grow over time, was effective. In August 1868, a new brothel quarter with twenty-one brothels officially opened in Nezu. A large sign posted on the gate that demarcated it from surrounding areas declared it to be the Syphilis Hospital District of the Western Medicine Institute. Unfortunately for Matsumoto, the syphilis exams had just gotten underway when the conflict between pro- and anti-Tokugawa forces moved from western Japan to Edo. As the civil war engulfed the city, the exams were suspended and Matsumoto later lamented in his memoir, "All I succeeded in doing was creating another brothel district."[18]

Meanwhile, another campaign to examine prostitutes was unfolding in the treaty port of Yokohama, only forty kilometers (twenty-five miles) from Edo. Unlike Nagasaki, Yokohama was a planned treaty port, and a brothel quarter was part of its design from the outset. When the port opened to foreign

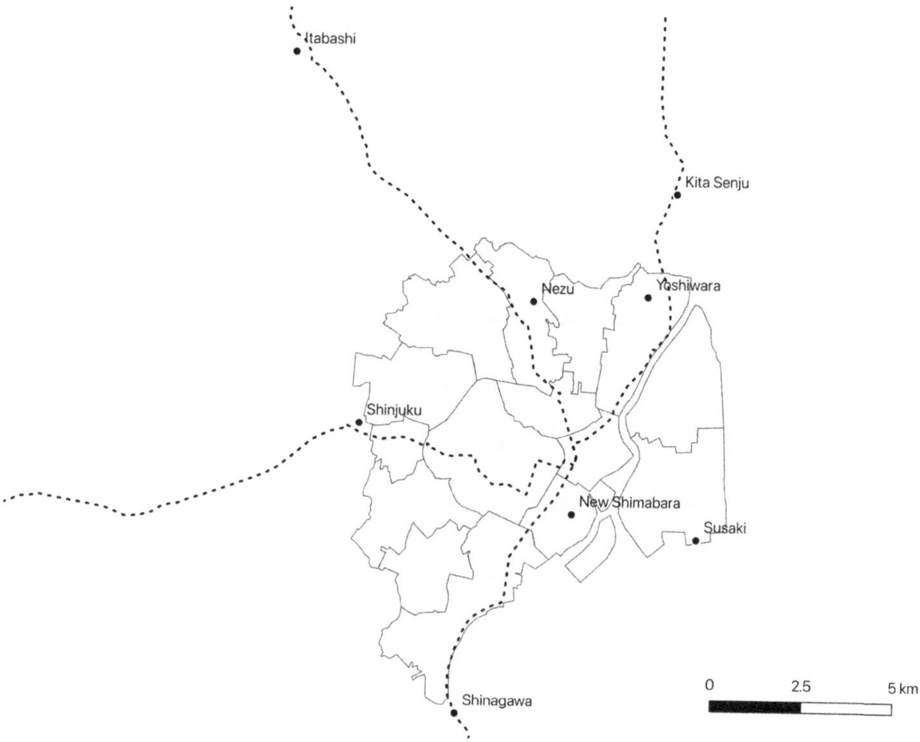

Figure 4.1. Brothel quarters in and near Tokyo. The Nezu District existed from 1868 to 1888; New Shimabara from 1871 to 1873; and Susaki from 1888 to 1958. Note the proximity of several of the quarters to the major roadways in and out of the city.

residents in 1859, the Miyozaki brothel district had fifteen brothels and three hundred prostitutes.[19] However, once Yokohama became one of the bases for Britain's China squadron, there was growing concern on the part of the British that Japanese prostitutes were infecting British soldiers and sailors, although, of course, it was just as likely that the reverse was true. In 1867 William Willis, a British physician employed by the British consulate, estimated that about a third of Yokohama's prostitutes died of syphilis during the term of their contracts, and he urged Sir Harry Parkes, the British consul general in Japan to pressure the Japanese government to authorize weekly examinations for syphilis and the isolation of infected women in a lock hospital for treatment. Willis planned for the examinations and hospitals to be in Japanese hands, but British military doctors soon objected, apparently unwilling to entrust the health of their country's sailors to Japanese doctors.[20]

Fortunately for those who wanted British control of the syphilis examinations, the civil war intervened, and shogunal officials had more pressing concerns than who should be responsible for the syphilis examinations. The task was entrusted to George Newton, a British naval surgeon, who began carrying out the exams in August 1868 in a two-story building adjacent to the brothel district, which by this time was known as Yoshiwara, after Edo's brothel district. Yokohama's Yoshiwara housed more than a thousand women in 1868, and the scale of the work required Newton to hire and train those he called "native doctors." With their help, he inspected every woman once a week. Those who were found to be infected with syphilis or gonorrhea were confined for treatment, which took the form of mercury fumigation and the application of salves containing nitric acid.[21] Newton carefully compiled statistics to demonstrate the effectiveness of his efforts. According to his reports, in contrast to 1867 when 90 percent of prostitutes were infected, by 1868 that number had fallen to 51 percent and by 1869, to 36 percent.[22] Of course, these data are unreliable, since Newton interpreted the lack of visible symptoms of the disease as evidence that it had been cured.

Syphilis and Prostitution in Post-Restoration Tokyo

Although Matsumoto concluded that his efforts to curtail the spread of syphilis had ended in failure, records in the Tokyo Metropolitan Archive indicate that an institution offering treatment was in operation in Tokyo during the chaotic first years of the new era. In March 1869 the new prefectural government granted five hundred gold ryō to fund medical institutions in the city, including the vaccination clinic, the medicinal garden, and what is described as the "syphilis clinic" (*baidokuin*).[23] Little information is available about this clinic or its relationship to Matsumoto's efforts in Nezu, but it seems to have been under the direction of the Eastern College, as the Western Medicine Institute had been restyled, suggesting that it was indeed the Nezu facility. Significantly, this institution no longer seems to have been solely concerned with the treatment of prostitutes. In 1871 a local official in Koishikawa wrote to the prefectural government to request that a widow and her son who had been treated and released from the syphilis clinic be transferred to the homeless shelter in Mita.[24] There is no suggestion that the woman in question was a prostitute, so the clinic apparently offered treatment to other residents of the city as well.

Even as this clinic was in operation, however, concern about prostitution and its role in the spread of syphilis was growing within official circles. In

1870 a petition authored by officials of the Eastern College and directed to the Council of State stated that "the harm caused by this disease is far greater than any other."[25] The anonymous author(s) of this document emphasized the economic and political threat posed by syphilis. The disease was sapping the strength of its soldier and sailors, imperiling the health of the children born to infected women, and rendering men in their prime unable to work and their families destitute.[26]

Two additional statements accompanied the college's petition. One was authored by George Newton, who by this time was overseeing the examination of prostitutes in the treaty ports of Nagasaki and Hyōgo (now Kobe), as well as Yokohama. He noted that while "governments of every country" were enacting laws to control the spread of syphilis, in Japan the disease went unchecked. Newton advocated for a system like that used in nearby Yokohama: every prostitute should be examined once or twice a week and those found to be infected confined for treatment until they recovered. Newton also addressed the funding of such a facility. He stated that a course of treatment for a single patient, including medicines, room and board, and nursing, would not exceed two kan two hundred bun per day, a very paltry sum. Based on the 1871 currency reform, this was less than five sen per day, at a time when a bath in a public bathhouse cost about one sen.[27] The Tokyo prefectural government also submitted a statement. Pointing to the perceived success of the lock hospitals in Nagasaki and Yokohama, it suggested that a hospital be established adjacent to Yoshiwara as a test case of the domestic use of the treaty port model.[28]

This apparently coordinated effort—between representatives of the new medical elite, the prefectural government, and a British naval surgeon—to lobby for an official policy to control syphilis that targeted prostitutes was successful. In April 1871 the Council of State issued a statement expressing concern for "the damage caused by the spread of syphilis that is the result of the increase in prostitution in every region," and it encouraged local governments to make efforts to control the disease.[29] In the months that followed, the examination of prostitutes was attempted in several brothel quarters outside of the treaty ports, including in the Senju post station located just outside of Tokyo and in Osaka.

In Tokyo, the prefectural government urged the owners of brothels in Yoshiwara to hire George Newton to oversee the examination procedure, but Newton's death later that year made this impossible. The failure to institute the examinations had other causes as well. In February 1872, the newspaper *Shinbun zasshi* reported, "There was a rumor last year that doctors in [Tokyo] prefecture would work together to establish a syphilis hospital in the brothel quarter. However, this was not accomplished because not only the women but also the owners of the brothels and teahouses all refused to agree." The newspaper was critical of this intransigence, noting that a syphilis hospital was "not only in the interest of the women themselves but also for the good of the ten thousand guests who come from all around the country," and it called for new regulations that would require the examination and treatment of prostitutes for syphilis.[30]

The brothel owners had good reasons for resisting the exams. The identification of the women in their employ as infected and the requirement that they be confined for treatment would have been a blow to business. Moreover, as a February 1872 *Shinbun zasshi* article noted, Tokyo Prefecture had not yet issued a law or administrative order requiring syphilis exams; it had only encouraged the brothel owners to take on this task—and its attendant costs.

The lack of cooperation did not necessarily signal a lack of concern. Early in 1872, the brothel owners allowed a school called Kyōkan Academy to establish a branch in Yoshiwara. The academy, which was based in Kyōbashi, was primarily an English-language school, but it also functioned as a cram school for those seeking to enter the government's medical school and for this reason it employed several doctors. The establishment of the branch was originally intended to facilitate teaching English to the prostitutes in Yoshiwara, in the hope of attracting international residents and visitors to the brothels.[31] The decline in the city's population, the economic contraction that followed, and the civil war had all affected the brothel quarters, sparking interest in the cultivation of a new clientele. In 1871 two men who operated brothels in Yoshiwara had petitioned the prefecture for permission to establish a new brothel district near Tsukiji, the area in Kyōbashi designated for foreign residences and businesses. Given the name "New Shimabara" after Kyoto's famous brothel district, it was located just west of Tsukiji and opened in November 1868 (see fig. 4.1). The new brothel district had sixty-five brothels at its height, but it failed to gain a following among the international residents and was abolished in the summer of 1873, less than three years after it had been established.[32]

It is unclear how the relationship between the English school and Yoshiwara came about, but the original Kyōkan Academy was located not far from the site of New Shimabara, and those associated with it were in a good position to know of the brothel owners' interest in attracting international visitors and residents to the brothels.[33] As a result, the Yoshiwara branch did more than just provide English-conversation instruction to the women of the quarter.

Eventually doctors on the staff of the school began to offer examinations for syphilis and treatment in the form of mercury injections.[34] Notably, the approach of Kyōkan Academy differed substantially from the coercive system in place in Yokohama. The examinations were offered on a voluntary basis, and those who were infected were treated as outpatients. This was apparently acceptable to the women, and brothel owners too seemed to have had no complaint, given their efforts to revive Yoshiwara. After all, the two services the academy offered would have produced a new kind of prostitute, one who was both English speaking and syphilis free.

Emancipation and Its Aftermath

Within a few years of the establishment of the new government, three models of syphilis clinics were available to Tokyo officials: the publicly funded clinic that provided treatment to city residents, the private clinic that offered treatment on a voluntary basis to prostitutes within the brothel district, and the coercive system used in the treaty ports that focused solely on prostitutes. The ultimate adoption of the treaty port approach followed a confluence of events that began in 1872. In the summer of that year, a Peruvian ship called the *Maria Luz*, which was transporting more than two hundred Chinese contract laborers to Peru, was forced by poor weather to enter Yokohama harbor. One of the Chinese took advantage of the unplanned visit to this port to flee the ship, and once in the hands of Japanese authorities, he complained of maltreatment at the hands of the ship's crew. New charges emerged when the Japanese investigated conditions on the ship. Some of the laborers claimed that they had been tricked into signing contracts they could not read, others that they had been kidnapped. The question of how to respond to the complaints of the Chinese laborers sparked an international conflict that involved not only Japan and Peru, but other countries as well.

The "*Maria Luz* Incident," as it was known, provoked new international scrutiny of brothel-based prostitution in Japan after Ōe Taku, the governor of Kanagawa who was also serving as a judge in the dispute between Japan and the Peruvian captain, ruled that the Chinese laborers could not be held in involuntary servitude and ordered their release. In response, the British lawyer representing the Peruvian side pointed out that Japanese women were typically indentured to brothels under contracts signed by their fathers or another male relative, meaning that they too were in a position of involuntary servitude.[35] Confronted with this uncomfortably accurate comparison, the Japanese government responded by issuing the so-called Entertainer and

Prostitute Emancipation Edict (Geishōgi kaihō rei) in October 1872. Declaring that indentured servitude was "the same as the buying and selling of human beings," it freed prostitutes and female entertainers (*geigi* or *geisha*) from their indentures.[36]

This "emancipation" was not intended to end the sex trade, but to counter foreign criticism of the long-standing practice of indentured prostitution. Even so, it led to new regulations: women entering prostitution were now required to be signatories to the contracts that consigned them to sex work and the term of employment had to be explicitly stated, rather than left open-ended.[37] These changes were intended to signal that young women were now free agents who voluntarily entered prostitution, a stance that ignored the realities of poverty and family pressure that propelled women into sex work. One result of the new requirements was that the sex trade came to be cloaked in a new vocabulary. Brothels were now termed "rental room businesses" (*kashi zashiki*), the brothel districts became known as "areas where rental rooms are licensed" (*kashiyashiki menkyo no chi*), and the "ransom" (*migawarikin*, *minoshirokin*, literally, "money for the body") that had to be worked off by the indentured prostitute or paid off was newly described as "advance money" (*maegarikin*).

The ostensibly emancipated figure of the prostitute that emerged after 1872 quickly became a source of anxiety for officials in Tokyo, where private prostitution had long been regarded as a threat to morality and public order and increasingly as a threat to public health. A year after the Emancipation Edict, a revision of the 1870 criminal code was issued. One of the new articles, Article 267 in the section on sex crimes, explicitly banned "private prostitutes," and set penalties for both women and their pimps. However, in a nod to the reality of sex work in this period, the new statute stated that when a woman entered prostitution at the order of her parents, it was they who should be punished, not the daughter.[38] The popular press was less sympathetic to the plight of prostitutes. An 1872 article in the *Tōkyō nichinichi shinbun* (*Tokyo Daily News*) castigated the newly emancipated prostitutes in moralistic terms, suggesting that they continued to engage in sex work out of greed and carnal desire: "Why, having received the right of independence, do they continue to act out of greed and . . . behave just like animals?"[39]

Amid growing concern about private prostitution, local officials began creating new regulations that essentially resurrected brothel-based prostitution, albeit in a form that responded to the concerns of the new era. In Tokyo, the prefectural government issued an administrative order in February 1873, introducing three new sets of regulations, for businesses that rented rooms to prostitutes (*Kashi zashiki tosei kisoku*), for prostitutes (*Shōgi kisoku*), and for female entertainers or "geisha" (*Geigi kisoku*). In a message addressed to "all the wards of the city," Ōkubo Ichiō, the prefectural governor, explained the need for these new regulations: "Recently I have heard that on every street in the city the number of women selling sex is increasing, and . . . this is damaging our customs and morals. Since this cannot be ignored, from now on, rental rooms and prostitution will not be allowed outside of Yoshiwara, Shinagawa, Shinjuku, Itabashi, and Senju."[40] In addition to confining prostitution to specific areas, the new regulations created a licensing system for rental room businesses, prostitutes, and female entertainers. The new licenses came with a hefty price tag in the form of fees that had to be paid monthly: five yen for rental room establishments, two yen for prostitutes, and three yen for entertainers.[41]

The regulations for rental room businesses and entertainers were relatively brief and straightforward. Rooming-house owners were now forbidden to rent rooms to unlicensed women, were tasked with ensuring that customers stayed no longer than one day and were required to report any suspicious behavior by clients to local authorities. Entertainers were subject to a similar reporting requirement, but the main concern of the regulations for them was the creation of a new distinction between entertainers and prostitutes: those licensed as entertainers were now forbidden to engage in sex work.[42]

In contrast to the brevity of these regulations, those for prostitutes were elaborate. In keeping with the ethos of emancipation, women (or rather, girls who were at least fifteen years old) were required to apply for a license in person and to affirm that they were entering the trade by their own volition. While licensed prostitutes could now live at home, sex work itself had to take place at a licensed rental room business, and it was forbidden to work out of one's home, an inn, or any other place. Moreover, the relationship with a rental room business had to be exclusive. Women were not allowed to "rent rooms" at more than one establishment. Most significantly, prostitutes who wanted a license were newly required to submit to syphilis examinations twice a month and to undergo treatment if infected. Hiding one's condition and continuing to see customers was strictly forbidden.[43]

The logic of the new licensing system is readily apparent. It created revenue for the cash-strapped prefectural government, placed the "emancipated" prostitutes under the supervision of both the local authorities and the rental room businesses, and provided a means to compel reluctant women to submit to syphilis exams. Still, the new regulatory scheme left many questions unanswered: Who would be responsible for the examinations, where would treatment take place, and how would recovery from the disease be verified? Initially, as with many aspects of public health policy in the 1870s, authorities expected the recently established prefectural hospital to fill this role. In May 1874, the governor announced that physicians on the staff of the hospital would be dispatched to the six brothel quarters (the five named above plus Nezu) within the prefecture to carry out exams. Those found to be infected would be treated in the hospital, with the costs covered by a special tax on the sex trade known as *fukin* (levy), which was created in 1874 when the Ministry of Finance directed local governments to tax prostitutes and associated businesses.[44] The ministry, however, cautioned that these taxes should not be comingled with other kinds of local tax revenue, presumably because this money was tainted by its association with immorality. The Tokyo government resolved the problem of how to use these funds by directing them to the prefectural hospital, providing a much-needed source of financial support.[45]

As the examinations got underway, problems soon arose. Tokyo's prostitutes intensely disliked the invasive exams and regarded them as humiliating and as prurient in intent. In some cases, women responded by harassing the doctors and others involved. In one case, a woman painted her genital area with lipstick to shock and embarrass the doctor conducting the exam. Other women directed expletives at the medical staff, insulted them in sexual terms, or discarded befouled bits of tissue, making use of what James Scott famously termed "weapons of the weak."[46] Newspapers reported that some women, when confronted with the reality of the examinations, simply refused to cooperate and announced on the spot that they were quitting the profession. This alarmed doctors and officials who seemed unable to understand the women's discomfort with the examination requirement. Instead, they assumed that the women were infected and were seeking to evade detection.[47] Women who were confined for treatment protested the requirement that they continue to pay the licensing fee even as they were prohibited from working.[48]

Eventually some of these issues were resolved, albeit in ways that ignored the interest of the women involved. Those who wanted to leave prostitution could do so, but only after submitting to an examination to verify they were syphilis free. Women who had difficulty paying the licensing fee during treatment were allowed to petition for relief, but the ultimate decision was in the hands of prefectural officials. Another problem proved more intractable.

Some women, it was reported, were turning to unlicensed prostitution to escape both the indignity of the exams and the burden of the licensing fees, an alarming development for Tokyo officials.[49]

In response to the growing number of private prostitutes, in April 1875 Governor Ōkubo issued yet more regulations, justifying them by referencing the familiar charge that private prostitution was damaging both the morals and the health of Tokyo residents. In an interesting move that reveals how much policy in this period could still be influenced by early modern practices, Ōkubo announced that women found engaging in unlicensed prostitution would be required to spend a year working in one of the city's rental room businesses, a punishment that reflected the Edo-era response to illicit prostitution that confined women to Yoshiwara as punishment. Of course, in this modern iteration, the women were required to undergo weekly syphilis examinations. In addition, substantial fines of from five to fifty yen were established for anyone found to be complicit with unlicensed prostitution, including parents, pimps, landlords, and innkeepers, with the provision that these funds be used to fund the reform of prostitutes in workhouses and their treatment for syphilis.[50]

The prefecture's willingness to revive Edo-era practices can be seen in another set of regulations issued in May 1875. Edo magistrates had long favored self-regulation by merchant guilds as best means to control commerce. We can recollect from chapter one that medicine wholesalers were charged with controlling rising prices during times of epidemic disease. At this juncture, prefectural officials similarly aimed to compel the brothel businesses to self-regulate. They ordered the so-called "three businesses" (*sangyō*) associated with prostitution (rental room businesses, the tea shops that introduced clients to prostitutes, and restaurants) to form an association that was subsequently charged with a broad range of new responsibilities that would reform prostitution by turning "private faults" into a "public good." Following up on Ōkubo's announcement the previous month, the association was required to take control of women found guilty of engaging in illicit prostitution, by assigning them to work in a specific rental room business. In addition, the association was to establish clinics where sex workers would be examined, workhouses where they could learn skills through piecework and save money for their post-prostitution lives, and classrooms where they could become literate. These endeavors were to be paid for by newly requiring the members of the association to create and contribute to a new fund overseen by the association.[51] Ironically then, the prefectural government ignored the overt interest of brothel owners in keeping women in prostitution and made it their responsibility to "reform" the women from whom they profited.

Policing Prostitution

The prefectural government's efforts to end illicit prostitution, control syphilis, and reform sex workers was cut short in January 1876, when the Council of State announced that the sex trade would henceforth be under the authority of the recently created Tokyo Metropolitan Police. Initially, the TMP focused on cracking down on conventional crimes such as burglary, theft, arson, and murder, prompting the city's newspapers to publish frequent reports celebrating its "achievements" (*jisseki, kōseki*) by citing the number of arrests and prosecutions.[52] Police control over prostitution unfolded gradually during the early months of 1876 as the TMP began to integrate itself into the civic administrative structure, a process that did not go smoothly. In the case of syphilis examinations, the TMP's claim to authority was twofold since it was charged with regulating both entertainment and public health. While the prefectural government took the position that the TMP's role was limited to enforcement and that it retained the power to make policy, Kawaji Toshiyoshi, superintendent of the TMP, asserted that its powers were more expansive, arguing that it could issue its own directives and enforce them. In addition, rather than working through or with the prefectural government to communicate with its lower-level officials, Kawaji's stance was that civil officials too were under the TMP's authority when it came to matters of the entertainment industry and public health.

As this suggests, control of prostitution, justified by the need to control syphilis, became a potent means of extending the authority of the TMP in relation to both civil authorities and Tokyo residents. In January 1876, the TMP issued the Regulations for the Punishment of Illicit Prostitution (*Baiin bassoku*), revoking the prefectural government's regulations of nine months earlier. Rejecting the prefectural government's recourse to Edo-era solutions, it adopted harsh "modern" sanctions. For example, the TMP regulations set heavy fines of up to ten yen for a first offense and twenty yen for each subsequent offense. For the women, many of whom likely charged less than twenty sen per customer (the fee of the cheapest prostitutes in Yoshiwara), these fines would have been devastating.[53] Those who were unable to pay faced an even harsher punishment, a jail term of up to ten weeks for a first offense and five months in jail for subsequent convictions. Upon their release from prison, destitute women were subject to further confinement in one of the city's public workhouses. Only a few days after the new punishments for unlicensed prostitution were issued, Kawaji released a sharply worded directive to ward and *machi*-level civil officials not only ordering them to report unlicensed prostitutes in their jurisdictions to the police but also instructing them to reprimand any woman whose behavior suggested she might turn to illicit prostitution.[54]

In relation to licensed prostitution, the TMP rejected the prefecture's attempt to create a system of self-regulation and dissolved the three-business association. Instead, the TMP required the businesses in each of the designated "zones" to choose representatives to assist TMP efforts to surveil sex work in the city. They were required to submit the names, photographs, and fees charged by the prostitutes in their districts to the police and to ensure that the rental room businesses properly maintained client rosters, to which the police could demand access at any time. In addition, the businesses were required to contribute 10 percent of their profits to create a new fund that was to be used to cover the cost of examining and treating women infected with syphilis. Prostitutes too were required to contribute, albeit at the slightly lower rate of 7 percent of their earnings. The aim was to ensure that no public funds were used for the police-mandated policy of syphilis prevention and treatment.[55]

As the TMP worked to extend its authority vis-à-vis the prefectural government, it took control of the licensing procedure, requiring women to apply for a license at designated police stations, and it made the syphilis examinations a police matter as well. According to the Regulations for Syphilis Examinations, doctors in the employ of the police were to be dispatched to the districts to conduct the exams, which were now to take place in purpose-built "examination centers" established by the rental room establishments. In addition, infected women would no longer be treated at the prefectural hospital. Instead, they were to be confined in syphilis wards established within the city's network of police hospitals. These wards were governed by strict rules. Not only were women denied the right to refuse treatment, but visitors were also not allowed, and amusements such as gambling, singing, and playing the shamisen (a banjo-like instrument) were strictly forbidden.[56]

Syphilis Exams as Urban Spectacle

It was not long before these new policies began to have an impact on the brothel quarters and their place within the city. As the syphilis examination centers were established, the TMP allowed the publication of their schedules in Tokyo's newspapers, a decision that transformed what should have been a private medical procedure into a public spectacle. In the spring of 1878, the *Yomiuri shinbun* reported that on the days when syphilis exams took place at Yoshiwara, a crowd of men, many in rickshaws, gathered outside the entrance of the examination center to watch the prostitutes come and go. They were, in the words of the author of this article, like "cats attracted by catnip." Each time a woman arrived for her required exam, the men excitedly shouted insults at her, "as if they had come from a land without women." Repelled by this boorish behavior, the reporter questioned why the police failed to restrain the crowd.[57]

The appearance of crowds of gawkers was not limited to Yoshiwara. Another report in the *Yomiuri* described how a group of pilgrims from Mie Prefecture, who were making their way to the famous Narita Temple in Chiba, stopped in Tokyo for some sightseeing. When they encountered a crowd outside the examination center of the Shinagawa licensed district, they asked a nearby rickshaw driver what was happening. He replied that the crowd was waiting for "the opening of a living Benten." This was an elaborate, sexually tinged joke. Benten, a Buddhist deity, was often depicted as a woman playing the lute and thus evoked the image of the shamisen-playing courtesans of the Edo-era brothel quarters. The reference to "opening" was a pun that referenced the practice of temples and shrines of occasionally displaying their prized statutes of Buddhist deities, which were typically stored in double-doored cabinets. These were opened on special occasions to display the image. "The opening of a living Benten" then was a salacious reference to the prostitutes spreading their legs during the syphilis examinations.[58] As this suggests, some in the crowd apparently eroticized the examination process—and perhaps the humiliation of the women involved, since their discomfort was well publicized.

As the syphilis exams started attracting spectators, the area in front of the examination centers began to be used for a variety of activities. In July 1878 members of the Divine Wind Congregation (Jinpūkō), a modern Shinto organization associated with the Ise Shrine, gathered in front of Yoshiwara's examination center. After the five-color flag of the organization was raised, a shrine official performed a ritual dance while holding a mirror, a sacred object at Ise, in a display that seemed intended to attract new members.[59] The proprietors of the rental room businesses also seized on the opportunity provided by the crowds. At the opening of Nezu's new examination center, prostitutes circulated among those gathered and distributed sweet confections to advertise their services, and in 1883, when improvements were made to the center, the proprietors of the brothels celebrated with a display of fireworks aimed to bring spectators to the brothel district.[60]

The examination centers were used for less commercially oriented events as well. In the mid-1880s they became a favored site for public "hygiene lectures" (*eisei kōenkai*). Widely advertised in the newspapers, these aimed to edify the populace about infectious diseases, presumably including syphilis. In some instances, the lectures were accompanied by magic lantern shows, which ensured they would draw a large crowd.[61] Major national events were also celebrated at the examination centers. In 1889, when Japan's constitution was promulgated, the brothel-related businesses in Shinjuku organized a celebration at their center that featured food stalls and a festive lion dance.[62]

The examination centers were also among the sites to which distinguished foreign visitors were brought. Initially, this provoked some controversy. In 1877, just before a planned visit by members of the royal family of Austria-Hungary, it was announced that Dr. Albrecht von Roretz, an Austrian physician on the staff of Aichi Prefectural Hospital, would accompany them on a visit to a syphilis examination center. The popular newspaper, *Kanayomi shinbun*, published a letter to the editor that was harshly critical of displaying Japanese women in this way, and asked rhetorically whether there was such a custom in any other country? Other newspapers responded by summarizing the letter and raising similar concerns.[63] It is unclear whether this visit took place, but others certainly did. For example, in 1896, when a representative of the recently established Republic of Hawaii visited Tokyo, the TMP gave him a guided tour of the examination center.[64] The TMP, it seems, was proud of its efforts to control syphilis and happy to show them off to distinguished visitors.

Print media contributed to the intense public interest in the syphilis exams by explaining and depicting the examination process. A case in point is the pamphlet-like work titled *Syphilis Examinations, Explained* (*Baidoku kensa no wake*, 1880), authored by Ajioka Yasuke, as part of a series of short, ostensibly educational texts on a variety of topics. *Syphilis Examinations, Explained* opens with a discussion of the transmission of syphilis very much in the manner of the home hygiene books (*katei eiseibon*) of the day. It explained that a syphilitic man could infect his wife via sexual intercourse, and the woman could then transmit the disease to their children either in the womb or postnatally via breast milk. This discussion is companied by an illustration of the examination procedure (fig. 4.2) that depicts a doctor using a magnifying glass to examine the genitals of a prone and draped prostitute, while two officials observe the procedure. Ajioka took note of the prostitutes' dislike of the exams but dismissed their discomfort. In his view, they were simply unhappy

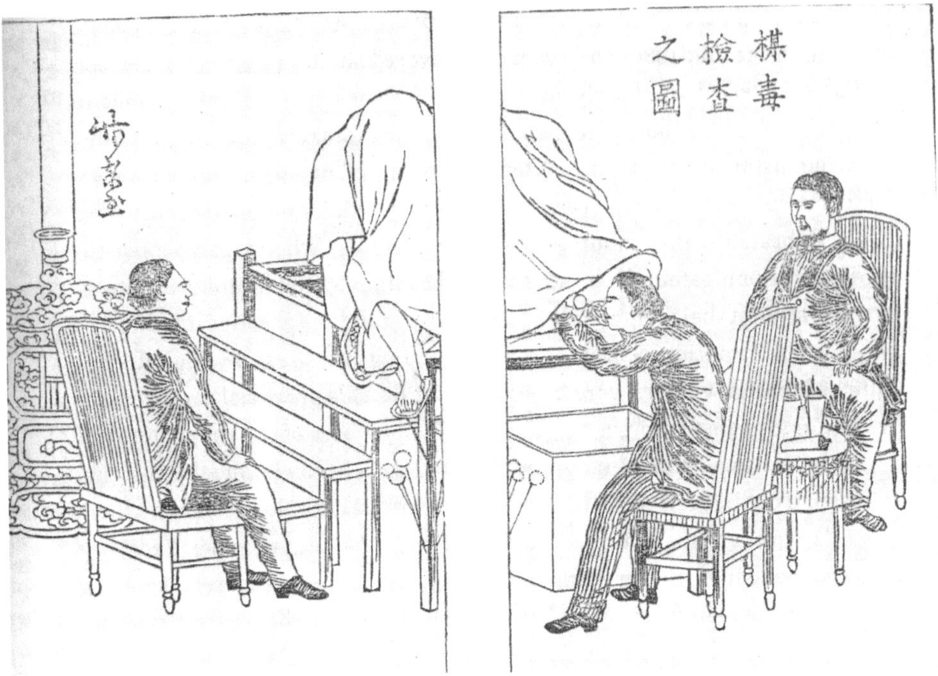

Figure 4.2. Examination for syphilis. Ajioka Yasuke, *Baidoku kensa no wake* in Yunomae and Akisada, *Baibaishun mondai*, 14:134.

because the lengthy hospitalization required for those infected would reduce their earnings.[65]

A different perspective was offered in *Conditions in the Brothel Districts* (*Karyū jijō*, 1880) by the satirical humorist Tajima Shōji (writing under the pseudonym, Suita Dōshi). Tajima claimed that he had always understood syphilis to be "an instrument of retribution to punish those who buy prostitutes," but the enlightened government of the new era had inexplicably decided to curtail this potent means of upholding morality.[66]

In keeping with this tongue-in-cheek criticism of "enlightened government," Tajima's sympathies were clearly with the prostitutes, who in his view not only had to endure the humiliating exams but also were required to pay for their compulsory treatment, even though they had already paid taxes, levies, and licensing fees. Moreover, he questioned the motives of the physicians involved. One of the illustrations (fig. 4.3) in the work depicts a woman lying prone on an examination table hiding her face while a doctor with the head of a catfish gazes at her genital area. It is accompanied by a satirical poem:

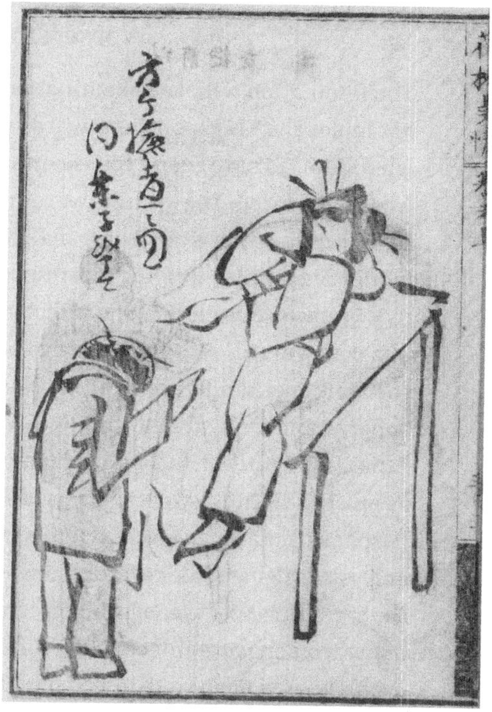

Figure 4.3. Satirical depiction of a syphilis examination. Suita Dōshi, *Karyū jijō*, 1:47–48. Waseda Kotenseki Sōgō Database, https://www.wul.waseda.ac.jp/kotenseki/html/wo06/wo06_00434/index.html.

"Six doctors one after the other, examine the same dancing girl." The depiction of the doctor as a catfish may be an allusion to the saying "slippery as a catfish," a description of a devious person. But Tajima's greatest scorn was reserved for those who gathered in front of the examination centers to catcall the women who were compelled to undergo the exams. In his view, they were penniless ruffians who, with nothing better to do, spent their time moving from one examination center to another to harass the women.[67]

Other representations of the examinations were less explicit but also took note of the women's discomfort. In 1883 the woodblock artist Utagawa Kuniaki II completed a triptych titled "An Illustration of the Examinations of Prostitutes at the Syphilis Hospital of New Yoshiwara" (*Shin Yoshiwara shōgi baidoku byōin kensa no zu*) (plates 10, 11, and 12). Unlike the other illustrations that depict the examination procedure, Utagawa's work focused on the waiting room, a richly decorated Western-style room that featured a colorful carpet, an ornate desk, a grandfather clock, and shelves of medicine. The officials and doctors overseeing the exams wear hakama, the wide trousers traditionally worn by men of warrior status, but also sport short modern haircuts, while the prostitutes who are waiting their turn to be examined are wearing elaborate kimono and multiple hair ornaments. While the men involved are not identified, each of the female figures is named by means of a small tag, identifying them as women who worked in Yoshiwara at the time. Confronted by the steady gaze of the men in the room, most look downward or sideways, perhaps out of embarrassment or distress. For at least some viewers, no doubt, it was the imagination of the examinations to come that made this scene interesting.

Worse Than a Prison

The fascination with the examinations lasted until the turn of the century, but under the TMP, policies toward syphilis continued to evolve. In 1880, in what seems to have been a cost-saving measure, the system of police hospitals was reorganized. The syphilis wards in police hospitals around the city were closed, and two hospitals, those in Kōjimachi and Hongō, were turned into facilities dedicated to treating prostitutes. Two years later, however, the hospital in Kōjimachi was closed, and infected prostitutes from Tokyo's six licensed districts were all sent to the Hongō hospital, which was officially renamed the Metropolitan Police Syphilis Hospital. Reports submitted to the TMP superintendent by the hospital's director reveal the poor health of Tokyo's licensed prostitutes. In 1885, for example, a total of 3,997 women were working as prostitutes in Tokyo's six licensed districts, and 2,751 were admitted to the hospital after a diagnosis of syphilis. Most were newly diagnosed cases, with only 130 designated as "readmissions." The large number of new cases reflects the rapid turnover among women employed in the districts and the fact that many women were infected soon after entering the profession. In 1885, for example, 75 women were infected with syphilis within a month of beginning work as prostitutes, most likely by one of their clients. Upon admission to the hospital, many women were found to be suffering not only from syphilis but also from other diseases, including gonorrhea, urinary and vaginal infections, lung infections, and what were described as "nervous" diseases. Even so, the duration of treatment was relatively brief (27 days on average) and in 1885 all but 183 patients (including 9 who died) were eventually released as cured.[68]

This compelling evidence of the poor health of Tokyo's prostitutes elicited little response from the TMP and the prefectural government, and in fact the health care available to infected women declined. In 1889, the central government reversed the tax-exempt status of the country's hospitals and began to tax the value of the land on which they were constructed, adding to the expense of operating a hospital. Initially, the TMP looked to the prefecture for aid and requested that the revenue derived from the levies imposed on the sex trade be used to cover this new expense. However, the prefectural assembly rejected this proposal and declined to transfer local taxes to the TMP. In response, the TMP decided to close its syphilis hospital and to require the rental room businesses to establish their own private syphilis hospitals adjacent to their respective licensed districts. This decision notwithstanding, the TMP retained considerable authority over the new privately financed hospitals:

for example, only doctors employed by the police were authorized to admit and release patients.[69]

The closing of the TMP's hospital initially found favor among its patients. Newspaper reports described some of their complaints, which included the high cost of traveling by rickshaw to Hongō from the various licensed quarters, the poor conditions within the hospital, and the many restrictions imposed upon them.[70] However, the new "cooperative hospitals" (*kyōritsu byōin*) established by brothel owners were even worse than the police facility they replaced. In 1903 the journalist Katsuragi Tenka, the author of several works on the sex trade, and his coauthor Furusawa Kodō, published *Yoshiwara yūkaku no uramen* (The Dark Side of the Yoshiwara Brothel Quarters). In the chapter "Yoshiwara Hospital and Hygiene in the Brothel District," they presented a disturbing picture of the hospital. In their words, "We wanted to compare it to a prison, but in fact Sugamo Prison is cleaner and better equipped." The hospital was overcrowded with as many as twelve or thirteen women sharing a ten-tatami room, a situation that required them to share bedding. In addition, patients were required to cook their own meals. The budget for this was only seven or eight sen per day per woman, so their diet was limited to rice mixed with other grains, miso soup, and pickled vegetables. To supplement their diet, women could pay the staff to buy them additional foodstuffs, but few women had the financial resources to do this. As a result, at mealtimes, hungry patients were like "dogs fighting over a bit of meat."[71]

By this time, the brothel district in Nezu no longer existed. In the years following its establishment in 1868, Hongō had been transformed into a center of elite higher education in Tokyo, and the Nezu brothel district was close to two of the most prestigious educational institutions in Tokyo, the University of Tokyo and the First Higher School, which functioned as a preparatory school for the university. This led to growing concern that the proximity of the prostitutes in Nezu posed a danger to both the bodies and the morals of the nation's most promising youths. To protect them, in 1888 Nezu's 97 rental room businesses, 44 teahouses, and 974 prostitutes were required to relocate to a site on the southwestern tip of Fukagawa Ward on a plot of low-lying reclaimed land in an area that was still largely undeveloped (fig. 4.1).[72]

The brothel and teahouse owners bitterly protested this decision, concerned that the remote location would deter potential customers. There were other problems as well. As we will see in chapter 6, Fukagawa was well known for the poor quality of its drinking water and its high rates of cholera during outbreaks of that disease. Newspaper reports in the late 1880s noted that there were complaints from brothel owners about water quality and quantity. In addition, the location adjacent to Tokyo Bay made it vulnerable to the high tides that accompanied high winds and typhoons, and the tsunami that were known to result from some earthquakes. In anticipation of the relocation of the brothels, the building of a sea wall to protect the new brothel district was discussed but it never materialized.[73] These concerns were justified. In 1911, fifty-four people, including prostitutes, clients, and others, died when heavy rains caused flooding on July 26.[74] The advantage of the new location—at least from the perspective of the TMP—was its location on the periphery of the city, and thus it effectively segregated what had come to be called the "shameful business" (*shūgyō*) from the rest of the city.

To attract customers, brothel owners sought to make the new district as attractive as possible. For example, the building that housed one of the largest rental room businesses, Honhachimanrō, featured an imposing clock tower, and one of its competitors followed suit. Woodblock prints of Tokyo's "famous places" (*meisho*) proliferated in this period, and those of Susaki emphasized its distance from the more mundane city proper, as well as its impressive towers (see plate 13). But the public image of the new brothel district concealed a darker reality. A report published in 1895 by Susaki's cooperative hospital reveals the dire health of the women who worked there. The year before, the TMP had issued a new directive requiring that the brothel district hospitals examine licensed prostitutes not only for syphilis but for all forms of infectious disease, specifically naming gonorrhea, chancroid (a sexually transmitted disease characterized by painful genital ulcers caused by the bacterium *Haemophilus ducreyi*), and tuberculosis. Susaki Hospital's staff responded by compiling information on cases of syphilis, gonorrhea, chancroid, and what it termed "miscellaneous diseases," that is, non-sexually transmitted diseases. It found that more than 50 percent of the women suffered from more than one sexually transmitted disease, and of these more than 70 percent had other infectious diseases as well, most often tuberculosis.[75]

In response to the growing body of evidence of the ill health of Tokyo's prostitutes, the high rates of syphilis, and poor conditions in the cooperative hospitals, the TMP reversed itself in 1911 and announced that it would again take control of the syphilis examination system. New police hospitals were opened in Yoshiwara, Susaki, Shinagawa, Itabashi, and Shinjuku, and these quickly gained the status of "famous places." Plate 14 is a picture postcard showing the "New Yoshwara [*sic*] Hospital," which is described as a "famous place of Tokyo." The TMP's direct authority over the health of sex workers

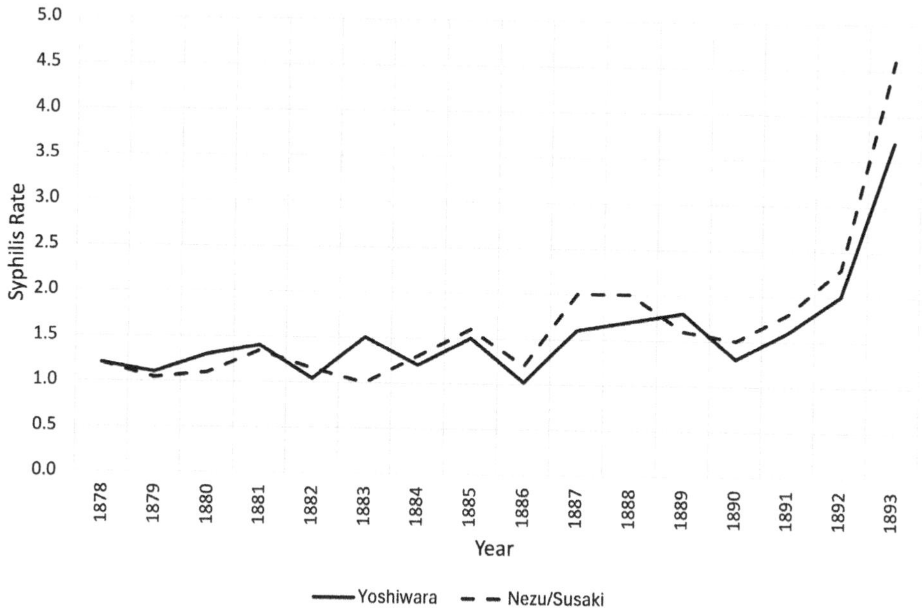

Figure 4.4. Number of syphilis diagnoses per 100 exams of licensed prostitutes in Tokyo's brothel quarters, 1878–1893. Data from Tōkyō-fu, *Tōkyō-fu tōkeisho, Meiji* 15–26.

would continue until 1942, when control reverted to civil authorities, apparently because the TMP was overburdened by its wartime responsibilities.

Syphilis Beyond the Brothels

The development of the syphilis examination system and the establishment of the syphilis hospitals adjacent to the brothel areas solidified the association of the disease with prostitution. Indeed, in the 1890s syphilis began to be routinely referred to as *karyūbyō* ("flower and willow disease" or "brothel disease"), referencing a metaphor for Yoshiwara that dates from the late eighteenth century. "Willow" referred to the large willow tree planted near the entrance to the quarter and "flowers" to the courtesan who resided within it. While the idea that syphilis was a "brothel disease" may have been comforting to some, data compiled by the TMP based on the syphilis examinations it conducted over fifteen years revealed the ineffectiveness of the policy of solely surveilling the bodies of prostitutes to control syphilis.

The number of cases of syphilis among licensed prostitutes in Tokyo did not decline even as the exams were routinized and treatment enforced (see fig. 4.4). Indeed, while the chart shows some peaks and valleys, diagnoses of syphilis trended upward after 1890. This was despite the expansion of the sex trade in Tokyo, which drew new, presumably uninfected women into prostitution year after year. In 1883, there were 3,156 prostitutes; five years later, that number had grown to 4,756. As we noted above, women new to the business were often infected within just a few months. The number of men who frequented the city's brothels also increased in this period. In 1883, Tokyo's prostitutes provided sexual services to 1.2 million men; by 1888 that number had increased by 65 percent to 2 million. With each sexual encounter came the risk of infection.[76]

The growth of the sex trade in Tokyo and the ineffectiveness of the examination procedure ensured that syphilis would spread among the city's general population. Even so, not until the mid-1910s was an effort made to investigate the spread of sexually transmitted diseases beyond the brothels. In 1916 the Hygiene Bureau decided to survey the rates of infection of syphilis, gonorrhea, and chancroid in each prefecture and in major cities. The method chosen for the survey was relatively simply. Hospitals and clinics were asked to retroactively review their records beginning in 1912 and report the number of cases of sexually transmitted diseases that they had documented for each year for the period between 1912 and 1915. However, the study was not comprehensive. In the case of Tokyo, it was based on patient records from some thirty hospitals at a time when more than eighty were in operation, and it is unclear which hospitals were selected for the study and on what basis.[77] This meant that the study was documenting the prevalence of the disease among a delimited patient population, although in the published report this figure was treated as a proxy for prevalence among the general population. In fact, it is likely that the number of cases was higher than the study revealed, since many sufferers, particularly those in stage two, did not realize that they were infected, and many city residents did not seek medical care because of its expense or their embarrassment.

The limitations of the survey notwithstanding, the situation it exposed must have alarmed Tokyo officials. The city had the highest rates of the three sexually transmitted diseases among the country's nine largest cities in the period 1912–1915. In the case of syphilis, for example, 42 percent of all patients within the Tokyo hospitals in the study were found to be infected, while in Osaka, the figure was 24 percent. The total number of infected patients in Tokyo identified during the four-year period was 265,510 or 13 percent of the city's total population. Most of the identified cases were men between the ages of twenty and forty, who worked in factories, commerce, or as company

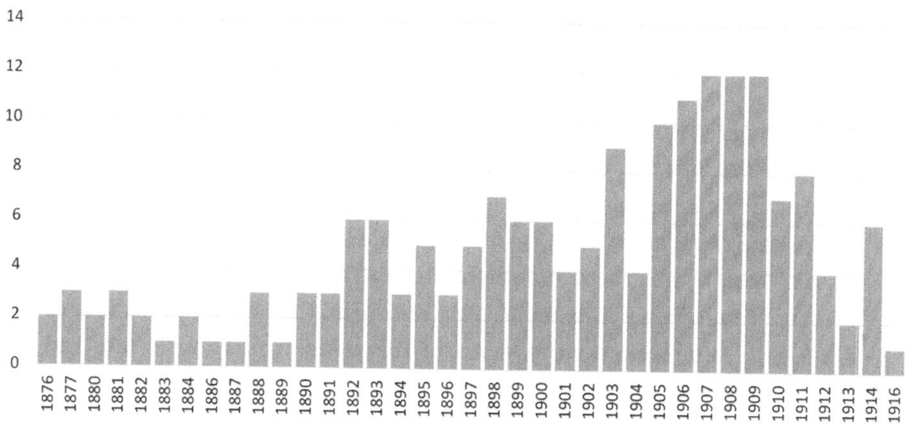

Figure 4.5. Number of hospitals and clinics advertising syphilis treatment by year in the *Asahi shinbun* and *Yomiuri shinbun* from 1876 to 1916.

employees, although a significant number of women, about 38 percent of the total, were among the infected patients. While the age range of the women was the same as that of the male patients in the survey, most did not work outside the home, making it likely that many were married women with children.[78]

Even before the survey was conducted, it was generally recognized that syphilis was common among the general population of the city, but the prefecture and the TMP took no measures to address this situation. Instead, it was the city's medical entrepreneurs who responded. As figure 4.5 indicates, between 1876 and 1914, at least 182 separate clinics and hospitals advertised in two of the major newspapers of the time that they specialized in the treatment of syphilis and other sexually transmitted diseases. The number grew over time with the largest number of advertisements appearing between 1905 and 1909. Between 1876 and 1914, at least 182 separate clinics and hospitals advertised in two of the major newspapers of the time that they specialized in the treatment of syphilis and other sexually transmitted diseases. The physicians who founded these clinics claimed expertise in a variety of medical subfields, including internal medicine, dermatology, urology, and obstetrics and gynecology.

Plate 15 shows the location of hospitals and clinics that advertised treatment for syphilis. It reveals that until 1896 most clinics were clustered in Kyōbashi and Nihonbashi, the densely populated central business districts of the time. As we saw in chapter 3, these areas attracted a large number of hospitals and clinics, with many clustered adjacent to the streetcar lines.

Considering the stigma attached to syphilis, it is possible that people preferred to seek treatment outside their own neighborhoods, so relative ease of access may have been a factor for patients.

There were also many hospitals and clinics in Kanda and adjacent areas in Hongō and Shitaya. This was, as we have seen, a favored location for all types of medical institutions due to the presence of several medical schools and large general hospitals. Like other private hospitals in the area, clinics offering syphilis treatment often employed staff doctors of major institutions on a part-time basis. For example, Dohi Keizō and Kinoshita Tōichi, both of whom graduated from the University of Tokyo Medical School in 1891 and became assistants (*joshu*) at the No. 1 University of Tokyo Hospital, served as medical directors of private dermatological clinics that specialized in treating syphilis. Kinoshita was the director of the private Dermatology and Syphilis Specialty Hospital while also serving as the director of the "cooperative" Yoshiwara Hospital established by brothel owners.[79] Until 1893, when he departed for study in Europe, Dohi was the director of the Tokyo Dermatological Hospital, which offered treatment for syphilis and leprosy. After studying at Vienna University for five years, Dohi returned to the University of Tokyo where he was a professor of dermatology and syphilology.[80]

After 1896, increasing numbers of syphilis hospitals and clinics were established beyond the areas where medical institutions were concentrated, in wards such as Azabu, Akasaka, and Yotsuya. These were still far less populated than the wards of the western part of the city and were residential rather than commercial centers. To understand this development, we need to consider the gendered nature of public health discourse. If prostitutes were identified as the source of infection, men were identified as their "victims," and specific categories of men were the objects of concern. These included those serving in the military and students of higher education, and by the 1910s members of the growing industrial workforce. It was of course a desire to protect the male students at the University of Tokyo and the First Higher School that had motivated the removal of the Nezu brothels to Fukagawa and concern about syphilis among the military dated back to the late 1860s.

While there is no information about rates of infection among industrial workers and university students, rates of syphilis among men in the military were carefully tracked. In 1906 the army published the first of many surveys that sought to reveal the extent of syphilis infection among the troops. Information on physical examinations of men conducted from 1897 to 1906 reveals that about 6 percent of the men in the Tokyo-based First Division were dismissed each year because of a diagnosis of syphilis, a rate of infection that was exceeded only by the Twelfth Division, which was based in Kyushu.[81]

Plate 16 shows the relationship between the areas of the city populated by the targeted male populations—military installations, universities, and large factories—and the hospitals and clinics that offered syphilis treatment. It reveals that in addition to the city center, these sites also attracted a significant number of syphilis clinics. A case in point is the cluster of military facilities on the border between Yotsuya and Akasaka, which included barracks, the Army University, an army weapons factory, and the headquarters of the Imperial Guard. Six clinics were established on the periphery of this extensive military complex. Another such site was Koishikawa Ward, one of the least populated at the time. Home to several military sites, some large factories, and not far from the University of Tokyo, it also contained a significant number of syphilis treatment facilities. The area around Keiō University in Shiba Ward is similar. Besides being the location of the university, it was home to several large factories and the naval arsenal. Here too we find a cluster of syphilis clinics. That said, clinics were lacking in other areas where they might be expected. Although Honjo and Fukagawa were home to many large factories, there were only a handful of syphilis clinics—although as we noted in chapter 3, these wards had few medical facilities or doctors of any type. There were, however, two clinics on Ishikawa Island. Located in the mouth of the Sumida River, it was the site of Japan's first modern shipyard.

It is worth noting that a substantial proportion of private syphilis clinics and hospitals, about 20 percent, were short-lived, with some surviving only a year or two before closing their doors, additional evidence of the highly competitive medical marketplace in Tokyo in this period. For example, a physician named Ōzaki Kenkichi opened Sen'yōdō Clinic in 1893 in Suwachō in Asakusa close to a major roadway, the old Nikko Highway. Despite its prime location, the clinic closed within a few months.[82] Other clinics and hospitals flourished, in some cases, for decades. An example of a successful enterprise was the Seishi Clinic, founded by Nagaoka Tenzō in Kanda in 1897. According to its many advertisements, Seishi Clinic specialized in "diseases of the reproductive organs," including syphilis. The first clinic must have been successful, because the next year Nagaoka opened branch clinics in Kyōbashi and Shiba and by 1900 there were branches outside of Tokyo, in Osaka and Nagoya as well. In that same year, the name of the original clinic in Kanda was changed to Hakuai'in. For six years, it was advertised as a syphilis clinic, until 1906 when it was rebranded as a clinic specializing in "rheumatism." All the other clinics continued to focus on syphilis and in 1907, the Shiba clinic was relocated to a new location near Ueno Station.

One of the keys to Nagaoka's success may have been his widely advertised policies of offering a free initial exam to potential patients and discounted treatment for students and soldiers. In 1911 Nagaoka's clinics were among the first facilities in Tokyo to promote the use of Salvarsan, and the characters for "606" (a reference to the fact that Salvarsan was known as compound 606 since it was the sixth of the sixth group of compounds to be tested) featured prominently in print advertisements at the time. The ads that offered treatment with Salvarsan described syphilis as "the nation-destroying disease" and promised (falsely) that a single injection was sufficient to achieve a cure.[83] In fact, patients typically required four to eight painful intravenous injections that had to be given at intervals of several weeks.[84]

Katō Tokijirō, who would become well known as a socialist activist around the turn of the century, was another physician who opened a successful clinic that specialized in the treatment of syphilis. Born the son of a Sino-Japanese physician in what is now Fukuoka Prefecture, he made his way to Tokyo while still in his late teens and in 1876 entered the Police Forensic Medicine School, which was a short-lived attempt to create a new corps of forensic physicians. The school closed the following year, and Katō began to study at Seisai Academy. He passed the licensing exam in 1882 and quickly found employment in the TMP's Hongō Hospital. In 1885 he resigned from that position and founded a private clinic in Senju that specialized treating syphilis. He also cared for patients from his home in Kyōbashi and made home visits for a substantial fee. Katō referenced his employment with the TMP in announcements of his new clinic, using his association with the TMP to enhance its reputation. The Senju Clinic was successful, and in 1886 it became an inpatient facility.[85]

In 1888 Katō left Japan for Europe where he intended to study medicine in Germany, and, after short stints at a couple of universities, he ended up at the University of Breslau. There he studied with Albert Neisser, a specialist in dermatology and sexually transmitted diseases, who identified the causative agent of gonorrhea, *Neisseria gonorrhoeae*, in 1879. After receiving his medical degree, Katō returned to Tokyo and in quick succession opened Katō Hospital in Kyōbashi, Takanawa Hospital in Shinagawa, and branch clinics in Kanagawa and Yokohama. Advertisements from this period trumpeted his lengthy period of study abroad and his German medical degree.[86]

Katō's public profile may also have contributed to his success. As a member of an organization called the Japan Popular Hygiene Association, he was a frequent speaker on matters related to public health, and he later ran for election to the Tokyo City Council, albeit unsuccessfully.[87] But the cost of care also undoubtedly came into play. Perhaps because of his socialist ideals, Katō's fees were significantly lower than those of many of his competitors. In 1910, he charged two yen for the initial examination and one yen for subsequent visits, with additional fees for medicines or inpatient care. In contrast, many other Tokyo clinics advertising syphilis treatment charged five yen or more for the first examination and as much as three yen for subsequent visits.[88]

Even Katō's relatively low fees would have been a stretch for many. As a result, many syphilis sufferers likely turned instead to patent drugs to treat themselves. The most famous of these was Dokumetsu ("poison extinguisher") produced by Morishita Hiroshi, whose Osaka-based pharmacy, Nan'yōdō, also produced Jintan, perhaps the most famous patent medicine of the day in Japan. Dokumetsu's primary ingredient was sarsaparilla root (*Smilax glabra rhizome*), a botanical closely related to chinaroot.[89] Morishita was a master at advertisement and Dokumetsu's trademark was the image of the German statesman Otto von Bismarck, which appeared in print media and on colorful signs that dotted the urban landscape, displayed in front of pharmacies and public places like streetcar crossings and entertainment venues (see plate 17). It was a far cheaper option than care from a physician, just 15 sen for two and half days of treatment in 1901, but it likely had little effect upon the infection.[90]

Syphilis and the Healthscape of Tokyo

By the early decades of the twentieth century, the public health campaign against syphilis had reshaped Tokyo's cityscape in significant ways. It propelled the relocation of the city's second largest brothel district to the periphery of the city, an area known for its poor, even dangerous living conditions. But prevention efforts also had unintended effects upon the cityscape. They led to the establishment of newly eroticized sites in the form of the syphilis examination centers and hospitals, where tourists and locals gathered to gawk at the women arriving for their compulsory exams. The syphilis exams created a new kind of urban spectacle in these spaces, which the TMP facilitated by allowing the publication of the examination schedules. Presumably, its intent was to demonstrate the pernicious role that prostitution played in the spread of the disease, but instead it allowed men within the city to demonstrate both their desire and contempt for women in the sex trade, while others sought to capitalize on these new "famous places" for their own purposes.

As prefectural officials and the TMP focused solely on prostitutes as the vector of transmission, the so-called brothel disease spread unchecked around the city, infecting women like Nakajima Yoshi, whose story began this chapter. While official policy left their plight unaddressed, the medical marketplace responded: syphilis clinics and hospitals began to line the streets and streetcar lines of central Tokyo and later clustered around military installations, universities, and factories. Meanwhile, advertisements for drugs like Dokumetsu filled the pages of newspapers and appeared on signs posted around the city. Ultimately, the inscription of syphilis onto the cityscape in these ways did little, however, to alleviate the spread of the disease, given the high cost of treatment and its ineffectiveness. But if surveilling prostitutes did not control the spread of syphilis, it succeeded in extending the authority of the TMP vis-à-vis the prefectural government and in publicizing its new and extensive powers to residents of the capital.

5

Psychiatric Care in Tokyo

Class and Social Order

In January 1886, police in Asakusa took a forty-eight-year-old woman named Mitsumura Hatsu into custody. An itinerant performer who made a living by chanting traditional stories while accompanying herself on the shamisen, Hatsu had attracted police attention after her odd behavior led to complaints that a mad woman was wandering the streets. When questioned by the police, she told them that she was possessed by a fox spirit named "Osaki" that had entered her body as she prayed at the popular Asakusa Kannon Temple. The police quickly transferred Hatsu to Tokyo's Prefectural Asylum, then located in Hongō. She would remain there for the next four years. The staff of the asylum tried various treatments, including sedatives and hydrotherapy, without success, but they also listened to and recorded her delusions, which were intimately connected to the politics of the day. Hatsu believed that Osaki had been sent by foreigners to compel her conversion to Christianity, targeting her because she was the aunt of the emperor and the mother of the nation. Eventually Hatsu refused to eat, and although efforts were made to force-feed her, she grew frailer over time. In July 1890 she passed away in the asylum.[1]

Hatsu was one of the first generation of Tokyo residents to experience the new scrutiny that the Tokyo Metropolitan Police (TMP) brought to bear on those viewed as mentally ill, and she was among the first to experience professional psychiatric care within asylum walls. But she was not alone. In 1890 almost four hundred people were confined in the prefectural asylum. Another two hundred or so were housed in three private asylums scattered around the city, and an unknown number were privately confined within their homes, an approach sanctioned by the TMP. Over the next two and a half decades psychiatric institutions in Tokyo continued to grow in both scale and number. By the 1910s, Sugamo Hospital, as the prefectural asylum had been renamed, had more than two thousand beds, and the thirteen private hospitals then in operation offered almost nine thousand more.[2] This meant that 70 percent of the psychiatric beds in Japan were in Tokyo.[3]

This chapter explores the events that led to psychiatric care becoming an important feature of urban life in Tokyo. Officials in Tokyo in the 1870s were deeply concerned about the perceived rise in poverty, crime, and vagrancy that followed the fall of the shogunate. The Tokyo Prefectural Asylum has its origins in this situation: initially, it confined impoverished people who were viewed as a disruptive and unwelcome presence on the streets of the capital. This institution evolved, as did the legal framework of confinement, but even as psychiatric hospitals (as they were termed after 1890) became medicalized spaces, concerns about social order continued, heightened by a new sense that urban life itself was contributing to increasing rates of mental illness. By the first decade of the twentieth century, a new spatial and economic order of psychiatric care had emerged, which reflected the growing economic divides within the city as well as the symbiotic relationship between public medical institutions and the modern medical marketplace.

"Disordered Hearts" and the Early Modern City

Early modern Japan had nothing like the insane asylums that began proliferating in Europe in the seventeenth century. There were, however, multiple modes of confinement for those viewed as unruly or delusional. An edict issued by the city magistrates in the mid-seventeenth century outlined the official policy toward those described as *ranshinsha* ("people with disordered hearts"). It required families with a member whose behavior had become "outrageous" (*furachi*) to confine the person in question at home but stated that if home confinement were difficult for any reason, the household head could request placement of that person in the city's jail in Denmachō.[4]

In this period, various terms were used to refer to madness, but *ranshin* was the term of choice in official records. It reflected the theory that the heart was the seat of consciousness and intellect and was used to describe the impairment of reason or will.[5] An edict of 1721 clarified the kinds of activities that were associated with the state of "disordered heart." These included often being drunk, being overly noisy in the streets, engaging in behavior that annoys neighbors, causing a public nuisance, and being careless with fire.[6] The final item, which is almost invariably cited in petitions for confinement, was prompted by the very real danger that fire posed in a city built largely of wood, bamboo, paper, and thatch. As the list of problematic behaviors suggests, a "disordered heart" was used to refer to socially aberrant behavior viewed as dangerous and disruptive. The aim of confinement was not to provide treatment or even to ensure the safety of those with "disordered hearts" but to preserve order in the city.

By the mid-eighteenth century, a well-defined process for the management of *ranshinsha* was in place. Families seeking to confine one of their members were required to submit to the magistrates a petition that included a description of the danger posed by the person to be confined and evidence of the consent of family members and *machi*-level officials to the confinement, along with a doctor's report confirming the state of *ranshin* and a diagram indicating the conditions of confinement.[7] Yamazaki Tasuku has argued that Edo officials required such information to ensure that families did not abuse home confinement to resolve family disputes over assets, succession, or other matters.[8] Even so, over time both the petitions and the doctors' reports became distinctly formulaic in content and language, suggesting a lack of consideration about the specifics of any case, and despite official concern regarding abuse, the conditions of confinement could be harsh. The diagrams attached to petitions suggest that "cages" could be as small as two square meters.[9] Some of those confined spent years in these cramped spaces: in one case, a family notified officials of the death of their family member after twelve years in confinement.[10]

The process for confining *ranshinsha* to the city's jail was less complicated. A collection of templates for official petitions from the 1830s includes one titled "Request to transfer a *ranshinsha* to jail." It consists of a brief statement that neighborhood officials know the person in question to be suffering from "disordered heart" and hence potentially careless with fire and thus they ask that the person be jailed.[11] Yamazaki suggests that from the perspective of Edo authorities, confinement in the city jail was the preferred approach to controlling *ranshinsha*, since it obviated the possibility of abuse by family members.[12] In addition to the jail, as discussed in chapter 1, *ranshinsha* were also confined within a third site in the city, the *tame* where the city's destitute and vulnerable were cared for by members of the beggar fraternity. The *ranshinsha* confined in the *tame* fell into two categories. Some were former prisoners of the jail whose condition required greater care; others came under the control of the fraternity via the periodic sweeps it carried out to remove the sick, dead, dying, and those viewed as disruptive from Edo's streets.[13]

Although confinement was the official response to socially aberrant behavior, there were alternatives to locking up one's family member at home, consigning them to jail, or abandoning them to the streets, and these reflected the complicated understanding of "madness" in this era. Despite criticism by Confucian intellectuals, doctors, and others, it was widely believed that madness resulted when an animal spirit or other supernatural entity entered the body.[14] This, of course, was how Matsumura Hatsu explained her condition. As a result, some families turned to temples and shrines to cure their afflicted members. By the late eighteenth century, as many as eighteen temples and shrines scattered around Japan were offering treatment to those viewed as suffering from madness; the care included prayers, exorcisms, and the ascetic practice of standing under a waterfall.[15] One of these sites was Yakuōin, a Shingon temple on Mount Takao, located about sixty kilometers from central Edo near the Kōshū Highway, which originated at Nihonbashi in the city center. In the early nineteenth century, two inns near the temple housed those who had come in search of a cure.[16]

The arrangement at Mount Takao reflects the durability of the idea of possession, but by the late Tokugawa period, it was challenged by the medical discourse on madness that asserted some somatic causes of "madness." For example, in his *Ryōji sadan* (Chats on Treatment, 1808) Tsuda Gensen, who practiced medicine in Edo, suggested that madness was the result of "heart disease" that developed when "poison" attacked the heart.[17] As the medical discourse on madness expanded, some physicians began offering to house patients for treatment, a departure from the typical practice of home-based medical care, but it was in keeping with the practice of removing those with "disordered hearts" from the community. In 1846 a physician named Narabayashi Ittoku established what he called a "madness treatment center" (*kyōeki chiryōjo*) in Komatsugawa, in Katsushika District (now Edogawa Ward), just outside of the city.[18] Trained in medicine by a domanial doctor in Edo, Narabayashi gained a reputation for treating the mentally ill after he took in the son of a local sake brewer who was acting strangely. After spending two months in Ittoku's care, where he was dosed with herbal medicines and shackled when agitated, the young man was released to his family as cured. More patients then followed and eventually Ittoku expanded his enterprise by buying up an adjacent residence, increasing the capacity of his clinic to about twenty patients.[19]

From the Poorhouse to the Asylum

Despite the existence of facilities like Narabayashi's clinic, the Japanese who encountered asylums in Europe and the US viewed them as novel but potentially useful institutions. An early description of asylum-based care came, predictably, from Fukuzawa Yukichi's *Conditions in the West* (*Seiyō jijō*). He coined the term "ten'in" as a translation for "asylum," using a character for "insanity" (*ten*), and explained that a *ten'in* was "a hospital where the mad are treated." According to Fukuzawa, the asylum he visited was a "quiet and serene" place where patients whose symptoms were not severe read books, painted, danced, and took walks.[20] Kume Kunitake, a member of the Iwakura mission that journeyed to the US and Europe in 1871, had a very different impression of the California State Insane Asylum in Stockton, which he toured in January 1872. Kume wrote, "There were more 1,500 patients there, both men and women. They were divided into different rooms depending on the severity of their sickness. Those who were very sick were locked in their rooms with restraints on their arms and legs and were soiled with excrement and urine."[21] Kido Kōin, another member of the same mission, was more favorably impressed by the institution. In his view, "its administration and cleanliness left nothing to be desired," and he requested a copy of the rules and regulations of the asylum, which he passed on to Nagayo Sensai.[22]

These encounters with modern institutional responses to mental illness, however, actually played little role initially in the founding of Tokyo's prefectural asylum. Instead, it took form gradually as the city's new leaders grappled with issues of poverty and social order in the aftermath of the fall of the shogunate. As discussed earlier, conditions in the new capital were chaotic after the city's traditional mechanisms of governance dissolved during the civil war of 1868–1869, and refugees from war-impacted areas and former samurai joined an already significant population of poor and homeless people in Edo. In response, the city's new leaders had hastily adopted measures designed to aid—and curb—the swelling numbers of the urban poor. Some were sent to Hokkaido, while others were housed and fed in hostels managed by the city's beggar fraternity.[23]

By 1872 these early relief efforts had largely lapsed as both the local and central government moved on to new priorities. In August 1871, the government had issued the "emancipation edict" that ended outcast status, meaning that in theory at least the beggar fraternity was no longer obligated to perform services at the behest of officials. This was also the period when the government abolished the positions of machi headman and *ienushi*, ending their role in providing poor relief and other aid at the neighborhood level. In June 1872, the Tokyo prefectural government dissolved the Machikaisho, the organization discussed in chapter 2 that had used "donations" from the city's landlords and householders to fund poor relief since 1792. The prefectural government took control of its remaining funds but repurposed them to finance infrastructure repairs in the city.[24]

The end of the early modern system of poverty relief contributed to the growing population of homeless people in the city, many of whom survived by begging on the streets and on temple and shrine grounds. However, when Grand Duke Alexei Alexandrovich, the fourth son of Tsar Alexander II of Russia, announced that he would visit Japan, officials grew concerned about displaying Japan's poverty, even in its capital, to the representative of a powerful and expanding empire. In anticipation of the grand duke's visit, Ōkubo Ichiō, the governor of Tokyo Prefecture, and officials in the Ministry of Justice worked together to ban mendicancy first in Tokyo and then in the whole country in October 1872. They also turned to Asakusa's beggar fraternity for support. At the time, the fraternity was still managing the *tame*, but it had been integrated, at least partially, into the city's new administrative structure. Regulations issued by the prefectural authorities now required ward officials to consign the sick and homeless to the *tame* for care.[25]

In anticipation of the grand duke's visit, Hasebe Senshichi, the headman of the beggar fraternity of Asakusa, was ordered to "hunt down" homeless beggars and corral them until the official visit was over. Hasebe agreed to take on the project of ridding the city of vagrants, but only for a fee of 385 yen, a substantial sum at the time.[26] On October 16, 1872, Hasebe and his compatriots rounded up several hundred people, who were then transferred to the grounds of the *tame* in Asakusa.[27] Although this was originally intended to be a temporary measure until the official visit was concluded, it was soon decided that "[releasing these people] would not be a good policy."[28] But what then should be done with them?

The long-term revival of the *tame* was an unpalatable solution considering both the celebrated "liberation" of the outcasts and the government's commitment to "civilization." Eventually it was decided to establish a new institution to care for the city's indigent. The Yōikuin (literally, "facility for care and education"), as it was termed, was to provide basic support for those incapable of work, while compelling the able-bodied to transition to wage labor. The new institution was established on land purchased from a temple in Ueno and made use of its existing buildings.[29] The transfer of people from the *tame* to the new Yōikuin was accomplished in December 1872. Numbering 245 in total, most were adults between the ages of sixteen and fifty, 94 percent were men, and 60 percent came from outside Tokyo Prefecture.[30]

Over the next few years, the number of clients of the Yōikuin grew, as the heads of the city's wards were instructed to transfer vagrants, abandoned children, sick travelers, and those who were impoverished and infirm to the new institution.[31] Although no explicit mention is made of those with mental illness, it seems likely that they too were among those housed in the Yōikuin. In 1872, the prefectural government had briefly experimented with the creation of what was known as the "Tokyo Watch" (Tōkyō bannin), an effort to recruit volunteers to aid in maintaining law and order in the city. In the "Rules for the Tokyo Watch" issued by the prefectural government, the auxiliary security officers (*bannin*) were ordered to turn over any mentally ill person they encountered on the streets to the police, who then presumably transferred them back to their families or to the Yōikuin.[32]

Further evidence of official concern for the mentally ill dates from 1875 when the prefectural government ordered the heads of the wards of the city to post the following warning on the public notice boards: "There are not a few cases in which those suffering from madness [*kyōbyō*] wander the streets alone and cause trouble to other people. In the worst cases, they commit arson or kill or injure someone. This ultimately arises from the failure of families to control their members. Hereafter, those who are judged to be suffering from mental illness, should be strictly confined within the household. If [families] are neglectful of confinement and allow [mentally ill family members] to wander the streets, there will be appropriate punishment."[33] With the new threat that they were to be punished for failing to control their unruly family members, some people turned to their local ward officials for help. In response, the prefectural government asked the staff of the Yōikuin to establish a special "madmen's ward" (*kyōjin shitsu*) to house them, with families to be charged a fee for their care. This was the origin of Tokyo's first public asylum.

According to the first official history of the Yōikuin, the new segregated unit for the mentally ill was established utilizing a building that had previously housed visually impaired people, who were moved to Tokyo's new residential school for the blind in 1876.[34] The new ward quickly proved successful, perhaps too much so from the perspective of the Yōikuin's administrators.

In 1877 the number of "madmen" in residence was forty (about 12 percent of the total number of residents of Yōikuin).[35] By early 1879, that number had reached sixty-eight, sparking concern from Shibusawa Eiichi, who had been appointed director in 1876. As a former government official who was making a name for himself in finance at the time, Shibusawa had already developed a reputation for public service and philanthropy. According to him, the Yōikuin was unable to offer the mentally ill appropriate medical treatment, and the cost of their care was straining the institution's budget, in part because unlike other residents, they could not perform piecework or cook for themselves, measures adopted by the Yōikuin officials to reduce the cost of running the institution. In Shibusawa's view, the care of the mentally ill threatened the financial viability of the Yōikuin. Kusumoto Masataka, who had replaced Ōkubo as governor, stepped in to resolve the crisis. He negotiated a new relationship with the prefectural hospital in Shiba, making it responsible for the care of the mentally ill.[36]

In late July 1879, the Yōikuin was moved to a new site in Kanda Izumi-chō, and the Ueno facility was renamed the Tokyo Prefecture Provisional Asylum (Tōkyō Furitsu Kari Tenkyōin). The name modified the translation coined by Fukuzawa two decades earlier by adding the character for "madness" (*kyō*) to the more obscure "insanity" (*ten*), but even this new term must have been unfamiliar to many Tokyo residents. In the 1870s the directors of newly established private asylums routinely advertised their facilities as "hospitals for the mad" (*kichigai byōin*), using a colloquial term for "madness." Notably, the founding of the new asylum was supported by a grant of 14,000 yen from the Imperial Household Agency, a gift implying that those confined were worthy of imperial compassion.[37] Donations from private citizens followed, typically small gifts intended for patients, such as fans, fruit, sweets, and hand towels, but also some larger cash gifts.[38] Such acts of private philanthropy were, as we have seen, part of a larger trend in Tokyo in this moment, as wealthy and middle-class people began using philanthropy as a source of social capital.

Japan's first public asylum had a capacity of one hundred, with thirty beds reserved for paying patients, who were charged seven sen per day. To encourage the admission of paying patients, the prefectural government actively sought to promote an awareness of the new institution, regularly publishing information about the application procedure in the newspapers.[39] Even so, most patients came from the city's poor and working-class residents and were admitted as charity patients through their local ward offices. Of thirty-eight applications for admission submitted to the prefectural government between July and December 1880, only three applicants indicated an ability to pay asylum fees themselves, while another four indicated the availability of support from landlords, neighbors, family, and acquaintances. The others, who listed occupations such as day laborer, rickshaw puller, and tofu peddler, described their financial situation as "without resources," "desperately poor," and "extremely poor."[40]

Class and the Care of the Mentally Ill

The prevalence of the poor within the asylum reflected the fact that wealthier city residents had alternatives to the new institution. In 1878, the TMP issued Police Ordinance no. 38, which authorized home confinement for "the care of the mentally ill and the admonishment of unruly young people." Addressed to ward and family heads, the ordinance outlined the procedure for "placing someone in a cage for discipline or treatment." The family head was to submit a detailed description of the circumstances that had prompted the application to the local police, including the names and seals of other family members in the case of a disobedient minor and a doctor's report in the case of a mentally ill person. The police were then to investigate to ensure that family members were acting in the best interest of the person to be confined. If the petition was approved, there were to be occasional checks on the conditions of confinement, and if the treatment was found to be overly harsh or cruel, the investigating officer was to report it for further investigation and action.[41]

The overlap with the Edo-era approach to *ranshinsha* is obvious. Targeting both the mentally ill and "unruly" youths, the decree was oriented toward maintaining social order, and as in the past, doctors played only a minor role in this procedure. However, important differences reflected both the state's sanction of the authority of the patriarchal family and the new power of the TMP. Under Police Ordinance no. 38, the care and control of the mental ill became one of a growing list of social responsibilities that family heads were required to assume, in their new role as a link between the state and civil society. This was in contrast to the Edo-era procedure, which required extensive community involvement in the form of five-person groups and machi officials. Now the decision to confine someone lay in the hands of the family head and the TMP.[42]

Confinement within the home thus required TMP involvement, but families with resources had another option. They could place their problematic parent, spouse, or child in one of the three private asylums that were in operation by 1879 (see plate 18). Initially, no regulations were in place to regulate involuntary admission to these institutions, meaning it was easier to commit someone to a private hospital than to confine them (legally) at home. Like most other private medical facilities established in the 1870s, the early private asylums were founded by physicians of Sino-Japanese medicine who had been trained in the pre-Meiji period. One of the private asylums was established by Narabayashi Genshun, the adopted son of Narabayashi Ittoku, who had established his "madness treatment center" three decades earlier. By the time of the fall of the shogunate, that facility had closed, but in 1878 Narabayashi Genshun applied for and received permission from the prefectural government to open a private asylum. He renamed his facility the Komatsugawa Asylum (*tenkyōin*).[43]

Unlike his competitors and most hospitals at the time, Narabayashi charged by the month rather than the day, suggesting that patients typically stayed for significant lengths of time. The asylum had forty rooms, with differing fees based on the quality of the room. In 1883 a superior room was 16 yen per month, while a standard room was 12 yen per month. These fees seem to have been more than the market would bear, and in the following years, they were reduced several times. In 1887 Narabayashi began charging by the day and the 25-sen daily fee made this the cheapest of the three private institutions then in existence: a thirty-day stay would have cost only 7.5 yen, less than half the cost of hospitalization four years before. Narabayashi worked hard to popularize his asylum, which initially struggled to find patients. He paid for newspaper ads, which included a promise of confidentiality, and for a time he partnered with a doctor in Honjo, who visited prospective patients in their homes and presumably facilitated their transfer to the asylum.[44] Still, patient numbers remained small, never rising above sixty patients per year for the first two decades of its existence, according to data in the *Tokyo Prefectural Statistical Handbook*.

A second private asylum, formally known as Katō Fūten Byōin, was more successful. Its founder Katō Teruaki (1822–1906) was born in a village in Echigo (now part of Niigata Prefecture) and received his medical education in Osaka and Kyoto. He moved to Tokyo in 1875 and established his asylum in Tamachi in Hongō. According to Katō, this endeavor was inspired by his sympathy for the mentally ill, "who had been ignored even as medicine had made great progress." Concerned about the plight of "these unfortunates," he vowed to help them to the best of his abilities.[45] In 1878, he moved his hospital to a new location, also in Tamachi, a quiet plot with fields on three sides. We get a glimpse into conditions at the Katō asylum in this period from a report written by

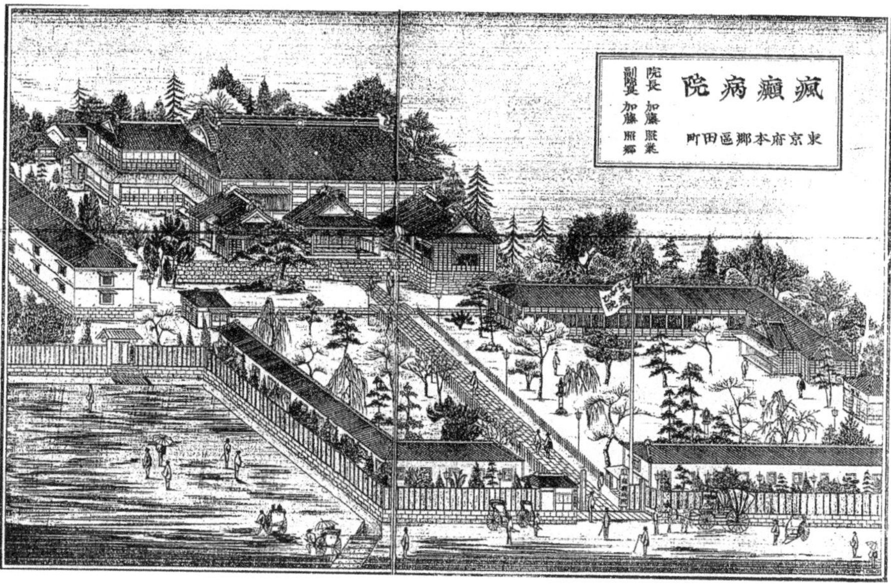

Figure 5.1. Katō Fūten Byōin. The text on the flag flying at the entrance reads "madman's hospital" (*kichigai byōin*). Arai Tōjirō, ed., *Tōkyō seikaku zuroku*, 7.

Sakaki Hajime, who would later become Japan's first professor of psychiatry. A recent graduate of the University of Tokyo Medical College, Sakaki had already been selected for a government scholarship to study psychiatry in Germany, one of many students in this era who was educated in Europe with the aim of introducing new forms of academic and technological expertise to Japan.[46]

Before his departure, Sakaki tried to familiarize himself with the state of psychiatric care in Japan and in 1882 he visited both Katō's hospital and the prefectural asylum. A few years later, while studying in Berlin, Sakaki published a report on asylums in Japan in a German medical journal. In describing Katō's asylum, Sakaki wrote that many of its patients were not suffering from serious mental illnesses. While some showed signs of what he described as "psychosis," many others appeared to be suffering from neuroses or neurological disease. Patients were treated by what Sakaki termed the "Chinese method," that is, herbal medicines, hot baths, and massage.[47]

Whether because of its familiar treatments, its location, or the fact that it was willing to take in even those with mild symptoms, Katō's asylum soon began to thrive. It was an impressive compound of Japanese-style buildings (see fig. 5.1). Like Narabayashi, Katō too advertised heavily in the city's newspaper, but he also worked to establish himself as a public figure. He put his philanthropy on display, offering to treat needy patients for free—a gesture that was duly reported in the newspaper, and this prompted an award for public service from the Tokyo governor.[48] These efforts seem to have paid off: by 1882, Katō's asylum was caring for almost 250 patients a year, although some of these were likely treated on an outpatient basis. In 1886 prefectural records began distinguishing between inpatient and outpatient care, revealing that while inpatient numbers at Katō's hospital hovered around 100 patients annually, the number of outpatients was typically about double that figure.[49] Clearly, many families were interested in treatment options that did not require confinement. Katō's hospital was successful even though its fees were high compared to both the other private asylums and the public option. Initially, Katō offered three levels of inpatient care, at 70, 15, and 40 sen per day. He soon reduced the options to two levels and lowered his fees to 60 and 45 sen per day, but he also began requiring a minimum two-week stay.[50]

The third private asylum was established in 1879 in what at the time was Kanasugi Village, although in 1889 the village would be incorporated into Shitaya Ward as Negishi-chō. Its founder was Watanabe Dōjun (1839–1900) who partnered with a successful tobacco merchant named Ishiba Bune'mon to establish the asylum.[51] Like the Komatsugawa Asylum, Watanabe's asylum struggled, treating only four patients in its first year, and although numbers gradually improved, they also fluctuated from year to year. This was despite its low fees: in 1882, the daily cost was 38 sen. In 1893, when patients numbered just five, Watanabe began advertising that his hospital specialized in surgical and internal medicine, in addition to psychiatric treatments, and this seemed to revive its fortunes, with more than six hundred outpatients treated in both 1894 and 1895.[52]

With the establishment of the private asylums, families could avoid placing their members in the Ueno asylum, where conditions were poor. Figure 5.2 reveals that at the public asylum patients were housed in multiple buildings that resembled the *nagaya* discussed in chapter 1, an arrangement that made both nursing and supervision difficult. To hinder their attempts to abscond, patients were issued deep blue cotton kimono modeled on those for prisoners but featuring the character *kyō* ("mad").[53] Initially, patient care was entrusted to seven or eight untrained men, who had been recruited from the residents of the Yōikuin, and they relied heavily on the use of constraints to control the patients.[54] In spite of such conditions, Kure Shūzō, considered by many to be the "father" of Japanese psychiatry, would later celebrate the temporary asylum as marking the beginning of the medical treatment of the mentally ill.[55]

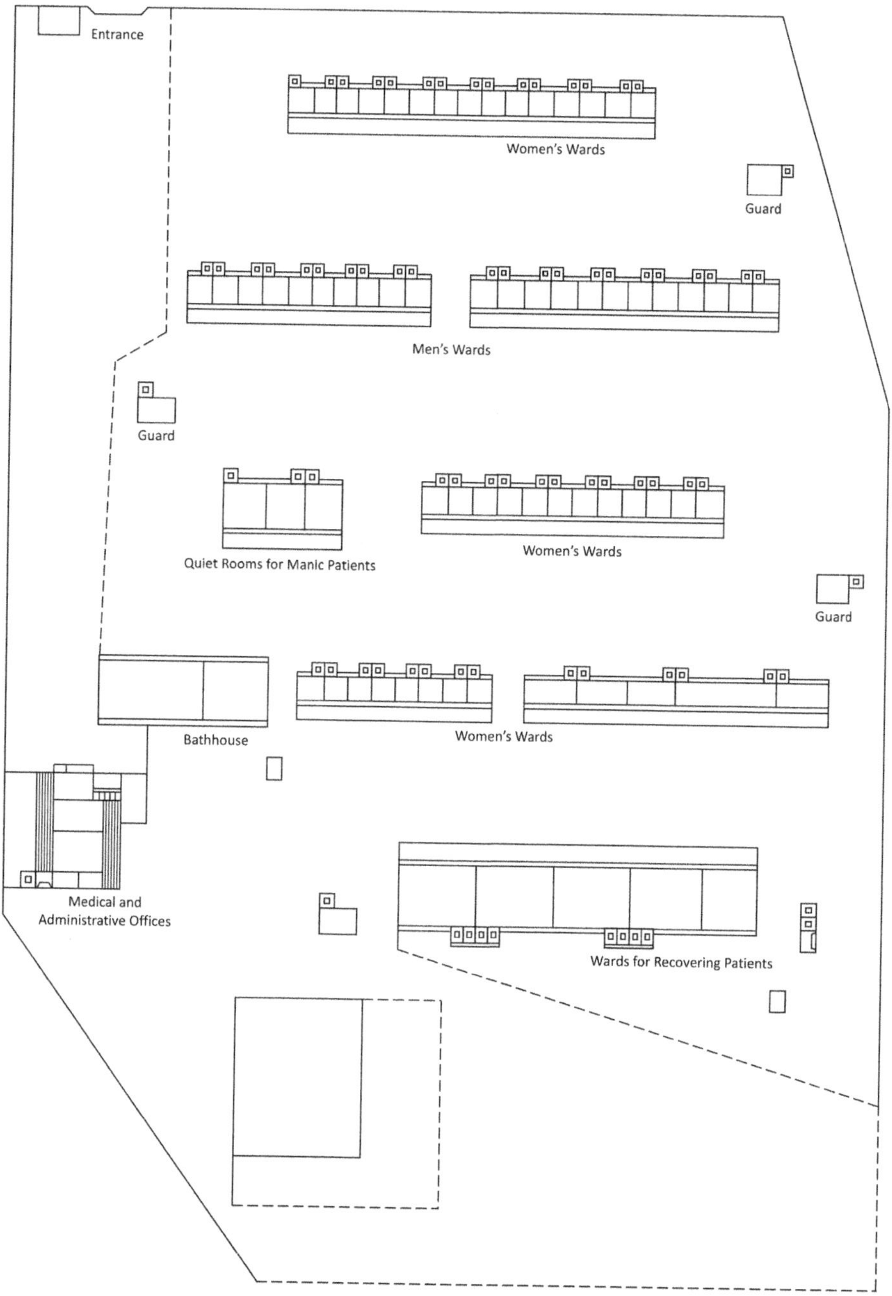

Figure 5.2. The Provisional Prefectural Asylum ca. 1879. Image by Hannah Tomio, based on Kure and Kushida, *Waga kuni ni okeru seishinbyō*, 176.

While this exaggerates the quality of care on offer, it was true that physicians had a role in the new institution. Hasegawa Tai, the director of the prefectural hospital, was appointed director of the asylum, and administratively the asylum was now a part of the prefectural hospital. As a result of this arrangement, physicians employed by the hospital assumed responsibility for the care of asylum patients as well.

In 1881 Hasegawa was replaced as director by Nakai Tsunejirō (1851–1914), then a doctor on the staff of the prefectural hospital. Like many other physicians of his generation, Nakai had been educated initially in a private Dutch learning academy, but in 1869 he left his home in Satsuma and journeyed to Tokyo to study at the government's medical school. In 1873, he was hired by the prefectural hospital, where he was involved in the founding of the prefectural midwifery school. He passed the licensing exam in 1876, and when cholera struck Tokyo in 1877, the prefectural hospital sent him around Tokyo to lecture ordinary doctors about how to treat the disease.[56]

The case notes compiled by Nakai and his staff on 130 patients offer a window into the patients and care within the early asylum. Patients were categorized using a rudimentary set of diagnostic terms that included "mania" (*kyōken*), "melancholia" (*utsukyō*), "manic-depression" (*sōutsu*), "idiocy" (*chisei*), "obsessive tendencies" (*hensei*), "tendency toward rage" (*kyōhakusei*), and "seizures" (*tankan*). As these terms suggest, the concept of "madness" in this period, even among elite physicians, included personality traits, symptoms of neurological disease, and intellectual disabilities as well as signs of mental illness. However, as might be expected given the concerns about social order that gave rise to the asylum, the most common diagnosis (for 40 percent of patients) was mania, with only 10 percent of patients given a diagnosis of depression. In addition, most patients were male (70 percent) and between the ages of twenty-five and forty-four (60 percent).[57]

The prefectural hospital's doctors experimented with a variety of treatments, including hydrotherapy (or hydropathy, as it was then known) and electrotherapy, both of which were also in use in European asylums at the time.[58] Hydrotherapy, essentially warm water baths, was used primarily to calm patients with mania, while electrotherapy—which involved placing electrodes on the body, sometimes the head, to shock the patient with electricity—was typically used on those suffering from melancholia to "stimulate" them.[59] Doctors also relied on a variety of sedatives to calm patients. These included potassium bromide (widely used as a sedative and anticonvulsant in the nineteenth century) and chloralum hydratum (a homeopathic medicine for sedation), as well as some herbal compounds based on traditional Sino-Japanese pharmacology.[60] Many patients stayed for a relatively short time, with 57 percent released within four months. However, many patients never left the asylum: 61 of the 130 patients whose cases were documented died while in confinement, a shockingly high figure given the youth of those confined, and evidence perhaps of poor conditions and lack of basic care.[61]

Medicalizing the Prefectural Asylum

The use of the Ueno site had always been intended as a temporary solution. Not only were the facilities too small for the growing number of patients but the Ministry of Education was pressing for the return of the Ueno property. After the establishment of Ueno Park, the area was gradually transformed into a cultural center, home to imperial displays of power, expositions, the first national museum, and a zoo.[62] The proximity of growing numbers of visitors to the asylum made Tokyo officials uneasy, so it was decided to move it to a new location. Various sites were considered, including, for reasons that are unclear, Yonbanchō in Kōjimachi, near the outer moat of the Imperial Place and adjacent to the Yasukuni Shrine.[63]

In the end, a large plot of land was purchased in Mukōgaoka-chō in Hongō. The site for the new asylum, ten hectares in area, was acquired from the Ministry of Education, and it had a number of attractive features (see plate 19). It was initially surrounded by undeveloped land, creating a buffer between the institution and residences and businesses, and it was within walking distance of the University of Tokyo Medical School and its affiliated hospital, a proximity that would soon become important. The new asylum had capacity for 150 patients, 50 of whom were to be paying patients, who would be charged 30 sen per day. This meant that the public asylum was only slightly less expensive than two of the private asylums at this time and about half the cost of the Katō Asylum.

With the new and improved facilities in place, the asylum gradually evolved from an institution primarily concerned with social control to a medical facility. This process began under Nakai Tsunejirō, who implemented changes to improve the level of care: he hired four staff doctors, two pharmacists, and increased the nursing staff to more than twenty. The latter included the first female nurses on staff at the asylum, and they were made responsible for the care of female patients.[64] Writing in the German medical journal, Sakaki Hajime described the public asylum in glowing terms. He noted its location in one of the "the better, healthy, and quiet" areas of the city, and the housing of

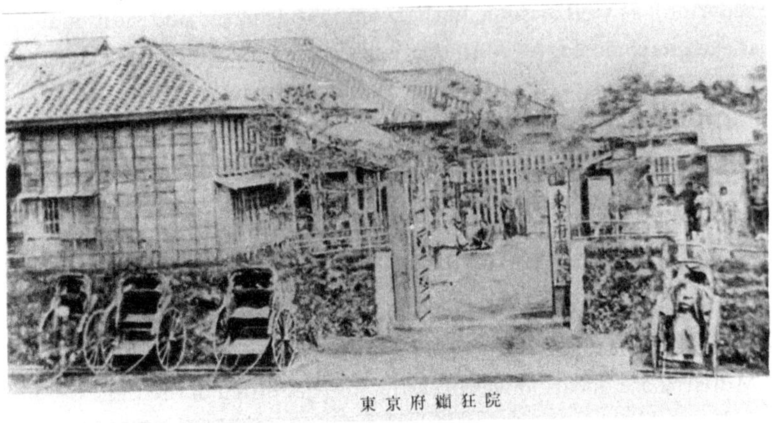

Figure 5.3. The Tokyo Prefectural Asylum in Hongō, ca. 1880s. Postcard from the author's collection.

its patients in one-story wooden pavilions, "like Japanese houses," that were joined by walkways. It even featured a large garden where patients could exercise (see fig. 5.3). According to Sakaki, patients were placed in wards based on their sex and the severity of their symptoms, and restraints were only used in the rooms housing those who were "agitated and unclean," although for security purposes, all the windows were fitted with iron bars and the institution was surrounded by a fence.[65] Sakaki's positive description of the new facilities was supported by other evidence that conditions had improved significantly. Mortality rates fell by 50 percent compared to the Ueno facility, and the number of patients released as "fully recovered" grew significantly.[66]

The use of the asylum for clinical training and research on mental illness also began in this period, and this was probably one reason for the relocation near the University of Tokyo. In 1882 Erwin Bälz, a German physician who taught at the medical school from 1876, began lecturing on psychiatry, referencing primarily Wilhelm Griesinger's textbook *The Pathology and Therapy of Mental Illness* (1861), arguably the most influential work on psychiatry until the 1890s.[67] In addition to his lectures, Bälz attempted to give his students clinical experience and instituted the practice of having medical students examine the patients at the asylum, albeit occasionally. But as was the case with the university's hospital, use of the asylum as a teaching facility had a darker side. Unless a family was present to object, charity patients who died in the institution were routinely subjected to dissection, an important tool considering the "brain disease" model of mental illness that prevailed at the time.[68]

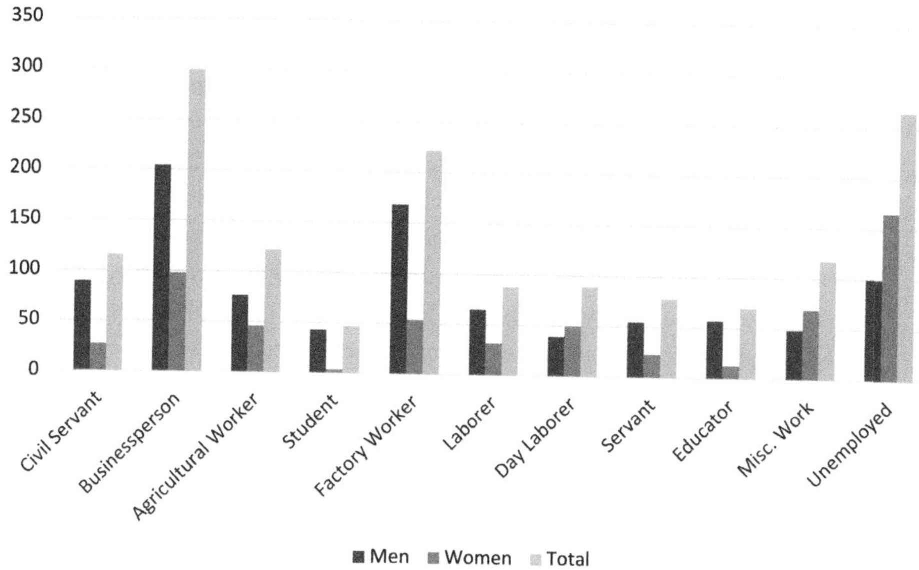

Figure 5.4. The occupation of patients in the Tokyo Prefectural Asylum, 1879–1887. Data from Sakaki, "Tōkyō-fu Tenkyōin no kanja . . . ," 1–7.

In 1886 Sakaki Hajime returned to Tokyo after three years at the University of Berlin, a well-established center of psychiatric research. He had attended lectures by Griesinger's successors, Carl Westphal and Emanuel Mendel, who both practiced at the nexus of neurology and psychiatry, and he undertook a study tour of asylums, visiting institutions in Germany, Switzerland, and Austria.[69] Sakaki never worked at the asylum while it was in Hongō, but he would later review more than 1,500 patient records and publish a series of articles in which he examined the patients' backgrounds and the potential causes of their conditions.[70] His work revealed the evolving nature of both the patient population and psychiatric practice. Sakaki's analysis reveals that young male patients continued to predominate within the patient population, but they were not necessarily poor or socially isolated. Most were married, and they came from a variety of occupations, many from business, the civil service, and factory work (see fig. 5.4).

While this may simply have indicated the embrace of the asylum by a wider swath of Tokyo residents, Sakaki made a bigger claim. He argued that personal and social-economic stresses played an important role in the development of mental illness among the patients. He classified mental illness as the result of either "tangible causes" (*yūkeiin*) or "intangible causes" (*muyūkeiin*). Tangible causes included overindulgence in alcohol, sex, or masturbation, head injury, gynecological disease, syphilis, febrile disease, seizures, and two catchall categories, "various brain diseases" and "physical changes." In contrast, Sakaki used "intangible causes" to refer to stressful or traumatic personal or social circumstances: household finances, educational or business difficulties, religious or political concerns, anxiety and heartache, psychological upset, and terror and shock. Sakaki offered no explanation for these two categories, nor did he clarify what he meant by phrases such as "anxiety and heartache, "psychological upset," and "physical changes." But whatever the weaknesses of his research apparatus, his conclusion challenged the well-established stereotype of the impoverished and homeless "wandering madman." According to Sakaki, the onset of mental illness in most patients (72 percent) was attributable to "intangible causes," such as "anxiety and heartache," household finances, and educational and business difficulties.

Sakaki's research on the asylum's population supported a growing belief that modern life, specifically urban life, was having a deleterious effect on both the physical and mental health of the Japanese people. In an 1892 essay advocating for the establishment of more asylums, Sakaki made this assessment explicit, writing, "As culture advances, it is unavoidable that the number of mentally ill people will increase."[71] This concern was, to be sure, not original to Sakaki. Many in Europe and the US in the nineteenth century also felt that urban environments were detrimental to both physical and mental health, and the earliest psychiatric texts translated into Japanese had made this point. According to *Seishinbyō yakusetsu* (On Mental Illness, 1872), the translation of a work by the British psychiatrist Henry Maudsley, "Insanity is a penalty which our present civilization necessarily pays" because of "the feverish activity of life, the numerous passions and the great strain of mental work incident to the multiplied industry and eager competition of an active civilization."[72] Another early translation of a psychiatric text, a work of the German psychiatrist Heinrich Schüle, made a similar claim about the conditions of modern life: "The progress of society's enlightenment encourages contact between people and the result is noise and activity, and people pursue lives that are fast-paced and full of change, and these conditions encourage the development of mental illness. Especially in the great cities, the majority of inhabitants live in crowded conditions and therefore their bodies are not sufficiently exerted, and this makes them susceptible to glandular diseases and lung disease, and so their bodies grow weak, and this encourages the development of a predisposition to mental illness."[73]

By the 1890s, Japan's first generation of psychiatrists agreed that the mental health of urban residents was under assault. Three years after Sakaki made his observation, his student and successor Kure Shūzō described "civilization" as one of the general causes of mental illness and claimed that this was proved by statistical data from "all countries." On urban life, he wrote, "As the population of the cities increases, hygiene and morality are impaired. . . . As the competition for survival grows more intense, it is easy for people to become overstimulated and as a result the brain and nerves become subject to delusions and pathological changes."[74] Modern life then—the very modernity that the state was pursuing—was now viewed as the source of mental illness, with higher education, factory work, and even riding in trains and streetcars blamed for rising numbers of cases of depression and other disorders.

From the Prefectural Asylum to Sugamo Hospital

Although the facilities in Hongō had been purpose built to house the asylum, in June 1886, after only five years in that location, the asylum was moved to a new site in Sugamo Kagomachi-chō in neighboring Koishikawa Ward. It would remain here until 1919, when the growth of the city forced another move, this time to Matsuzawa Village in Ebara District (now Setagaya Ward), where it remains today. According to Kure Shūzō, the move to Koishikawa was necessitated by the proximity of the Hongō asylum to the Yayoi Shrine, and this was also the explanation publicized in the newspapers at the time.[75] The shrine, which fell under the jurisdiction of the Imperial Household Agency, was founded in 1885 to honor the spirits of fallen firefighters and police officers, and its grounds housed a shooting range. The noise of the gunfire was said to be a source of distress to the asylum patients, and this necessitated the relocation of the facility to another site.

This explanation is not entirely satisfactory since the shrine itself would be relocated to Shiba just a year later. A more likely reason for the asylum's relocation was that the University of Tokyo was expanding, and the asylum occupied what had become prime real estate within the most important educational zone in the city. In fact, the site of the former asylum soon became home to the elite First Higher School, a preparatory school for the university established in 1886. As noted in chapter 4, the emergence of Hongō as a center of elite higher education also propelled the relocation of the Nezu brothel quarter to Fukagawa.

The asylum's relocation reveals again the prefecture's ongoing need to negotiate the priorities of the national government, but the site for the hospital in Koishikawa, on the border between the city ward and neighboring Kita-Toshima District, was well chosen, especially given growing concerns about the effects of modern urban life on Tokyo's residents. Contemporary maps reveal that at the time of its founding, the hospital was surrounded by fields in a quiet part of the growing city. At this time, Koishikawa had the lowest population density of all the wards and the greatest number of households involved in agriculture.[76] The ward then offered relatively cheap land, and few neighbors who could have protested the presence of the institution.

In addition, Koishikawa was home to several national and prefectural institutions, and their number was increasing. In 1886, the year the new asylum was established, Koishikawa already housed an army hospital and an army veterinary hospital, as well as an army artillery depot. Sugamo Prison was established in Sugamo Village just outside the ward in 1895, and the Yōikuin, which by this time was devoted to housing orphaned children, was relocated here in 1896. Additionally, Komagome Hospital, a prefectural hospital dedicated to infectious diseases, was established in 1897 quite close to the asylum in neighboring Komagome Dōaka-chō in Hongō. The cluster of these institutions, which housed populations regarded as problematic, on the margins of the city reflects a logic like the one that prompted the relocation of the Nezu brothel district to Fukagawa. That is, it was designed to protect the central area of the city from those who were poor, sick, criminal, and mentally ill.

The new asylum was initially constructed as four pavilions surrounding a central courtyard with the buildings joined by covered walkways. As the patient population grew over the years, more wings were added, and so were amenities such as a patient library and recreation rooms (see fig. 5.5). When Frederick Peterson, a professor of psychiatry at Columbia University and chairman of the New York State Commission in Lunacy, visited the asylum in 1911, he found much to admire in its facilities. Peterson described the asylum as "a series of one-storied pavilions scattered in a considerable park" with buildings that were "airy, neat, and clean." While some patient rooms had beds, Peterson observed that "for the most part the furnishing is Japanese." In addition, by this time, the institution was fully electrified and equipped with modern plumbing. Peterson noted that patients bathed daily, and the hospital continued to use hydrotherapy as a primary mode of treatment.[77]

In March 1887 Sakaki Hajime was appointed professor of psychiatry at what was the University of Tokyo and medical director of the asylum, replacing Nakai Tsunejirō. This resulted in a curious bureaucratic arrangement: although the asylum continued to be funded by the prefectural government,

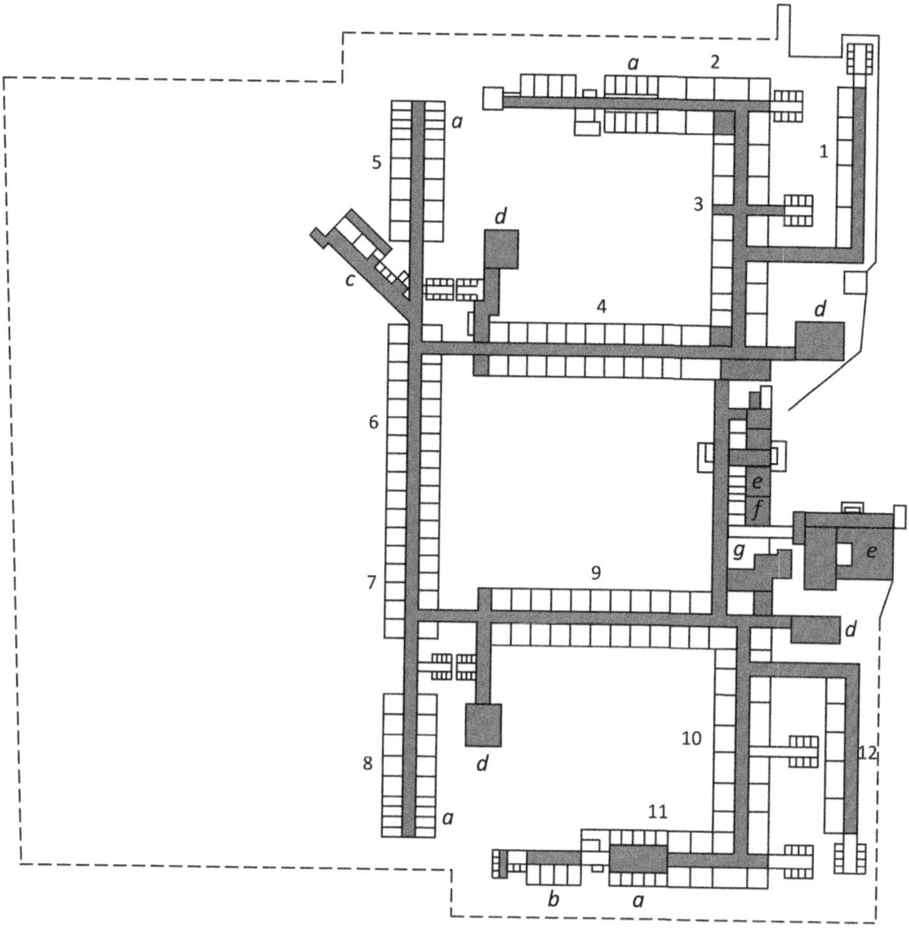

Figure 5.5. Sugamo Hospital, ca. 1897. Buildings numbered 1–12 were patient wards. Other facilities included (a) isolation room, (b) infectious disease unit, (c) Sōma Tomotane's former quarters, (d) bathhouses, (e) administrative office, (f) medical staff office, (g) pharmacy, and (h) medical director's office. Image by Hannah Tomio, based on Kure and Kashida, *Waga kuni ni okeru seishinbyō*, 1.

it was placed under the direct administrative control of the national university through its representative, Sakaki. The aim was to facilitate the clinical training of psychiatric professionals by normalizing Bälz's practice of using the asylum for occasional medical training and research. One of Griesinger's innovations in Berlin had been to transform the public psychiatric ward from a warehouse into a site of teaching and research, and Sakaki quickly set out to make the prefectural asylum function in the same way.

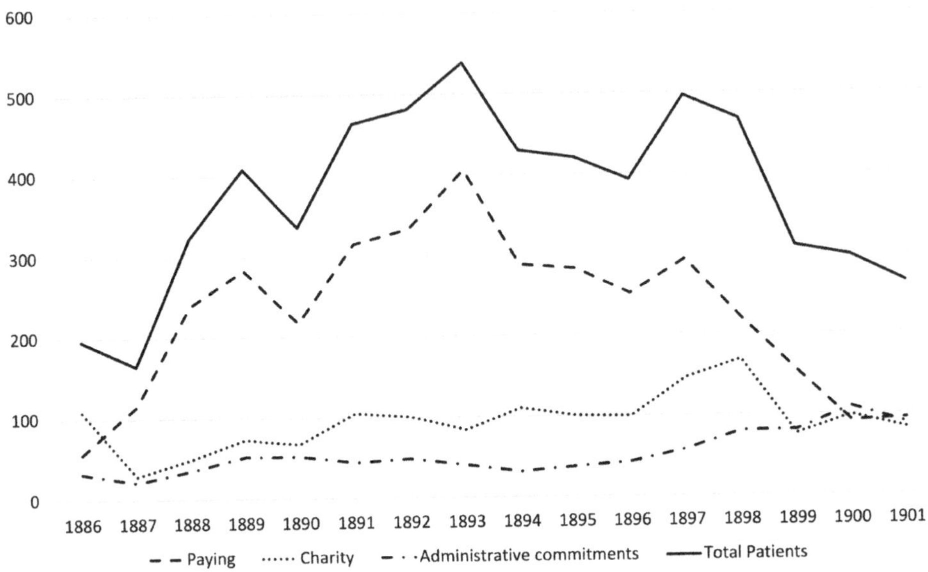

Figure 5.6. Patient numbers and categories within the prefectural asylum, 1885–1901. Data from Kure, "Meiji 12-nen naishi 34-nen Tōkyō-fu Sugamo Byōin iji hōkoku," 1086–87.

In May 1886, he began conducting clinical lectures in the asylum and integrating his students into the diagnosis and treatment of those confined there.[78] He required students and staff to compile voluminous case notes on each patient, which included discussions of potential hereditary factors, other health concerns, and social and familial factors. Some of these case notes were edited and published in the *Journal of the Tokyo Medical Society* (*Tōkyō igakkai zasshi*) and other medical journals. We know about the case of Matsumura Hatsu, with which I began this chapter, because she was the subject of one of these published studies. By 1889, the institution had been thoroughly medicalized, and it was renamed Sugamo Hospital.

The affiliation with the medical school improved staffing by incorporating faculty and students into patient care, but Sakaki also implemented reforms designed to improve conditions in the asylum. He restricted the use of shackles and other restraints, provided art supplies and musical instruments to patients, and allowed them access to the asylum grounds for recreation and exercise.[79] As conditions improved in the asylum, the makeup of the patient population began evolving. Figure 5.6 shows that paying patients became the majority, comprising more than 60 percent of total patients between 1886 and 1901, although that proportion declined around the turn of the century as more private psychiatric hospitals were established. In this period, the hospital charged thirty-five sen per day for a second-class room and seventy-five sen for a first-class room, making it affordable, if barely, for Tokyo's middle class in this era when a junior-level civil servant made about fifty yen a month.[80]

Charity patients made up the second largest category of patients. This group consisted of people who entered the asylum on a voluntary basis, although they lacked the means to pay for their care. In a third category were so-called *itaku kanja*, patients who were committed at the request of ward officials or the police because they were presumed to be a danger to themselves and others. The case reports published by Sakaki and his students offer a window into how these patients came to be involuntarily committed. Like Hatsu, many were picked up on the streets, homeless, and seemingly in a delusional state, but others were sent to the asylum after committing an act of violence while in a state of apparent mental illness. One such patient was an impoverished rickshaw puller who attacked his wife and child in what was described as a fit of despair over their financial situation. His family survived and after the man had spent months in the asylum, he was released as cured.[81] Not every violent act that led to confinement was so serious: a thirty-one-year-old former geisha named Yone was confined after she attacked a stranger on the street whom she believed had mocked her as a madwoman.[82] Other patients were admitted due to chronic alcoholism, and a few after failed suicide attempts.[83] We know far less about the circumstances that brought paying patients to the asylum. They do not appear in published patient records, since status as a paying patient brought a measure of privacy denied to poor patients.

The Sōma Incident

As the use of committed and charity patients for teaching and research purposes suggests, there was little regard in this period for what would later be termed "patients' rights," especially when the patient was both poor and mentally ill, and this lack of concern extended to the process of asylum admission. Writing in 1912, Frederick Peterson noted that "the method of commitment is very simple. . . . When a case of insanity develops, a member of the family reports it to the police. A doctor then goes to the house with the police officer to examine the patient and reports his findings to the head of the police who issues an order of commitment."[84] In the 1880s and early 1890s, the process for admission was even "simpler," to borrow Peterson's language: with little regulation or oversight, families, the police, and ward officials were able to compel the confinement of vulnerable people.

This changed when the plight of Sōma Tomotane, arguably the most famous person with mental illness of the Meiji era, became public and made involuntary confinement an issue of public debate for the first time. Sōma Tomotane was born in 1852, the son of Sōma Michitane, the lord of Nakamura Domain (now part of Fukushima Prefecture) and a concubine. After the Meiji Restoration, Michitane and Tomotane, like other former daimyo and their heirs, were required to reside in Tokyo. Tomotane attended Fukuzawa Yukichi's Keiō Gijuku (now Keiō University) and later married the daughter of another former daimyo. All seemed well until 1876 when Tomotane began having violent angry outbursts, prompting his family to ask Totsuka Bunkai, the surgeon-general of the navy, to examine him. Totsuka concluded that Tomotane was "mentally ill" (*seishinbyō nari*) and in addition to prescribing medicines, suggested that travel, exercise, and a change of climate might help.[85] According to Tomotane's family, despite their best efforts, his condition continued to decline, until one day in 1879 he attacked a family retainer with a knife, severely wounding him. Fearing further violence, his family decided to confine him within their home.

Things might have ended there, with Tomotane privately confined, but for the intervention of Nishigori Takekiyo, a low-ranking former vassal of the Sōma. In the early 1880s Nishigori apparently heard rumors of Tomotane's confinement, and this prompted him to go to the Sōma mansion in Kōjimachi where he demanded to speak with Tomotane. When he was rebuffed, Nishigori declared to other former Sōma vassals that Tomotane was not mentally ill.[86] In 1883 he made his way to the Tokyo Minor Crimes Court and lodged a complaint that Tomotane was being unlawfully confined.

Nishigori had had no contact with Tomotane at the time when he made his charges and thus had no way of knowing anything about his mental state, and both his contemporaries and later scholars have puzzled over his motives, wondering whether he was sincerely concerned, delusional himself, or a fraudster seeking financial gain. Whatever Nishigori's motives, the Tokyo Minor Crimes Court took his report of unlawful confinement seriously and launched an investigation, which soon exposed several irregularities. Rather than going through ward officials and the police as required by Police Ordinance no. 38, the family petitioned the Imperial Household Agency for permission to confine Tomotane, and it granted permission without consulting the TMP. In response to Tomotane's case, over the course of 1884, Ordinance no. 38 was revised. It was newly required that an application for confinement be supported by at least two family members and include a doctor's report, rules that were also applied to admission to a private psychiatric hospital.[87]

Seven months later, the TMP issued "Instructions for the Treatment of the Insane" (*Fūtennin toriatsukai kokoroe*), which further revised the requirements for involuntary confinement. According to a new procedure, when a local police station received an application for confinement, its officers were to work in tandem with a doctor to investigate by visiting the home. If confinement was approved, both the prefecture and the TMP were to be notified. In addition, after this approval, the police were to visit the home or hospital once a month to ensure that the patient was being treated appropriately. The treatment of the "wandering mad" was also addressed. When people believed to have a mental illness were taken into police custody, they were immediately to be sent to the prefectural asylum for evaluation. The local police station was to inform the prefectural authorities and the central TMP bureau and work to identify the patient's household head and ward head. In addition, private asylums were prohibited from admitting patients on an involuntary basis unless their families had followed the procedure outlined in the "Instructions for the Treatment of the Insane."[88]

The Sōma family attempted to follow the revised regulations. They submitted a new application to the Kōjimachi Police Station for Tomotane to be confined. Attached to the application was a statement of diagnosis signed by Iwasa Jun, the personal physician of the Meiji emperor, which confirmed that Tomotane was insane.[89] This document would later prove an embarrassment to all concerned when it was revealed that Iwasa had never actually examined Tomotane. Instead, he had sent a young aide in his place and in return for his services Iwasa had received a very generous gift of one thousand yen.[90] The doctor's involvement thus revealed the weakness of the revised ordinance, which allowed families to shop for a physician who, for a price, would produce the requisite certification that confinement was appropriate.

Even before the news of Iwasa's "blind diagnosis" became public, the police had decided to investigate the case and dispatched a delegation to the Sōma home that included additional medical luminaries of the time, Hasegawa Tai and Nakai Tsunejirō. To the undoubted dismay of Tomotane's family, they concluded that Tomotane was mentally ill, but not so severely as to require home confinement. Tomotane was then briefly placed in the Katō Asylum, but once Nishigori learned of Tomotane's location, he began a campaign of harassment, prompting Dr. Katō to discharge Tomotane and send him back to his family.

They then decided to move him to the prefectural asylum, where special quarters were hastily constructed.[91] There, a second team of elite doctors, including Julius Scriba, a German physician, and Miyake Hayari, one of the first neurosurgeons in Japan, both of whom were faculty members at the University of Tokyo Medical School, examined Tomotane over a four-month period. Their report confirmed the diagnosis of insanity. In response, in January 1887 Nishigori and several compatriots broke into the prefectural asylum and abducted Tomotane. Although he was quickly found and Nishigori was criminally charged with unlawful entry, what the media now dubbed "the Sōma Incident" continued to unfold. Tomotane was moved to the university hospital, where he was examined by a third group of doctors, including Erwin Bälz, and Sakaki Hajime, who had just returned from Germany. They too concluded he was mentally ill, but rather than confinement, they outlined a plan for treatment that included access to books, exercise, and a diet of nutritious food, and the use of medications to keep him calm. Under their care Tomotane lived quietly and apparently more or less happily for five years until he died suddenly at the age of thirty-nine.

This unexpected event ushered in the most frenzied moment of the Sōma saga. Nishigori now claimed that Nakai, Miyake, and Sakaki had conspired with the family to murder Tomotane with poison. After months of relentless media speculation about Tomotane's death, the TMP arrested Nakai, Sakaki, and several members of the Sōma household in August 1893. Tomotane's body was disinterred the following month, but when an autopsy revealed no evidence of poison, the charges against the doctors were dismissed. Nishigori was subsequently convicted of making a false police report and sentenced to four years in prison.

The sensational and lurid claims that propelled the Sōma Incident and the involvement of many members of Tokyo's elite fascinated the public but the resulting reportage in the form of newspaper articles, books, and trial transcripts shined a harsh light on Tokyo's psychiatric institutions and professionals. The debates over Tomotane's diagnosis and the question of whether confinement was justified, the dubious ethics of elite doctors, the poor security at the prefectural asylum, and the lax rules regulating home confinement seemed to erode confidence psychiatric institutions. In the aftermath, the number of paying patients at Sugamo Hospital decreased sharply, although involuntary commitments rose. At the same time, the scandal eventually led to the establishment of new private psychiatric hospitals, presumably to capitalize on the declining reputation of the public asylum.

The controversies surrounding Sōma Tomotane's death prompted new regulation. In 1894 the TMP issued a new ordinance called "Instructions for the Treatment of the Mentally Ill" (*Seishin byōsha toriatsukai kokoroe*). The title of the law signaled the adoption of a new normative vocabulary: terms such as "the mad" and "the insane" were replaced by references to "mentally ill people," and the term "asylum" was abandoned in favor of "psychiatric hospital," "brain hospital," or simply "hospital." But more significantly, the TMP seized this moment when medical knowledge and ethics were under scrutiny to strengthen their authority over the confinement of mentally ill people. The first article of the 1894 ordinance required those who wanted to confine someone either at home or in a public or private hospital make an application for permission to the police and authorized the police together with a police doctor (*keisatsu'i*) to carry out a "detailed examination" of the patient and decide whether commitment was warranted. The police were also authorized to visit the patient, whether at home or in a hospital, at any time. Finally, in the cases of those who appeared to be violent, the police physician could unilaterally order confinement to the Sugamo Hospital, even if the patient or his family objected.[92]

Tokyo, as we noted in chapter 2, was intended to be a testing ground for medical policies, and in this case it was. The TMP ordinance became the model for a new national law in 1900— the "Law for the Protective Confinement of the Mentally Ill" (*Seishin byōsha kango hō*). Home Ministry bureaucrats initially drafted the law in 1898 with input from members of the Central Sanitary Committee (*Chūō Eiseikai*), a parastatal organization founded in 1880 as cholera raged in Japan. Consisting of prominent physicians and officials, it was founded to advise the Hygiene Bureau about policy, but notably none of its members had psychiatric training.

According to the new procedure defined by the 1900 law, when someone applied to confine a family member, local authorities were to investigate the patient's circumstances and could appoint a doctor of their choice "if necessary" to examine the person. If permission for home confinement was denied, the guardian of the mentally ill person was then prohibited both from attempting to transfer the patient to a psychiatric hospital and from reapplying for permission for a period of three years. The law also included a lengthy list of punishments for those who did not follow its provisions, including public officials, physicians, and family members. The law's most striking feature was that it included no requirement for treatment or even medical oversight if confinement was approved.[93]

In the following decades, this law and its exclusion of medical authority in favor of that of the police would be harshly attacked by Japanese psychiatrists, with Kure taking the lead.[94] He devoted considerable energy to exposing the terrible conditions endured by many of those in home confinement. He also denounced the 1900 law, writing, "For the tens of thousands of mentally ill in our country, their misfortune is not only to have fallen victim to this disease; they have had the additional misfortune to have been born in this country."[95] Home confinement became the default option for many families, in part because there was simply no alternative. In areas outside of Tokyo, Osaka, and Kyoto, psychiatric beds did not exist or were few in number. Some have argued that the intent of the law was in fact to relieve the public sector of the necessity to construct psychiatric hospitals by making home confinement easy and affordable.[96] Certainly, the construction of psychiatric hospitals proceeded slowly, and it was not until 1937 that the number of people in psychiatric institutions surpassed the number of those in home confinement for the country as a whole.[97]

Private Psychiatric Hospitals and Economies of Care in Tokyo

In Tokyo, the situation was different. Between 1889 and 1913, thirteen private psychiatric hospitals were established within and just outside the city.[98] These were in addition to two of the three private asylums founded in the 1870s, excluding Kātō Hospital, which had closed in 1898.[99] Writing in 1908, the journalist Nagao Setsuzō noted that these hospitals attracted patients beyond Tokyo. In major train stations, one often encountered people who had come to the capital from the countryside, escorting their "mad" son or daughter, husband or wife, intending to install them in one of the city's psychiatric hospitals. They were met, he noted, by agents employed by the hospitals, which were competing for this valuable new commodity.[100]

Plate 20 shows the distribution of the hospitals circa 1912. Unlike in the 1870s, when hospitals established outside the city struggled to attract patients, in this era most hospitals were located on the periphery of the city, with six located outside the city's wards in what, at least administratively, were still considered villages. As the map shown in plate 20 reveals, the most popular location for psychiatric facilities was in the general area of Sugamo Hospital—that is, in the northeast corner of Koishikawa Ward and in neighboring Kita-Toshima District. Eight of the thirteen private hospitals were located within three kilometers of the public institution. This spatial order reflected a variety of factors including the availability of cheap land, the growing concern about the impact of the urban environment on mental health, the development of the city's transportation network, as well as concerns that the mentally ill posed a danger to the city and its residents. During this period, a series of fires broke out in psychiatric hospitals in Tokyo and elsewhere, reinforcing the long-standing perception that the mentally ill had a proclivity for arson. Katō Hospital was closed after a fire killed six patients, and the prefectural hospital also suffered fire damage in 1889.[101] The involvement of patients in these events was disputed, but this went unacknowledged in much of the reportage at the time.

But important too in creating this cluster of institutions was the symbiotic relationship that emerged between the prefectural institution and private psychiatric hospital. The proprietors of the private facilities recruited physicians from among the students and staff of Sugamo Hospital, and the hospitals absorbed patients who could not be housed in the public institution, either because of lack of beds or because they did not meet the requirement that patients be residents of Tokyo Prefecture. Sugamo Hospital was notorious for the poor salaries it offered junior doctors (reportedly just twenty-six yen a month), making additional part-time work necessary and often prompting employees to leave the public institution when more lucrative jobs in private hospitals were available. Administrative staff were also poorly paid, which led some, it was rumored, to accept bribes to refer potential patients to private hospitals.[102]

The Tokyo Brain Hospital (Tōkyō Nōbyōin) is an example of the complicated relationship that tied the private institutions to Sugamo Hospital. It was founded in 1898 in Tabata in Kita-Toshima, an emerging suburb well-known for its tranquility and fine scenery, conditions that attracted many literary figures and artists. The hospital itself was established by a group of investors, which was typical of the new psychiatric hospitals. They hired Gotō Shōgo to be its medical director. A graduate of the University of Tokyo Medical School, Gotō had worked as a staff doctor at Sugamo Hospital for some years, but he left when the private hospital offered him the very generous salary of 250 yen a month.[103] According to one contemporary report, the architecture of the Tokyo Brain Hospital was modeled after Sugamo Hospital, and the owners even erected a sign near the latter institution offering to provide "guidance about psychiatric hospitals" (*seishin byōin annai*) in order to direct patients to its doors. It quickly became the hospital of choice for those who could afford its high fees.[104]

The situation was similar at Tokyo Psychiatric Hospital, which was established in 1901 in Kōshinzuka in Kita-Toshima by Machida Yasumichi, a former prefectural official, and Nonaka Gibei, a Nihonbashi businessman. In 1907 it was renamed the Rest Home (Hoyōjo), a term that had gained favor as a euphemism for psychiatric care facilities, especially those catering to the wealthy. Its medical staff would eventually include Kadowaki Masae and Ishikawa Teikichi, both of whom were formerly employed by Sugamo Hospital.[105] Another institution that eschewed the use of terms such as "psychiatric hospital" and "brain hospital" was the Otowa Yōjōen ("rest garden"). It was established by none other than Kure Shūzō, the director of Sugamo Hospital. Kure lived in Otowa-chō in Koishikawa Ward, about four kilometers from his workplace, and in 1908 he founded a private hospital that offered "family-style care" to about fifty patients near his home. Kure's frustration with the lack of psychiatric beds in Japan and the poor quality of care offered by home confinement prompted his interest in alternative models of care. His patients apparently had relatively mild symptoms, and the atmosphere in the rest home was described as "open" compared to other hospitals of the day.[106]

Initially, there were some outliers to the pattern of establishing hospitals near Sugamo Hospital or on the periphery of the cityscape. Kanda was, of course, a popular site for hospitals generally, but the psychiatric hospitals established here did not endure for long. The Imperial Brain Hospital (Teikoku Nōbyōin) established in 1903, is a case in point. Its founder, Saitō Kiichi began his medical training in a prefectural medical school and then came to Tokyo to study at Saisei Gakusha. After he passed the licensing exam, Saitō quickly proved to be a successful medical entrepreneur, first opening a clinic in Asakusa and later a hospital in Kanda, both of which prospered. In 1900 he departed for Germany to study psychiatric medicine, one of the growing numbers of privately funded medical students and doctors who went abroad. Upon his return in 1903, he rebranded his Kanda hospital as the Imperial Brain Hospital, and he opened another psychiatric hospital in the far quieter area of Akasaka. As figure 2.2 (in chapter 2) indicated, as late as 1920, Akasaka was one of the least populated wards in the city. In 1907 Saitō moved the Imperial Brain Hospital to the grounds of the Akasaka hospital, presumably because this location was more successful, and eventually the two institutions were combined to form the Aoyama Brain Hospital.[107]

The situation with Kanō Hospital was similar. It was originally established in Izumi-chō in Kanda in 1901 by Kanō Kengo, a native of Miyagi Prefecture and a graduate of what would later be the medical school of Tōhoku University. Within just a few years, however, Kanō Kengo moved his hospital to Hara-chō in Koishikawa, a pleasant area quite close to the former shogunal medicinal garden, now a botanical garden and part of the University of Tokyo. The hospital had ten rooms and three staff doctors and was advertised aggressively as specializing in the treatment of neurasthenia or "nerve weakness," a favored diagnosis at the time, especially among male intellectuals. Bolstering this claim of expertise were Kanō Kengo's many publications on neurasthenia, which included works like *How to Prevent Neurasthenia* (1904) and *Self-Treatment of Neurasthenia* (1907).[108]

Questioning Home Confinement

In 1906 Ishikawa Teikichi noted the growing number of psychiatric hospitals in Tokyo and examined the question of the comparative popularity of home confinement versus admission to a psychiatric facility. A graduate of the University of Tokyo Medical School, where he studied under Sakaki, Ishikawa was employed for some time at Sugamo Hospital. In 1906, however, he was working in the medical office of the TMP, a job that gave him access to the records on home confinement, although he admitted that he also "had a relationship with a private psychiatric hospital," a circuitous way of acknowledging that he had side employment in at least one of them. As noted above, he would eventually serve as the medical director of the Rest Home, and later in 1913 he founded his own psychiatric hospital, Sugamo Brain Hospital (Sugamo Nōbyōin).

Ishikawa examined the records for both home confinement and admission to psychiatric hospitals in the period from 1894 to 1906 and found that the number of hospitalized psychiatric patients more than doubled over this twelve-year period. By 1901 the annual number of patients in the eight psychiatric hospitals he examined (Sugamo Hospital, Toyama Psychiatric Hospital, Negishi Psychiatric Hospital, Tokyo Brain Hospital, Ōji Psychiatric Hospital, Tokyo Psychiatric Hospital, Komatsugawa Hospital, and Aoyama Hospital) numbered over a thousand. In contrast, in the same twelve-year period, the number of those in home confinement exceeded one hundred in only two years. In fact, over the course of the entire period he examined, the number of those who were hospitalized in psychiatric facilities was ten times the number of those in home confinement.[109]

Ishikawa used the apparent preference of Tokyo residents for hospital care to criticize the system of home confinement, arguing that those who had the financial resources to place family members in psychiatric hospitals did so, as did the poor who could have their family members admitted as charity patients or as *itaku kanja*. The problem was the fate of the mentally ill from the working and middle-class families, who could not afford to pay for hospital-based care but were neither poor enough to qualify for charity nor dangerous enough to be forcibly confined.

Ishikawa was no doubt correct about the prohibitive cost of long-term hospitalization. In about 1905, Sugamo Hospital had two classes of rooms that cost two yen and sixty sen, respectively, per day. Some private hospitals, including

Toyama, Ōji, and Komatsugawa were considerably less expensive, charging between one yen and one yen fifty sen for their first-class rooms. The least expensive rooms in the private hospitals (typically communal tatami-style rooms) were priced similarly to the second-class rooms at Sugamo Hospital at 50–60 sen per day. However, even these would have been far beyond the means of Tokyoites, in an era when skilled artisans made 40–85 sen per day.

Like Kure, Ishikawa was a critic of home confinement. He noted that the 1900 law had two purposes, the protection (*hogo*) of the mentally ill and the preservation of law and order (*hōan*), but he argued that home confinement failed to ensure either. Not only did mentally ill people suffer under the poor conditions of home confinement and the lack of treatment, but ordinary homes also typically had none of the security safeguards (barred windows and continual surveillance, for example) used in psychiatric institutions. The current system thus failed both patients and the public. More psychiatric hospitals and favorable fee structures were needed to make these institutions accessible to more people. Interestingly, as evidence of people's desire for additional treatment options, Ishikawa pointed to the situation at Mount Takao, where he estimated that ninety people were receiving care in the warmer months, residing in two inns situated near the waterfalls that had been used therapeutically for at least a century.[110]

In contrast to Ishikawa's affirmative view of Tokyo's psychiatric hospitals, a far more critical perspective was offered in a lengthy report serialized in the *Yomiuri shinbun* in 1903. Writing under the title "The Darkest World of Mankind" (*Jinrui no saiankokukai*), the anonymous author(s) took up the hospitals Ishikawa would discuss three years later, with the exception of Aoyama Hospital, which was yet to be established.[111] The report reflected the then popular genre of muckraking journalism (exemplified by the reportage on the Sōma Incident), and its title hearkened back to Matsubara Iwagorō's 1893 *In Darkest Tokyo* (*Saiankoku no Tōkyō*), an exposé of conditions in Tokyo's slums that catered to the voyeuristic gaze of middle-class readers via its vivid descriptions of the squalid lives of the poor. "The Darkest World of Mankind" offered a critical view of the hospitals, focusing on the corruption, avarice, and personal foibles of their directors, physicians, and staff.

Of the seven hospitals described, the author found only the Negishi and Komatsugawa institutions acceptable, writing approvingly of their small scale, comparatively low fees, and what he described as the "devoted love" of the directors for their patients.[112] In the case of the Negishi Hospital, the director at the time was Matsumura Seigo, who had revived the hospital's failing fortunes after taking over from Watanabe Dōjun. Matsumura studied medicine at Seisai Gakusha and passed the licensing exam in 1881. He then worked with Sakaki Hajime in some capacity, although he does not seem to have been a formal student.

The situation at Koishikawa Hospital was similar. It too now had a new director with psychiatric training. Narabayashi Asajirō (Genshun's adopted son) was a graduate of the university medical school and a former student of Sakaki. Although the author of "The Darkest World of Mankind" approved of the compassionate care offered by the hospital's staff, he was critical of its facilities, which he described as cramped, shabby, and unclean. This situation likely improved when Narabayashi Asajirō oversaw the hospital's relocation to Kameido-chō, just outside Honjo Ward, where it was housed in a newly constructed Western Japanese syncretic-style building with 60 rooms and capacity for 150 patients.[113]

The author of "The Darkest World of Mankind" was far more critical of what he described as "enterprise-style" private hospitals, which in his estimation were primarily concerned with maximizing profits. He included the Tokyo Brain Hospital and Tokyo Psychiatric Hospital (later, Rest Home) in this category. While some of these hospitals targeted the wealthy, others exploited the *itaku kanja* system, in which patients were committed involuntarily by ward and police officials. Pursuing these patients made good business sense, since they tended to be hospitalized for far longer than fee-paying patients, and private hospitals typically priced the rooms for these patients to compete with the fee charged by Sugamo Hospital.

A prime example of this "enterprise-style" facility was Toyama Hospital, which was established in 1900 in Ushigome Ward by Yoshiyama Takezō and Sugimura Masakane, both former members of the Tokyo Metropolitan Police. According to the authors of "The Darkest World of Mankind," the founders made use of their connections with police and ward officials to recruit significant numbers of *itaku kanja* but once ensconced in the hospital, these patients were subjected to inferior care and poor conditions. To keep salaries low, the hospital was staffed by physicians who had no training in psychiatric medicine; the ratio of nurses to patients (1:11) was inadequate; there was no pharmacist on staff; and while the Japanese-style building looked "splendid at first glance," conditions inside were deplorable, with patients housed in filthy, unheated rooms.[114]

Ōji Hospital was another institution that capitalized on the availability of *itaku kanja*. It was founded in 1901 by Komine Zenjirō, who operated an inn in Hongō near the University of Tokyo Medical School. He had prospered by offering accommodation to would-be patients and their families who had journeyed to Tokyo in search of treatment. According to both "The Darkest World of Mankind" and a memoir written by his grandson, Komine was approached by a former staff member of Negishi Hospital who suggested that they join forces and funds to establish a hospital of their own in Takinogawa Village, a location near Sugamo Hospital that was described as "extremely well suited for a hospital." Unfortunately for Komine, running a psychiatric hospital turned out to be more challenging than operating an inn. Initially, the hospital had difficulty retaining staff due to its low salaries, and it employed at least seven physicians as the medical director in just twelve years. Kadowaki Masae was briefly employed by the hospital for a salary of forty yen, less than 20 percent of the salary paid to Gotō Shūgo at the nearby Tokyo Brain Hospital. To recruit paying patients, the hospital resorted to positioning staff outside the more popular hospitals to steer potential patients toward Ōji Hospital. When this proved unsuccessful, Komine began work with the Hygiene Departments of Hongō, Shitaya, Asakusa, Honjo, and Koishikawa, the wards with the largest numbers of impoverished residents, with the aim of receiving more *itaku kanja*.[115]

Psychiatric Care, Social Class, and Tokyo's Healthscape

Institutionalized psychiatric care had its origins in the concerns over public safety and public order that erupted following the collapse of local governance with the end of the shogunate. For that reason, tensions between the TMP and civil authorities were more muted than in the case of either syphilis or cholera. Under the TMP in the 1870s, confinement at home or in an asylum became a police procedure that involved little medical oversight. The Soma Incident exposed the vulnerability of the mentally ill, even those who were part of the city's elite. Although Japan's first generation of psychiatrists worked hard to improve conditions at Sugamo Hospital, the facility lacked the capacity to house growing numbers of potential patents. As a result, private institutions proliferated as the TMP began using them to house those who were confined by police order. The business of warehousing the mentally ill proved profitable, particularly for those with connections to the TMP.

By the early twentieth century, Tokyo was home to a multitiered system of psychiatric care. Elite hospitals like Kure's "rest garden" offered comfortable accommodations and the care of trained doctors, but at a price beyond the reach of many. In contrast, in many other private hospitals patients lived in squalid conditions with little in the way of medical attention, behind the modern veneer of a "psychiatric hospital." At the center of it all was Sugamo Hospital. The doctors and nurses it employed circulated through the private hospitals, and its fee structure influenced theirs as well. Most important, its policy that charity patients and those who were involuntarily confined had no right to privacy and could be used for research and teaching purposes contributed to the culture of indifference toward those, who—to borrow the words of Kure Shūzō—had the misfortune to be both poor and mentally ill.

As psychiatric hospitals proliferated in the early 1900s, they become an important aspect of Tokyo's healthscape even as they were relegated to its periphery. They were mentioned in guidebooks and illustrated magazines, which presented them to readers far beyond Tokyo as urban landmarks worthy of notice.[116] Women's magazines also explored the hospitals, offering readers a window into the new institutions with articles like "A Visit to the Tokyo Brain Hospital and the Female Patients I saw There" and "The Strange Lives of Women in the Asylum."[117] One enterprising author even put together a guidebook, complete with photographs, of Tokyo's psychiatric facilities and offered advice on the procedures for admission.[118] Thus, while psychiatric hospitals had been removed from the city's center, they assumed a powerful place in the imaginary of the city.

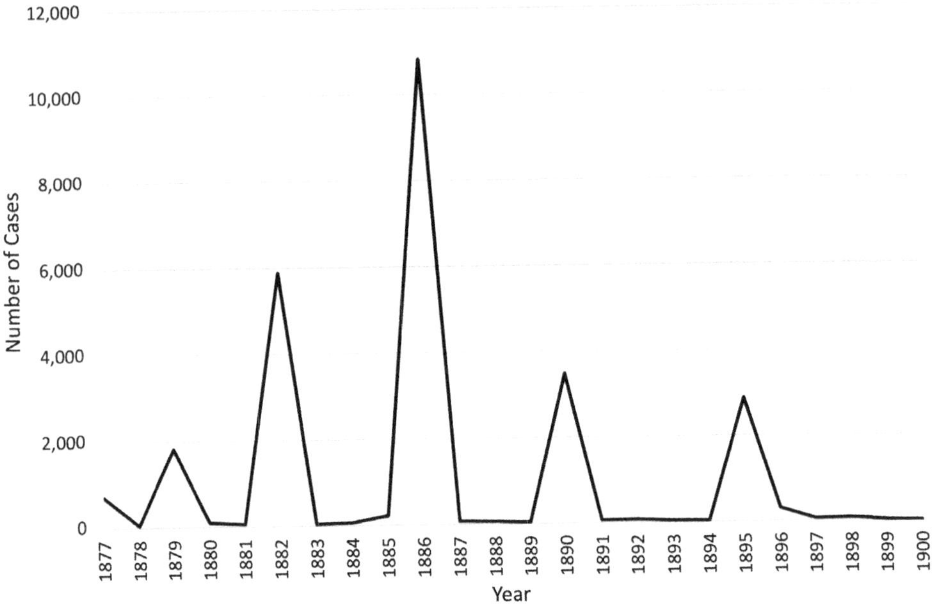

Figure 6.1. Cholera cases in Tokyo by year. Data from Tōkyō-fu, ed., *Tōkyō-fu tōkeisho Meiji* 15-nen.

6

Cholera in Tokyo

Waste, Water, and Poverty

In late July 1879, a fifteen-year-old boy named Horii Naokichi, who lived in Honjo Ward with his parents and siblings, fell ill with cholera. Having heard rumors of the boy's condition, a hygiene officer promptly made his way to the Horii home, where he ordered Naokichi's transfer to a quarantine hospital, as cholera prevention regulations required. However, his parents, Tsunejirō and O-Man, refused to comply. As neighbors and the officer argued with the parents, Naokichi's condition continued to worsen and within hours he was dead. In the days that followed the family's tragedy deepened, as did their intransigence. A second son fell victim to cholera, followed by a daughter. Both children passed away as the parents barricaded their home, refusing to allow either the removal of their children's bodies or the disinfection of their home. It was only when O-Man developed symptoms that Tsunejirō finally relented and allowed quarantine officers to take her to one of the four quarantine hospitals in the city.[1]

The three Horii children and their mother were just four of more than 160,000 people in Japan who would be infected with cholera in this single year, and the outbreak of 1879 was but one of a series of devastating cholera epidemics that struck Japan in the late nineteenth century—others took place in 1877, 1882, 1886, 1890, 1891,1895, and 1896. Cholera caused more than 400,000 deaths nationwide during these years. Tokyo was particularly hard hit (see fig. 6.1). In the 1882 epidemic (the first for which we have infection and mortality rates for the city's wards), more than 11 percent of all cases were in Tokyo, although the city's population was only 3.2 percent of the country's total population. The share of cases in Tokyo in subsequent epidemics was lower, 4–7 percent of the national total but continued to be disproportionate in relation to city's population.[2]

We know about the terrible toll that the disease took on the Horii family because the *Yomiuri shinbun* reported on it, albeit as a cautionary tale. In the newspaper's account, Tsunejirō is depicted as both arrogant and ignorant for putting his family and community at risk by refusing to respect public health regulations. However, it is unlikely that his compliance would have saved his children. The mortality rate inside Tokyo's crowded and understaffed quarantine hospitals was shockingly high. Indeed, cholera patients were more likely to die in a quarantine hospital than outside one.[3]

This chapter explores the impact of cholera on the cityscape and people of Tokyo. The repeated epidemics in the city alarmed officials at all levels of government, and over the course of three decades they sought to understand why cholera flourished in the city and to develop policies to control the disease. As Japan's capital and the epicenter of the project of modernization, Tokyo was intended to showcase the accomplishments of the new government, but cholera exposed the city's vulnerabilities. Although it was recognized early on that the city's aging water supply and sewage removal systems contributed to the spread of the disease, the government was slow to act to improve the city's infrastructure. Instead, public health measures focused on the city's residents, their domestic spaces, and their daily habits. Such measures were posed as the solution to cholera, but in fact they revealed and deepened the city's spatial and social divisions.

Encountering Pandemic Cholera

The 1879 epidemic was the second to strike Japan following the establishment of the new government. In the summer of 1877, news reached Japan that cholera had broken out in Amoy, Shanghai, and Hong Kong. In response, the Home Ministry attempted to establish a system of maritime quarantine to prevent the spread of the disease to Japan, a strategy deployed in European ports from the 1830s after the first appearance of cholera in Europe.[4] Prefectural authorities in Kanagawa, Hyōgo, and Nagasaki were instructed to create quarantine stations near their open ports and appoint medical officers to inspect all incoming ships, and Japanese consuls in Chinese ports were ordered to ensure that ships bound for Japan were free from cholera. This plan, however, was short-lived. When both the British governor of Hong Kong and Sir Harry Parkes, the British consul general in Japan, complained that such measures were unnecessary, the Japanese government backed down, turning its efforts instead to instituting measures to control the domestic threat of the disease.[5]

In the spring of 1879 when cholera broke out again, it quickly engulfed much of western Japan and ushered in what would be the greatest epidemic of the late nineteenth century on the national level. In desperation, the government attempted to establish a limited system of maritime quarantine to prevent the spread of the disease from the infected areas to the capital. Tokyo and Yokohama were closely connected, not only by Japan's first rail line but also by the many cargo ships that moved goods between Yokohama and Koami-chō in the heart of Nihonbashi near the Sumida River. On July 1, at the instruction of the Home Ministry, prefectural authorities issued a new regulation requiring ships coming from the ports of western Japan to stop at Nagaura in Kanagawa for inspection and disinfection. Within days, this requirement was made more rigorous: ships coming from infected areas were required to dock at Nagaura for ten days before being allowed to proceed to Yokohama.[6] The government also established quarantine stations near the three highways that provided land access to Tokyo, the Tōkaidō, Nakasendō, and Kōshū Kaidō, requiring anyone who hoped to enter the capital to quarantine for five days.[7]

The attempt to enforce a maritime quarantine was challenged almost immediately. On July 11, a German merchant ship, the *Hesperia*, entered Tokyo Bay, having left cholera-infected Kobe the day before. Japanese naval vessels approached the ship and ordered it to quarantine at Nagaura. Initially, the captain of the *Hesperia* complied. However, when the German consul at Yokohama informed his government of these developments, it ordered the ship to proceed to Yokohama and on July 14, after only three days in quarantine, the ship entered Yokohama harbor where its passengers disembarked, and its cargo was unloaded. The "*Hesperia* Incident," as the affair became known, quickly escalated into a major diplomatic conflict, with the governments of Germany, Britain, and France arguing that Japan could not enforce quarantine regulations without their consent while the US, Russia, and Italy agreed to accept Japanese measures.[8]

Amid this conflict, also on July 14, the government issued its first quarantine regulations for all ports. The "Cholera Prevention Regulations for Seaports" authorized the establishment of regional quarantine facilities staffed by officials from the Home Ministry, Foreign Ministry, and army doctors, who were charged with enforcing the ten-day quarantine rule and the disinfection of incoming ships.[9] However, in an attempt to assuage foreign concerns and avoid international conflict, the government authorized the involvement of representatives of foreign governments in the new quarantine stations. In 1879 the staff of the Nagaura Station included members of the Yokohama international community: a British and an American doctor, a German naval surgeon, and a Dutch pharmacist.[10] As this suggests, the quarantine stations were the site of conflicting national interests, and the treaty ports continued to be important gateways for the introduction of cholera. It is believed that the 1882 epidemic began in Yokohama and the outbreak of 1891 in Nagasaki as ships carrying infected passengers or crew continued to arrive in Japan's ports.[11]

Water and Waste in the Capital

Preventing the introduction of cholera into the country was thus an elusive goal, making it even more crucial to curtail its domestic spread. Beginning with the epidemic of 1877, Tokyo's prefectural government ordered doctors, family heads, owners of inns, shops, and factories, and the staff of schools to notify the local authorities of any suspected case of cholera. From 1882 this information was compiled at the level of the ward, revealing that cholera did not affect all parts of the city equally. Outbreaks were centered in wards in the eastern part of the city, particularly Kanda, Asakusa, Nihonbashi, Fukagawa, and Kyōbashi (see figs. 6.2 and 6.3). In fact, more than 60 percent of cases in the city between 1882 and 1890 were in these five wards. These were, to be sure, in some of the most densely populated areas of the city, but this does not account for the higher incidences of the disease in these wards, since cholera, a waterborne disease, is not transmitted via casual contact.

By this time, officials had an understanding, albeit not an entirely accurate one, of how the disease was spread. *Vibrio cholerae* was first identified in 1854, but knowledge of this discovery went largely unnoticed until 1884 when the German microbiologist Robert Koch independently identified it and successfully publicized his discovery. However, three decades earlier, the British physician John Snow had demonstrated the spread of cholera via contaminated water when he traced the source of a cholera outbreak in London to the Broad Street pump.[12] The theory that human waste was responsible for transmission was introduced to Japan by at least 1871, when Ishiguro Tadanori published the Japanese translation of a European text under the title *Korera ron* (On Cholera). This work explained that human waste spread the disease and emphasized the need to keep toilets clean and carefully dispose of the waste of those infected.[13] During the 1877 cholera outbreak, medical officials in the city acted

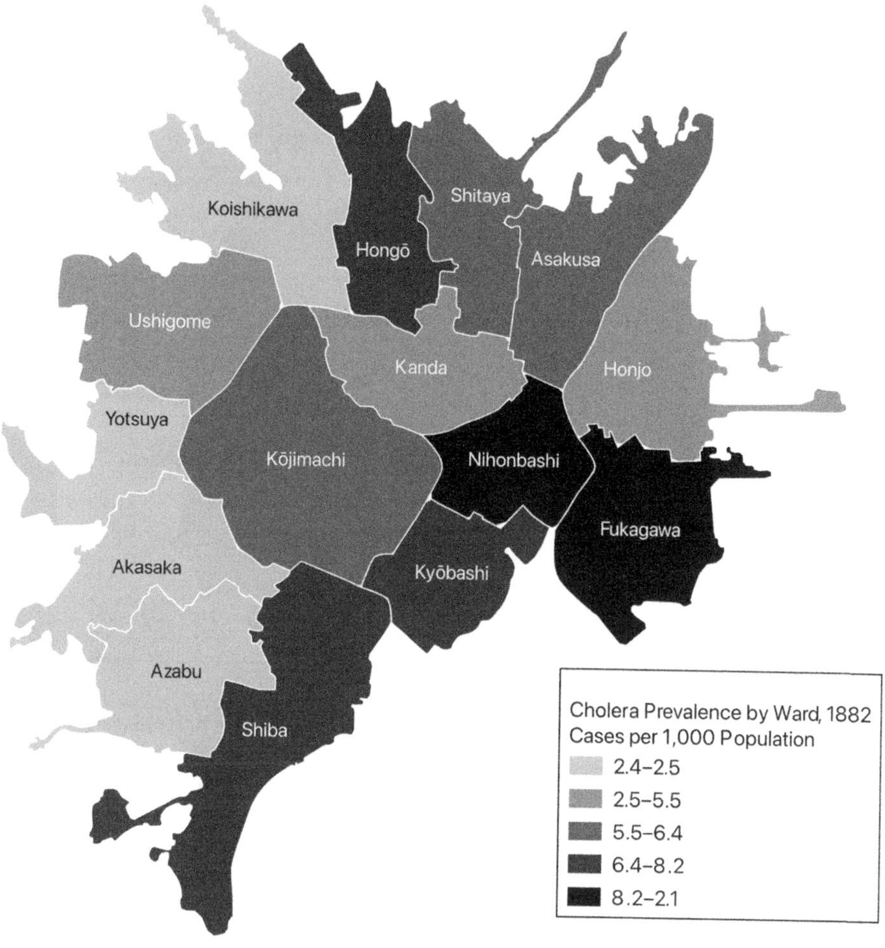

Figure 6.2. Distribution of cholera cases in Tokyo by ward, 1882. Data from Tōkyō-fu, ed., *Tōkyō-fu tōkeisho Meiji* 15-nen, 25–26.

on this information: the prefectural hospital issued multiple warnings in the newspapers urging people to exercise caution in relation to drinking water.[14]

In 1880 the Home Ministry officially recognized the waterborne nature of the disease and the role of human waste in transmission. It informed the Tokyo Metropolitan Police (TMP) and the Tokyo prefectural government, which shared responsibility for public health in the city, that "the disease poison is contained in the vomit and diarrhea of the sick person . . . and if it enters into dirty and polluted water or soil, its propagative power increases as it moves. It enters drinking water and from there into the human body where

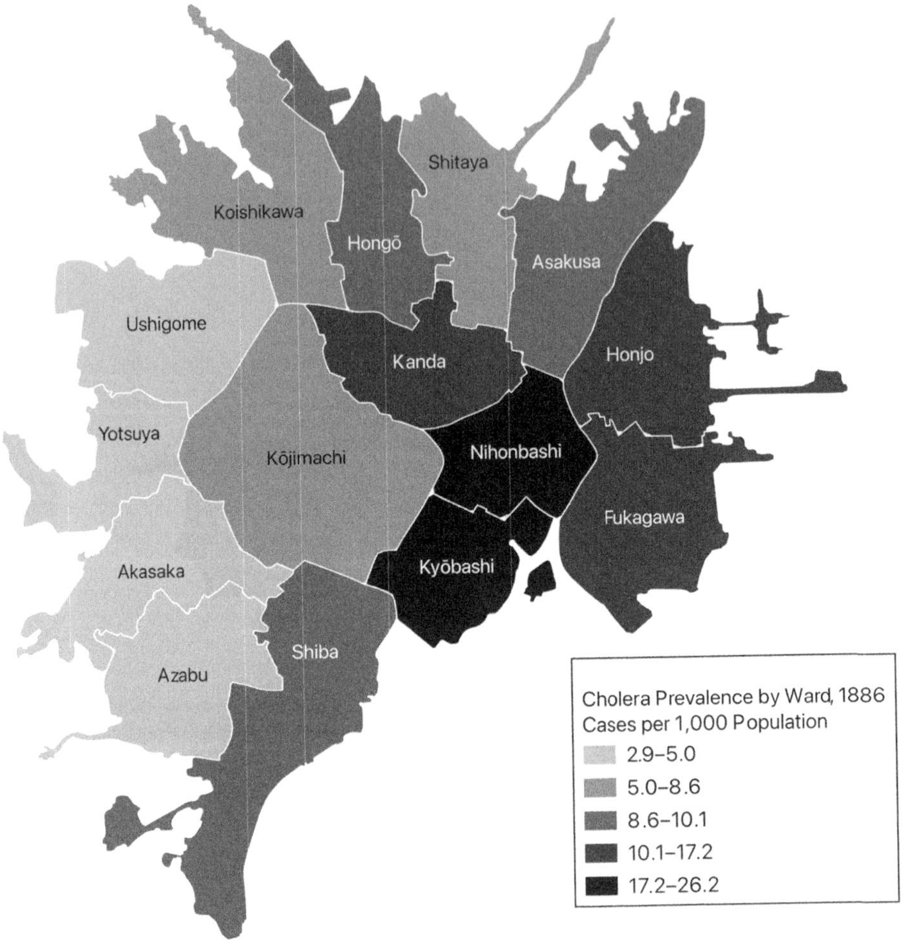

Figure 6.3. Distribution of cholera cases in Tokyo by ward, 1886. Data from Tōkyō-fu, ed., *Tōkyō-fu tōkeisho Meiji* 19, 273.

it multiplies, causing the symptoms of explosive diarrhea and vomiting."[15] The notion that the virulence of the "disease poison" increased due to exposure to other forms of contamination was, to be sure, mistaken, but the new knowledge that cholera was spread via the water supply reinforced growing concern about Tokyo's drinking water and sanitation.

At this time, Tokyo still relied upon the antiquated system of aqueducts constructed in the late sixteenth and early seventeenth centuries for its drinking water. In the 1870s, as before, large swaths of the city had little or no access to aqueduct water (see fig. 6.4). The aqueducts had never been

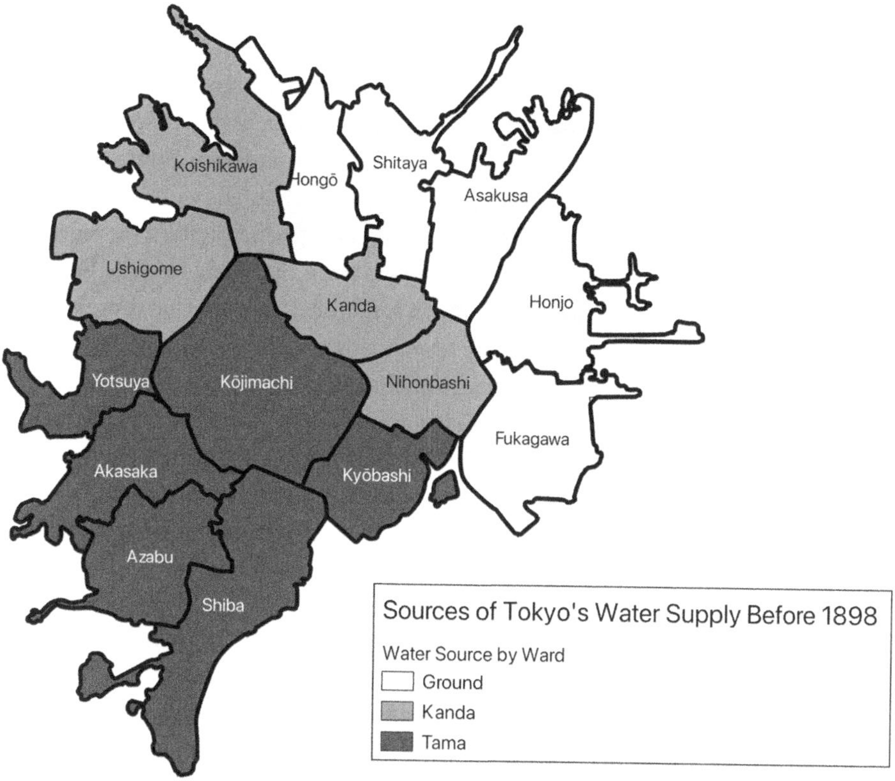

Figure 6.4. Tokyo's water system in the mid-nineteenth century.

extended beyond the Sumida River, and residents of Honjo and Fukagawa relied on wells that tapped into groundwater. These wards were in the lowest part of the city (and portions of Fukagawa were reclaimed land), and much of the groundwater was brackish and unsuitable for drinking, forcing residents to buy water from water vendors. Some of this water was in fact drawn from the runoff of the aqueducts, which testing in the late 1870s and 1880s would reveal to be contaminated. Parts of Hongō, Shitaya, and Asakusa too had no access to aqueduct water until 1880, when an abandoned aqueduct created in the late seventeenth century was repaired and reopened by a private company in preparation for the 1881 Domestic Industrial Exhibition, which took place in Ueno Park.[16] Also reliant on groundwater were elevated areas in Banchō in Kōjimachi and Surugadai in Kanda. The Edo-period water system relied solely on gravity to move water, and the higher elevation of these areas of the city made it impossible to tap into the aqueduct system.[17]

By the 1870s, new problems arose as well. In the Edo period, considerable effort was made to maintain the safety of the water supply, which was managed jointly by the city magistrates and their commoner counterparts, the city elders. Early on, three ken (approximately 5.5 meters) on both sides of the open channels of the aqueducts were set aside as a buffer from agriculture and other uses, and villagers residing in the proximity of the channels were prohibited from using them for fishing, washing clothes, and other activities. Moreover, as part of their corvée requirement, villagers were also made responsible for regularly dredging and cleaning the open conduits. To ensure that these rules were followed as well as to adjust the flow during times of heavy rain, a system of "water guards" (*mizu bannin*) was established at points along the conduits and at the weirs within the city.[18] The maintenance of the water system was costly, and the magistrate's office funded its upkeep by taxing landholding Edo residents. Warriors paid based on their *kokudaka*, the income (paid in rice) imputed to them by the shogunate or the daimyo whom they served, while commoners paid based on the number of rooms in their homes.[19]

By the 1870s, many of these safeguards had been abandoned. Reports from this period attest to the dismal state of the channels: garbage dumps were found on their banks, considerable quantities of household refuse and other waste, including animal corpses, were routinely found in the water fences outside the city, and local people were using the conduits to wash their clothing and perform other domestic tasks. In many areas, farmers had appropriated the buffer lands and were growing crops up to the banks of the channels, with the result that runoff from the fields (including human manure and other forms of fertilizer) was contaminating the water.[20]

Part of the problem was that the aqueduct system was no longer being maintained. The regular cleaning and dredging of the conduits fell into abeyance during the turbulent years leading up to the 1868 revolution. Lack of funds contributed to the decline of the aging waterworks. After the end of alternate attendance in 1862, many warriors had left the city and could no longer be taxed, and as the economy of the city declined, commoner residents also stopped paying. It was not until 1872 that the prefectural government announced its intention to require payment, which led to protests from city residents. Officials backed down for several years, but in 1875, collection efforts began in earnest. Initially, the prefecture relied upon the Edo-era system for commoners, but in 1876, a new yearly tax was imposed on each well, with the result that that some landlords filled in the wells on their properties or attempted to hide them to avoid the water tax.[21]

Concern about water quality thus predated the first cholera epidemic of the modern era, and in 1874, the Ministry of Education ordered Georg Martin, a German chemist who was on the staff of the recently created Pharmaceutical Testing Center (Shiyakujō) to carry out the first tests of Tokyo's water supply. He found the water at its source in the Tamagawa River to be "incredibly pure" and of far better quality than the headwater of the Kanda aqueduct. However, water supplied by both sources was contaminated by high levels of organic matter by the time it reached city residents due to waste that entered via both the open channels and the decaying pipes that lay beneath the city. According to Martin's analysis, the Tamagawa headwater contained no significant evidence of contamination by organic matter such as human waste, only naturally occurring minerals. In contrast, samples taken from within the city found significant levels of nitric acid (0.46 grams per liter), a substance that results from the oxidation of human and animal excreta, as well as other organic and nonorganic compounds that were not present in the headwater.[22]

Although the causal relationship with Martin's conclusions is unclear, in 1874, the Home Ministry ordered another "hired foreigner," Cornelis Johannes van Doorn, a Dutch civil engineer employed by the ministry to draw up a plan for modernizing Tokyo's water supply. Van Doorn's proposal, which he said was aimed at "supporting the health of the city's residents" and "making Tokyo a great city," would have kept the two Edo-period aqueducts in place. It envisioned the development of a system of reservoirs to bring water to areas not serviced by the aqueducts, the establishment of steam-powered water-purifying facilities, and the gradual replacement of the deteriorating subterranean pipes with cast iron ones.[23] As an employee of the government, Van Doorn was perhaps aware of its strained finances, and he developed this plan with economy in mind. Even so, he estimated the cost of the renovations he proposed to be 1.5 million dollars (approximately 1.47 million yen) with an additional 185,000 dollars required per year to maintain it.[24]

In response to this plan, in 1877 the prefectural government created a "waterworks improvement committee." The following year, the committee issued a report that confirmed Van Doorn's plan but attached a much higher price tag. It estimated that to implement it would cost a total of 1.8 million yen, which included expenses that Van Doorn had left unaddressed, such as the cost of purchasing land for the new reservoirs. In 1879 Tokyo Prefecture's total tax revenue was 268,939 yen, and as noted in chapter 3, by the late 1870s the prefecture was struggling to fund the prefectural hospital.[25] Improving the water supply would have been impossible without funds from the central government, but in 1880 it issued the Waterworks Ordinance making the improvement of water systems a local responsibility.[26]

Studies of water quality continued, although the absence of a defined methodology for evaluating water quality and agreed upon standards of potability complicated this analysis. In 1877 Robert Atkinson, a British scientist who was teaching applied chemistry at the University of Tokyo, analyzed the water in wells connected to the aqueducts and in the groundwater wells around the city, with the assistance of his students. At the time, 3,989 wells drew water from the Kanda aqueduct, and 2,432 wells were connected to the Tamagawa aqueduct, while more than 40,000 wells tapped into groundwater.[27] Atkinson and his students found that the quality of aqueduct water progressively declined as it moved through the city's underground pipes. In regard to the Tamagawa aqueduct, Atkinson concluded that contamination was "much more marked in those districts towards the end of the supply where water was more sluggish." The situation was more dire in the parts of the city served by the Kanda aqueduct, which consisted of some of the most populous areas of the city. Atkinson noted that samples taken at the end of the supply near Ryōgoku Bridge were "very largely contaminated with organic matter, [with] the amounts of albumenoid ammonia being very large."[28] Albumenoid ammonia is an indicator of sewage contamination. The quality of water drawn from wells that tapped into groundwater was also alarming. Atkinson noted that "the number expressing 'the previous sewage contamination' is very high," with the worst water found in Surugadai. He concluded that "most of the surface waters are dangerous, and some are exceptionally bad."[29]

A follow-up study conducted by Oskar Korschelt, a German chemist and instructor at the University of Tokyo, elaborated on Atkinson's analysis of groundwater wells. He did not object to Atkinson's conclusion that Tokyo's "well water should . . . be condemned," but he argued that by failing to take into account the depth of the wells, Atkinson had missed an important point: "The high ground water of [Tokyo] is twice as impure as the low ground water." Korschelt suggested that shallow wells that tapped into contaminated groundwater should be replaced with deep ones that drew from an aquifer that he believed lay deep beneath the city. He admitted, however, that in the lowest parts of the city, the wards east of the Sumida River, it would be impossible to sink a sufficiently deep well, and another solution was necessary.[30] Korschelt's study was not without some flaws. He examined seventy-eight wells, but twelve of these were actually supplied by the aqueducts, one was supplied by spring water, and a third was a deep well albeit one in a site of high elevation.[31]

In 1884 the Home Ministry commissioned a new study, this one solely in the hands of Japanese researchers. Tawara Yoshizumi, an employee in the Home Ministry's Hygiene Bureau and one of Atkinson's former students, oversaw the project, and he sought to differentiate his approach from earlier research. According to Tawara, limited testing at a single point in time and a limited number of sites was not sufficient to reveal the quality of the water from Tokyo's aqueducts. He and his staff collected water samples from a far larger number of sites once a month over the course of twelve months. Some of his results surprised even Tawara. He had assumed that the aqueduct water would be more polluted during the agricultural season due to the runoff from surrounding fields, but the results did not bear this out.

In the end, however, Tawara's analysis confirmed the results of previous research: the water from the Kanda aqueduct was considerably more contaminated than water from Tamagawa. Tawara suggested that this was explained by the superior quality of the wooden piping used in the Tamagawa system, the faster flow of the water, and the relative cleanliness of the area around the open channels. He also confirmed that the water became progressively contaminated as it moved through the system, acquiring more and more organic matter, which he believed originated from human and animal waste.[32] One of the outcomes of Tawara's study was a series of color-coded maps that illustrated the extent of Tokyo's water problem. One of these is presented in plate 21, which depicts the state of the well water in Nihonbashi and Fukagawa, with red indicating areas where well water was "not good" and orange indicating "bad."

The contamination of the city's water supply was intimately connected to other aspects of Tokyo's urban infrastructure. Japan's farmers had long utilized human waste as fertilizer, but as the population in Edo swelled over the course of the seventeenth and eighteenth centuries, farmers in surrounding villages sought to increase food production through intensive agriculture. When waste produced locally was no longer sufficient to meet their needs, farmers turned to the city itself for this resource and the "human manure" (*shimogoe*) produced by city residents became a valuable commodity.[33] Agents from agricultural villages outside the city forged contracts with specific landowners that gave them the right to remove the waste from the wooden or earthenware containers placed under the flooring of toilets in this period. Since farmers in villages around Edo preferred solid waste undiluted by urine, toilets often had a separate container for urine, although it was also common for men and women alike to urinate in the open wastewater gutters that ran

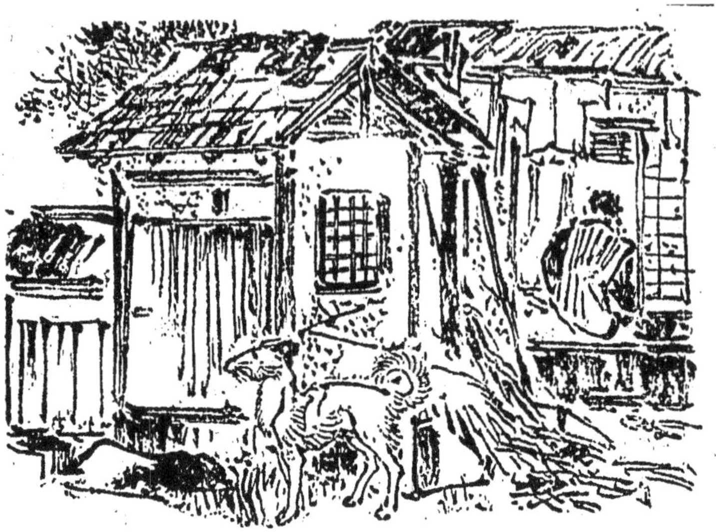

Figure 6.5. Public toilet on a Tokyo street. From Matsubara, *Saiankoku no Tōkyō*, 12.

through the city.[34] The actual work of removing waste from the toilets of specific homes was carried out by villagers, who traveled to Edo in the mornings with produce to sell in local markets, and in the afternoons cleaned the city's toilets and returned home with buckets of excrement suspended from poles or loaded on horseback. Villages with good access to waterways had another option: they could transport human manure via boat. This was the method used for waste collected from Fukagawa, Honjo, Asakusa, Nihonbashi, and Kyōbashi into the twentieth century.[35]

Officials in Tokyo looked askance at the human waste that was carried through the city's streets, but they were even more concerned about the movement of waste that could not be seen, that which occurred underground, when waste from toilets seeped into groundwater and aqueduct water. In an edict issued in 1878, the TMP announced that "drinking contaminated water is a danger to human health" and asserted that "polluted water naturally infiltrates the wells."[36] Beginning in the 1870s, public health officials became particularly concerned about two types of toilets: the *gaitō benjo* (also known as *ōrai benjo*), which stood on the city's streets for the convenience of passersby, and the shared communal toilets used by residents in so-called *ura nagaya* (back-alley tenements).

In the Edo period and early Meiji period, street toilets were typically constructed by human manure agents on private property (see fig. 6.5). These benefited the property owners in two ways: they were not only paid for the excrement gathered from the toilets but also received a small fee for the use of the toilets. These "public toilets" were certainly necessary given that half of Tokyo's *machi* lacked toilets. As a result, the number of street toilets grew steadily over time, from about 160 in the late eighteenth century to 1,300 in the 1870s.[37] Officials of some wards began forging new contracts in the 1870s with the human manure agents for the construction and maintenance of street toilets, evidence of the new understanding of toilets as a public service for urban populations.

Their utility notwithstanding, the street toilets were often crudely constructed and notoriously filthy, although the reasons for their generally poor condition are not entirely clear. It may have simply been that with little oversight by the ward officials, human manure agents who were tasked with waste removal gave priority to the maintenance of toilets in private homes. Or it was possible that scheduled cleanings did not keep up with the frequency of their use (and thus the amount of waste that accumulated). In any case, as early as 1873, the prefectural government ordered ward authorities to regularly inspect the street toilets in their jurisdictions, and if they were found to be dirty, residents were to be ordered to clean them.[38]

Officials in the city were perhaps even more concerned about the communal toilets in the back-alley tenements. These "long houses" (*nagaya*) were one-story wooden structures built to house poor and working-class people in small, single-room apartments with raised tatami flooring. As we saw in chapter 1, these buildings were typically sandwiched between parallel streets lined with the homes and businesses of more prosperous city residents, and residents shared communal toilets and a well. As figure I.1 in the introduction indicates, pockets of poverty (more than seventy by the 1890s) were scattered around the city, and slum districts were often located near more prosperous neighborhoods. Some of the slum areas, like Shin'ami-chō in Shiba, which was discussed in chapter 3, were originally the site of early modern outcast communities but were transformed as they absorbed new impoverished migrants to the city. Others like Samegabashi in Yotsuya had been home to day laborers in the late Tokugawa period but expanded as former warrior properties were sold off and the investors who purchased them built new tenements.[39]

A survey of back-alley tenements in Kanda carried out in the early 1880s reveals the living conditions of about half the city's population. It found that the population density in the ward's poorest neighborhoods was 2,121 per hectare, almost four times the population density of Kanda Ward as a whole. In one area, seventeen families occupied an area of 178 square meters. The apartment buildings themselves occupied about 80 percent of a given property, meaning that shared facilities—toilets, wells, and garbage dumps—were crammed tightly together in the remaining area. As a result, the space between the well and toilets was often less than 4 meters. In addition, toilets in the tenements were both crude and heavily used. Typically, waste was collected in repurposed wooden oil casks, and a single toilet was used by 5.3 households, consisting of perhaps twenty people or more. Under such conditions, according to the report, "there is no doubt that dirty water from the garbage and excrement is seeping into wells."[40]

Tokyo officials were certainly concerned about the proliferation of slum areas in the city, but the strength of traditional property rights and the city's complicated pattern of land tenure impeded efforts to address slum conditions.[41] A case in point was Hashimoto-chō in Kanda, an impoverished neighborhood from the Edo period, but one that expanded during the 1870s. After a fire in January 1881, the prefecture adopted the extraordinary measure of buying up all the property in Hashimoto-chō in order to displace the tenement landlords and their tenants. No provisions were made, however, to rehouse those who had lost their homes, and it seems likely that former Hashimoto-chō residents then moved to other impoverished neighborhoods in the city, leaving the overall problem of substandard housing and sanitation unaddressed.[42]

The view that poor neighborhoods with a high concentration of tenement housing were responsible for the spread of cholera would shape the response to the disease over the next several decades. In 1886, for example, the prefectural government engaged in another project of "slum clearance," utilizing the same strategy deployed in relation to Hashimoto-chō. This time its object was Samegabashi, a tenement area that stood close to the Akasaka Detached Palace, the residence of the crown prince. In this instance, the prefectural government was aided by the Imperial Household Agency, which was uncomfortable with the proximity of tenement housing to an imperial residence. With funds from the agency, the prefecture purchased almost three hectares within Samegabashi for 24,700 yen. This land then became part of the Detached Palace grounds. In explaining this purchase, the prefecture argued that it was necessary to prevent the spread of contagious disease.[43]

In fact, it is unclear whether these areas had higher rates of cholera. Data were collected only at the level of the ward, thus making comparisons at the level of the machi impossible. Nonetheless, the claim that cholera was a disease of the unhygienic poor, whose waste seeped into the water supply and threatened the city, came to prevail, even though those who were so stigmatized had little control over their living conditions.

Policing Everyday Life

In August 1877, anticipating that cholera, then raging in Chinese ports, would make its way to Japan, the Home Ministry issued "Instructions for the Prevention of Cholera" (*Korera yobō kokoroe*) to the prefectural governments. It laid out a detailed plan for controlling the disease, beginning with a reporting requirement directed toward doctors and others. Once a case was reported, it triggered a cascade of new responsibilities for local officials. First, they were to post a notice on the home or facility in question, clearly stating that a cholera patient was on the premises. Next, they were to ensure that the home and environs of the patient were properly disinfected. Any waste from patients was to be disposed of in designated locations, where it could be properly incinerated. Toilets, garbage dumps, and drainage gutters were to be inspected, and people living in the vicinity could be ordered to clean and repair those in poor condition. Local officials were also required to oversee the transfer to quarantine hospitals of those who had no one to care for them, and in the case of a death, to oversee the transfer of the corpse to a designated burial site. Additional articles detailed the prescribed process of disinfection, including which chemicals were to be used (various forms of carbolic acid) and which items and areas of the home were to be disinfected, including the patient's room, toilet, clothing, bed linens, newspapers and books, dishes and utensils, and anything else with which the patient had direct contact. Finally, local governments were to secure an adequate supply of carbolic acid and make it accessible to residents for purchase.[44]

This lengthy list of directives likely proved difficult for cash-strapped local governments around Japan to implement, but the situation in Tokyo was exacerbated by the ongoing tensions between the prefectural government and the TMP. At the time, both the TMP and the prefectural government claimed authority to issue orders to heads of wards and households as well as to ordinary citizens. Moreover, there was no mechanism for collaboration between the two bodies.[45] It was not long before jurisdictional tensions emerged. The first case of cholera in Tokyo in 1877 was reported on September 14, and over the next month the TMP issued a series of orders that reflected the "Instructions for the Prevention of Cholera."[46] The measures put into place by the TMP soon came into conflict with the prefecture's efforts, leading to, for example, the creation of two systems of quarantine hospitals, one established by the TMP and the other by the prefecture, an issue we will examine later in this chapter.

Nothing proved more contentious than the regulation restricting the removal of human waste from the city to the hours between 6:00 p.m. and 7:00 a.m. and requiring that it be transported in covered containers. Those involved in waste removal, primarily villagers from outside of the city, complained to prefectural authorities that the new restrictions not only interfered with their usual schedule of bringing produce to market early in the day, collecting waste, and returning home in time to do agricultural work but also increased the cost involved by requiring them to travel and work by lamplight, which, in addition, exacerbated the danger of fire within the city. The prefecture instructed those involved in waste removal to address their complaint to the TMP, which promptly rejected their request to loosen the time restrictions.[47]

The time constraints on waste removal would become a feature of subsequent epidemics as would the protests of villagers engaged in the human waste trade. According to Andō Yūichirō, during the 1879 epidemic, more than half the villages outside of Tokyo petitioned the prefectural governor to end the ban on daytime waste removal. In 1888–1889, there was a prolonged discussion of the issue among prefectural officials, the TMP, and village representatives with the latter arguing that if waste was removed in rigid, covered containers it posed no risk. In this instance, the Tokyo governor Takasaki Goroku weighed in with support for the TMP's position that the temporal restrictions were necessary—but not for reasons of cholera prevention. Instead, he cited the ongoing process of treaty revision, suggesting that the traditional system of waste removal was an embarrassment, given the growing international population within the city.[48] Public health measures, then, were once again mediated by international tensions.

In the aftermath of the 1877 outbreak, the Home Ministry attempted to clarify the spheres of civil and police authority in Tokyo in relation to public health matters. In March 1878, the ministry noted the tensions of the previous year and ordered the TMP to "confer with the prefecture about all matters great and small." Two months later, the ministry issued a clearer delineation of the authority of the two agencies. It made the TMP responsible for (1) the implementation of preventive measures, (2) the enforcement of bans on traffic on vicinity of patients' home or lodgings, (3) the inspection, quarantine, and disinfection of ships, and (4) the patrol of the quarantine hospitals. Tokyo Prefecture was given authority over the treatment, burial, and cremation of victims, and the establishment and administration of quarantine hospitals.[49] This did not settle the matter, however. The prefecture took the position that the TMP was responsible for "implementing" policies formulated by the prefecture.

The prefecture's position would be tested when cholera returned in March 1879, for what would be Japan's most devastating outbreak of the post-1868 period. In June, the Home Ministry responded by issuing "Temporary Regulations for the Prevention of Cholera" (*Korera yobō kisoku*), which supplanted the 1877 "Instructions for the Prevention of Cholera." The change in terminology from "instructions" to "regulations" is revealing of the evolving approach of the ministry, which gradually adopted a more top-down approach to infectious disease control, giving local officials little opportunity for innovation. In the "Temporary Regulations," as in the "Instructions" of two years earlier, doctors were required to notify authorities of a case of cholera—and this prompted additional measures designed to contain the disease. To ensure the compliance of doctors, the ministry now endorsed fining those who failed to report a diagnosis of cholera. These were important changes, but even so the day-to-day management of cholera prevention was largely left in the hands of local officials. For example, addressing the issue of how to handle the corpses of cholera victims, the Home Ministry directed that "local officials of each place should develop an appropriate procedure."[50]

In Tokyo, things were different. The TMP immediately assumed control of efforts to manage the disease and issued a flurry of orders beginning in June and continuing until December. These included the temporal restrictions on the human manure trade and requirements for posting notices on the residences where a case of cholera had occurred and banning traffic near these homes. There were new directives as well and many of these disproportionately affected the city's poor. Even before the 1879 outbreak, the police had issued "Regulations for Street Cleaning" and "Regulations for the Construction of Toilets and Removal of Waste." The former made the residents of tenements (not the property owners or landlords) responsible for the regular cleaning of streets and drains and the weekly cleaning of toilets. Thus, much of the day-to-day labor of cholera prevention became the responsibility of renters, rather than the propertied residents of the city. The new regulations for toilets required that household toilets be inspected and leaky wooden waste containers be replaced, preferably with more expensive ceramic ones, and the area around the new receptacle was to be packed with sand or ash as a further measure to prevent the contamination of water.[51] In this case too, the new regulations did not clearly designate that the property owners were responsible for these renovations, a significant issue in a city where the majority of residents lived in some form of rental housing.

As cholera cases proliferated, the poor bore the burden of other new restrictions as well. A case in point was a new regulation banning the sale of the clothing and bedding of cholera patients. Clothing and bedding were often the only assets of the poor and were valued not only for use in everyday life but also because they could be pawned or sold to raise cash in times of need. Another new regulation forbade members of a household where someone had been infected with cholera from working in any business involving food or drink for a period of seven days, a regulation that affected a broad swath of working-class Tokyo residents who made tofu and other foodstuffs, ran food stalls, and peddled vegetables or fish.[52] To carry out the expanded role of the police in enforcing these regulations, the TMP ordered each police station to designate three to five officers to work solely on public health.[53]

As the numbers of the sick and dying surged in the early summer of 1879, the Home Ministry created a new, nominally civic organization to aid the government in responding to the epidemic. The Central Sanitary Association (Chuō Eiseikai) was headed by Nagayo Sensai, then director of the Hygiene Bureau, and was intended to function as an advisory committee on policy. Its thirteen original members included eight doctors, a chemist, a civil engineer, and representatives of the Hygiene Bureau, Home Ministry, and police. The doctors in the association came to include the surgeons general of the army and navy, professors from the University of Tokyo Medical School, the emperor's personal physician, and even prominent foreign physicians such as Erwin Bälz.[54] The Home Ministry, in turn, encouraged the prefectures to oversee the formation of similar organizations at the local level. This prompted the founding of the Tokyo Local Sanitary Association (Tōkyō Chihō Eiseikai, TLSA) in December 1880.

Made up of members of the prefectural assembly, the governor, and prominent physicians, the TLSA's self-described role was to "investigate the entirety of public health for the greater Tokyo area and maintain the health of its people." To that end it would "aid the police and the prefecture."[55] While this implies that the organization was an adjunct to the prefecture and the TMP, the TLSA soon took on many of the responsibilities formally belonging to the prefectural government. It was involved in determining the sites for quarantine hospitals and cremation and burial sites for cholera victims, took control of communications with the public and the various consulates located in Tokyo, and carried out surveys of hygiene standards in homes and other buildings.[56] While it included representatives of the prefectural government, the TLSA was in principle a civic organization with limited powers. Its establishment and the diminishing role of prefectural officials set the stage for the TMP's assertion of primary authority over disease prevention, and in 1881 it created the Office of Hygiene Police (*eisei keisatsu jimu*) to enforce public health regulations.[57]

The previous year, the Home Ministry had issued the Regulations for the Control of Infectious Diseases (*Densenbyō yobō kisoku*), which defined punishments for failing to abide by public health regulations. A family head could be fined as much as 50 yen for failing to follow regulations, while others faced fines of 1.5 yen.[58] Failing to follow public health regulations was now part of a category of minor crimes known as "offenses against police regulations" (*ikeizai*), which did not have to be adjudicated within the regular court system. Those who wanted to contest a charge had no option but to pursue the case in special police-run courts and there was no mechanism for appeal. The power to fine city residents for such offenses was thus a powerful extension of police authority.[59]

Quarantine Hospitals as Contested Places

Efforts to prevent and control the spread of cholera were compromised by bureaucratic tensions, conflicting priorities, public resistance, and the policy of shifting the burden of cholera prevention to the city's poorer residents. As a result, the isolation of the sick in quarantine hospitals became the most visible and sustained method of cholera prevention over the course of the Meiji period. The use of quarantine hospitals to control cholera was, to be sure, by no means unique to Japan. In 1831–1832, during the second cholera pandemic, German cities such as Stetten, Memel, and Hamburg had attempted to confine victims to special cholera hospitals but were forced to abandon these efforts in the face of public outrage. In Stetten, for example, crowds tried to prevent cholera victims from being removed from their homes and then turned their anger toward the official in charge.[60] The same epidemic prompted the New York City Board of Health to establish five cholera hospitals in 1832, using schools, an abandoned work shed, and an old bank to house patients. This initial effort seems not to have provoked much resistance, but when cholera returned to the city in 1849, the board found it almost impossible to rent space for cholera hospitals; landlords either refused to rent their buildings or demanded exorbitant rents. Eventually, the board managed to secure the second floor of a tavern but was forced to abandon this plan after an angry mob threatened to burn down the building.[61]

It is unknown whether Japanese officials were aware of such events, but the initial guidelines for quarantine hospitals issued by the Home Ministry in the 1877 "Instructions for the Prevention of Cholera" suggest that at this point they were primarily concerned with using quarantine to prevent cholera from entering Japan or moving from one part of the country to another via the port cities. Article 3 directed that temporary quarantine hospitals be established on islands or in other secluded places near harbors for the isolation of shipboard passengers with cholera. However, it also authorized local officials "when appropriate" to compel the confinement of cholera patients in quarantine hospitals, although it offered only a few directions for the establishment of these facilities. The construction of the hospitals was to be "extremely simple." There had to be three wards so that patients could be separated based on the severity of their symptoms; hospitals had to display a yellow "Q" flag; and no one was to be released unless completely recovered and all their belongings had been disinfected.[62] The term chosen for the new facilities, *hibyōin*, which meant "facility for the avoidance of disease," strongly implied that their role was not to care for the sick, but to protect the uninfected.

In Tokyo, local officials quickly moved to establish quarantine hospitals as soon as the first case of cholera in the city was reported. On October 3, 1877, the prefecture announced the opening of three facilities for cholera victims on the grounds of the prefectural hospital and in the commoner neighborhoods in Fukagawa and Asakusa, near the branch clinics of the prefectural hospital. It seems likely that clinic staff were tasked with providing care for patients. The next day the TMP responded with a terse announcement that it had established four hospitals of its own. In contrast to the prefecture's quarantine hospitals, the placement of which suggested that they were, at least nominally, medical in nature, the TMP facilities were located on sites associated with state power: the grounds of the Ichigaya Prison, property held by the military in Shinagawa and Hongō, and school grounds in Honjo. The TMP's choice of sites likely reflected its position within the Home Ministry, which gave it easy access to state-held properties within the city. Whether intentionally or by happenstance, the hospitals formed a ring around the city (see fig. 6.6). Four hospitals were located adjacent to major highways into the city: the one in Shinagawa, situated on the site of a former battery, and that in Shiba were both adjacent to the Tōkaidō Highway, which linked Tokyo and western Honshū.

In addition, the facility in Asakusa was near the Nikkō Highway and the one in Hongō was adjacent to the Ōshū Highway.

It was initially unclear who was to be confined in the new institutions, but, gradually, from late September into October, the TMP issued a series of decrees to address this issue. On September 28, the first such decree announced that people infected with cholera who made use of communal toilets, including those who lived in *nagaya*, worked in backstreet shops, or resided in inns for travelers, should all be transferred to the closest quarantine hospital "regardless of wealth or poverty." A week later, another decree was issued. It required that students and others living in boardinghouses or similar communal lodgings were also required to be transferred to a quarantine hospital if they fell ill. A subsequent edict added travelers, those without a fixed residence, and boat workers and others in jobs on the water to the list of those subject to confinement. This was followed on October 11 by an edict reiterating the types of individuals specified previously but adding "poor people who have no property." The next day, the TMP expanded its list to include "those who lack caution" as well as people whose living situation meant that they could not be cared for adequately.[63]

Despite the initial statement that wealthy cholera victims could also be quarantined, clearly, Tokyo's poorer residents were far more likely than others in the city to face quarantine. The procedure in place required doctors or the family to notify local police if a case of cholera were suspected; the police then had the authority to decide whether a patient could be quarantined at home or had to be removed to a quarantine hospital. The rules for home quarantine, announced on October 10, were elaborate. The patient had to be isolated from the rest of the household in a private room with access to separate toilet facilities and with care provided by a single family member, who would have no contact with anyone but the patient. Meanwhile, other family members were forbidden to leave the house.[64] Needless to say, those living in the city's tenements, where families typically occupied one room and used a communal toilet, would not have been able to abide by such rules.

In Tokyo as elsewhere, the quarantine hospitals provoked fear and suspicion from urban residents. The early facilities were hastily constructed wooden structures that housed only twenty to thirty people at a time, many of whom already severely ill on arrival. From the outset, the hospitals adopted several unpopular restrictive measures. No visitors, including immediate family members, were allowed, and patients were forbidden to leave, unless a doctor certified that they had recovered. To ensure that no one entered or left without permission, a guard was posted at the entrance. In addition, patients were required to turn over all personal belongings when they were hospitalized, and these were returned only after they had been disinfected, a process that often left clothing discolored and damaged.[65]

Those who were discharged stinking of carbolic acid were the lucky ones. Of the 889 patients confined in the TMP hospitals in 1877, 614 or 70 percent died. The prefecture's hospital did only slight better, with a mortality rate of 67 percent.[66] It was not long before sensational rumors began to circulate about quarantine facilities. A TMP directive on November 2, 1877, warned Tokyo residents to cease spreading "baseless rumors" about the quarantine hospitals, giving as examples claims that patients were drained of blood or had their livers stolen.[67] In at least one instance, suspicion of the hospitals led to violence. Late on the night of November 18, the hospital at Midori-chō was firebombed. The flames were quickly extinguished, but the *Yomiuri* newspaper speculated that the perpetrator had to be someone "with a grudge against the hospital."[68]

The quarantine hospitals were intended to be temporary facilities and by early January 1878 all seven of Tokyo's hospitals had been burned to the ground together with their furnishings and any remaining supplies. The practice of destroying the hospitals meant that with each subsequent epidemic the prefecture—with sole authority over quarantine hospitals after March 1878—was able to experiment with their placement. Plate 22 shows that in 1879 the hospitals were located on the periphery of the city, with three situated outside the fifteen wards in Shinagawa, Ōkubo, and Komagome. It is unclear what the rationale for this choice was. Certainly, the distance from some of the hardest hit wards (Kanda, Nihonbashi, Kyōbashi, and Shiba) must have posed difficulties at a time when only stretchers or rickshaws were available to transport the sick.

Of course, it may have been that officials purposefully chose less populated areas, hoping to avoid the rumors and violence evoked by the hospitals two years earlier. If so, their hope was not realized. Articles in the *Yomiuri* newspaper reveal the growing unease of residents about the quarantine facilities in their midst. The Shinagawa Hospital was not far from the entertainment district where brothels were located. According to the complaint made by the brothel owners, the hospital was so close to their businesses that customers were disturbed by the moans of cholera sufferers. Other articles relate that Shinagawa innkeepers petitioned for the closing of the hospital and that residents of Ōkubo and Komagome Villages had also complained to the prefecture about the hospitals near them.[69]

The newspaper also noted individual cases of resistance, like that of the Horii family described at the beginning of this chapter, and described a troubling new trend. Some people were choosing to conceal cases of cholera in their households lest it lead to the transfer of their family member to a quarantine hospital.[70] In late August, brothel owners within the city petitioned the prefecture to allow them to establish their own quarantine hospitals, at their own expense, for stricken prostitutes, so that they could avoid transfer to the public institutions.[71] A group of doctors also seized upon the idea of creating an alternative to the public facilities, petitioning the prefecture for permission to open a quarantine facility where they would offer treatment based on Sino-Japanese medical principles.[72] None of these efforts to circumvent the system of public quarantine hospitals came to fruition, but they reveal the growing antipathy many felt toward these facilities.

In the aftermath of the 1879 epidemic, the Home Ministry issued new guidelines designed to improve the quarantine hospitals. In the "Instructions for the Prevention of Epidemic Disease" (*Densenbyō yobō kokoroe*), issued in September 1880, local officials were advised to establish the hospitals in unoccupied areas that were easily accessible but not near wells, springs, waterways, or heavily traveled roadways. In addition, they were to avoid sites such as prisons, graveyards, and crematoria grounds, presumably because of their unsavory associations with imprisonment and death. In constructing a hospital, local officials were advised to ensure good ventilation and large enough facilities for each patient to have 2 tsubo of space (6.6 square meters). Wards for severely ill patients were to be staffed by one nurse for every two patients, while in the ward for less severely ill patients that ratio could be one to four. When someone passed away, their family was to be notified immediately and given an opportunity to view the corpse upon request.[73]

While well intentioned, these instructions would prove difficult to adhere to amid the confusion and fear that accompanied an epidemic, as Tokyo's experience in 1882 revealed. Cases of disease appeared in the city in May, but the first quarantine hospitals did not open until July. Two were established in Honjo and Ōkubo on the sites utilized in 1879, while a third was in Shiba using the buildings of the now closed prefectural hospital. The latter quickly became an object of contention. Shiba, with its mix of slums, temples, shrines, and government offices, was far from the kind of unpopulated site envisioned by the Home Ministry. In 1882 its population density was less than half that of wards such as Kyōbashi, Nihonbashi, and Kanda but significant, nonetheless.

In a series of petitions submitted beginning in late July, Shiba residents asked repeatedly that the hospital be closed. One such document, dated July 24 and signed by representatives of thirty-nine of Shiba's machi, describes the conditions residents confronted. Throughout the day patients were carried through the streets toward the hospital, their moaning making it difficult to sleep or eat, while at night dozens of corpses were removed for transfer to local crematoria. Many residents were overcome by anxiety, fearful that they too would be infected. Those who could had fled, leaving local businesses struggling in their wake.[74]

Individuals too submitted petitions. Horibe Zenkichi, who lived near the hospital, wrote to plead that the prefecture buy his property, arguing that its proximity to the hospital had made it worthless. He described the foul odor that emanated from the hospital's mortuary, which mingled with the pervasive smell of carbolic acid and "pierced his nostrils."[75] Another petition from a man who identified himself as a former samurai (*shizoku*) and an employee of the Ministry of Doctrine (Kyōbushō) was less self-interested. He called upon the prefecture to ensure better treatment of patients. Rumors of their mistreatment led many to avoid the hospitals, which had been established with "a great deal of money" from the "Imperial Court" (*chōtei*).[76]

The petition submitted to the Tokyo governor Yoshikawa Akimasa by Miyaishi Chōnosuke, a resident of Atago-chō, in contrast, made an argument based on the intertwined problems of water and waste and thus reflected the same understanding of the disease that was the foundation of the government's policies of cholera prevention. Miyaishi pointed out that the prefectural hospital was situated on low-lying ground, making it a natural drainage site for surrounding higher areas, such as Atago-san, the site of the Atago Shrine, and the hills of nearby Azabu. Flooding was common and when it occurred, the contents of the area's toilets mixed with rainwater and flowed through the streets and into homes, contaminating the whole area, including the former shogunal villa known as Hama Rikyū, the many military installations in Shiba, and schools with hundreds of students. Given this situation, Miyaishi argued, establishing a quarantine hospital in Atago was a dangerous choice that threatened to spread, rather than contain the disease and, in an aptly chosen metaphor, he described the residents of Atago as akin to beans in a boiling pot of water with no means to escape.[77]

The flood of complaints notwithstanding, the Shiba facility continued to function throughout the 1882 outbreak and would even be reopened in 1886. But discussions within the TLSA reveal that its members were acutely aware of the problems surrounding the quarantine hospitals. In early August, the TLSA met and discussed at length the public's antipathy toward the quarantine hospitals. In attendance were influential physicians such as Hasegawa Tai and Sasaki Tōyō, as well as the chairman of the prefectural assembly, Numa Shuichi, and Governor Yoshikawa. Participants explicitly noted the seeming contradictions in the policies. Did it make sense to halt traffic around a residence where a cholera victim resided, only to carry other victims through the street to a quarantine facility? Why refuse to allow family members to visit patients in the quarantine hospitals, when patients who remained at home were cared for by their family?

Participants also discussed the quality of care on offer in these facilities. One TLSA member pointed out that the root of resistance to the quarantine hospitals was their high mortality rate, which led many to believe that death awaited those who were transferred to these facilities. Sasaki Tōyō agreed that improving the care would help mitigate public resistance, and he suggested that putting a high-profile physician in charge—perhaps someone from the medical faculty of the University of Tokyo—might restore confidence. Others pointed out that the doctors who staffed the quarantine hospitals on a day-to-day level were the problem. They were described as physicians in private practice, who held their poor and working-class patients in contempt. In response, another member noted that it was difficult to hire better-qualified physicians given the low compensation they were offered.[78] This latter point is borne out by the many newspaper advertisements for quarantine hospital staff published during cholera outbreaks.[79]

This was not the only meeting of the TLSA where the quarantine hospitals were discussed at length. On August 9, 1882, the group met to discuss the need to open additional facilities. At the time, the highest rates of disease were in Kanda, Nihonbashi, and Hongō, all of which were a significant distance from the three hospitals established earlier. It was proposed that two additional hospitals be opened, one in Sakamoto-chō in Nihonbashi on the site of a former police hospital, and another in Hongō on the site of the former prefectural beriberi hospital, both in densely populated parts of the city. TLSA members acknowledged that establishing quarantine hospitals in crowded neighborhoods was less than ideal but they concluded that this was preferable to transporting patients a considerable distance to any of the existing hospitals. The choice of these sites also illustrates the ongoing practice of making use of publicly held properties. Governor Yoshikawa raised a concern about the proposed site in Sakamoto, which was adjacent to an elementary school, but Sasaki Tōyō brushed his concerns aside. Not only was cholera not an airborne disease but almost twenty meters would separate the school and the hospital.[80]

Numa Shuichi raised a more fundamental opposition, protesting not the placement of the hospitals but their effectiveness. He noted, correctly, the scant evidence that the quarantine facilities were helping to control the disease. In addition, the cost of opening more hospitals would undoubtedly require raising the prefectural tax, a tremendous burden on a city already suffering under the weight of repeated epidemics. In his view, it would be better to allow people to remain at home, and to make cash grants to their families to help them fund appropriate care. This approach would save money, respond to public sentiment, and provide for better care. Numa's proposal, however, found little support among the TLSA members. Yoshikawa, for one, responded that the central government's policy required the establishment of quarantine hospitals, and neither he nor the other members of the association expressed any interest in pushing back on this position. However, although they approved the opening of the two additional hospitals, the TLSA also tacitly acknowledged Numa's assertion that the availability of medical care in the hardest hit areas of the city could help alleviate the need for more quarantine hospitals. To that end, members approved the appointment of two to four temporary ward doctors in the hardest hit areas of the city.[81]

The year 1886 saw the worst cholera epidemic in Tokyo. More than ten thousand people in the city died over the course of several months. At the outset, the prefectural leadership seemed ready to act on the lessons learned during previous outbreaks. The initial plan was to utilize the former prefectural hospital as a quarantine facility for the whole city, but this was rejected by Mishima Michitsune, the head of the TMP, who asserted that transferring patients through the streets of the city would be dangerous both for them and the city since it would "scatter the disease poison in four directions." In response, the city came up with a new plan. Rather than temporary "facilities for avoiding disease," they now envisioned a system of "provisional prefectural hospitals." The change in nomenclature was clearly intended to counter the negative associations of the widely reviled quarantine hospitals, but there were to be other changes as well. These were to be purpose-built medical facilities that would provide a better level of care for victims of infectious disease. Four sites were chosen for the new hospitals, Honjo, Komagome, Ōkubo, and Shibuya, and it was specifically recommended that the sites in Nihonbashi, Shiba, and Hongō not be utilized.[82]

This plan was quickly abandoned, however, as the epidemic exploded, leaving little time to construct new facilities. In the end, quarantine hospitals were reopened in all the sites used in 1882 except for Hongō. Instead, a hospital was opened in Komagome Village, on a site utilized in 1879. In addition, no doubt to the dismay of Shiba residents, in mid-August a second hospital was established on the grounds of a former police hospital, not far from the former prefectural hospital. Despite the concerns expressed during the previous outbreak, there is little evidence that conditions in the hospitals improved. Indeed, the mortality rates were the highest of the era: at the Komagome hospital, for example, 77 percent of patients died.[83]

The devastating 1886 epidemic revealed the futility of many of the policies for cholera prevention and marked the end of an era. In its aftermath, the prefecture followed through with its earlier plan and established four dedicated "infectious disease hospitals" (*densenbyōin*) on the periphery of the city, in Honjo, Komagome, Ōkubo, and Shibuya. In 1895 the recently established Tokyo City acquired the hospitals from the prefecture. Decades later they would become a system of general public hospitals, the first in the city since the closing of the Atago Hospital in 1880. There were other changes in the practice of quarantine. Since 1879 it had been forbidden for general hospitals to treat cholera patients, but this rule was relaxed and private hospitals in the city began to advertise their infectious disease wards. Although hospitalization was expensive, with many extra fees for disinfection and special nursing, this option freed families from the burdensome restrictions of quarantine at home and spared patients from the danger of the public quarantine hospitals.[84]

Missed Opportunities

These changes were certainly important, but the most important legacy of the 1886 epidemic was renewed interest in improving the built environment. In cities around the world, including London, New York, Paris, Berlin, and Hamburg, fear of cholera had prompted expensive improvements to urban infrastructure, most notably the construction of underground sewer systems designed (albeit with varying degrees of success) to safely remove human waste. In Tokyo, however, improvements to the city's infrastructure came slowly, and some initiatives probably did more harm than good. In 1886, for example, the prefecture announced its plan to remove the bulk of the city's

1,300 street-side toilets, citing both their lack of hygiene and their interference with the movement of people and goods. The following year about 80 percent of the toilets were dismantled, and although some were later rebuilt, the number of toilets was substantially reduced to only 261.[85] It seems that no one considered what the lack of public toilets might mean for the overall cleanliness of the city.

The value of human waste as fertilizer and the high cost of constructing a modern sewage system meant that the reliance on the traditional method of waste management went largely unchanged. In 1883 the home minister, Yamada Akiyoshi, had acknowledged the intertwined problems of waste and water yet again when he instructed the Tokyo governor Yoshikawa Akimasa that "the improvement of the water supply, sewers, and gutters is your urgent duty."[86] In response, Yoshikawa oversaw the development of an ambitious plan to improve the roads, parks, sewers, and water supply of the city. At this juncture, however, the only part of the plan that was implemented was limited improvement of the city's sewers, with the national government and prefecture sharing the cost. In 1884 the construction of new sewers began in Kanda, the site of the devastating report that had led to the "clearance" of Hashimoto-chō. Over the course of five years and at a cost of 110,000 yen, eleven kilometers of new underground brick sewers were laid, but then the project ended abruptly. With no further funds available from the central government, the prefecture found it impossible to continue.[87] As a result, human waste continued to be removed by village agents well into the twentieth century. It was only in the 1930s, when the collection of human waste was no longer profitable due to the widespread use of chemical fertilizers, that it was transformed into a municipal service.[88]

Attempts to improve other aspects of the built environment languished as well. Between 1886 and 1890, prefectures around Japan enacted building codes (*kenchikuhō*) that established minimal standards for residential housing. The focus of many of these codes was specifically the *nagaya* that in Tokyo and other cities was the typical housing for poor and working-class residents. Interest in improving housing dated back to the late 1870s. In 1876 Nagayo Sensai had traveled to the US, where he learned of growing interest in regulating the construction of tenement housing to improve the poor health of urban residents. Prompted by the new view that housing could be a legitimate object of public policy, the TLSA had undertaken the survey of tenement housing in Kanda referenced above. In 1883 the Hygiene Bureau directed the prefectures to investigate the circumstances surrounding recent cholera outbreaks. The order included detailed questions regarding housing. Did those who were infected live in a single-family home or tenement housing? Was the home on the street front or in a back alley? How many people did they live with and what was the area of the living space? Did they rely on communal toilets? What was their source of drinking water?[89] Based on the information gathered, in 1886 the Home Ministry directed prefectures to issue regulations for the construction of tenements and homes. In most cases the Hygiene Departments of the prefectural governments took the lead in drafting these regulations.[90]

In Tokyo, however, the situation was once again complicated by the contentious relationship between the prefectural government and the TMP. Spurred by the death toll of the recent epidemic, the prefectural government took the lead in drafting the "ordinances for the construction of rental tenements" (*Kashi nagaya kenchiku jōrei*) in 1887. Several of the ordinances reflected concern about the contamination of the drinking water. Toilets and garbage dumps were to be at least 3 ken (about 5.5 meters) from wells, and the waste containers within toilets were to be made of stone or ceramic. Household wastewater was to be disposed of via ceramic pipes that were to be laid at a suitable incline to ensure proper drainage. Other articles were concerned with ventilation and sunlight. Every room was to have access to fresh air to ensure proper ventilation and the wall space given over to windows must be at least 20 percent of the floor area.

If enacted, the ordinances would have improved, albeit slowly, the living conditions of many in Tokyo. However, Mishima Michitsune, the powerful head of the TMP, rejected the draft ordinances. Tanaka Yoshio, who has written extensively on the history of building codes in Japan, suggests that there were two reasons for Mishima's resistance. First, at the time, he was deeply involved in crushing the popular activism for representative government known as the "freedom and people's rights movement," which had become increasingly violent during the 1880s. In 1887 he had advocated for an imperial edict that would allow him to crack down on activists in the capital.[91] The "ordinances for public order" (*anji jōrei*) empowered the TMP to ban activists from the capital, and within two days of its promulgation on December 26, 570 people had been ejected from the capital. Clearly, Mishima valued public order over public health.

Second, Mishima also had a different vision of the capital, one that prioritized showy projects over infrastructural improvement. In the early 1870s, while serving as a "counselor" (*sanji*) to Tokyo Prefecture, Mishima had participated actively in the rebuilding of Ginza as Tokyo's showcase "bricktown" and later he advocated for other flamboyant improvements, including moving the Ise Shrine to a new location near the imperial palace.[92] Although this plan went unrealized, Mishima had little interest in the time-consuming work of enforcing building ordinances in Tokyo's slums, a project that would have done little to improve what he called "the face of the capital."[93]

Modernizing Tokyo's Water Supply

Mishima's priorities notwithstanding, the devastating epidemic of 1886 brought significant changes to Tokyo's aging waterworks. One response came from Shibusawa Eiichi, the entrepreneur who had played an important role in the founding and administration of the Tokyo Poorhouse. In 1887 he joined forces with other businessmen in Tokyo to establish the Tokyo Water Company, which planned to raise private capital to carry out needed improvements to the water supply. There were international precedents to this approach: London's water was supplied by multiple private companies until the establishment of the Municipal Water Board in 1904, albeit with mixed results.[94] Shibusawa and his allies turned to Henry Spencer Palmer, a British engineer, and asked him to develop a plan for modernizing Tokyo's water supply. Palmer had overseen the construction of the Yokohama waterworks in 1887, the first modern system in Japan and one that had been financed entirely by the central government. The use of state funds for an ostensibly local project was justified as necessary because Yokohama was a port city of "national concern." It not only was a gateway for the introduction of cholera to the capital and the rest of the country but also, as the home to a substantial foreign community, it offered an opportunity to demonstrate Japan's modernity, a pressing concern in the era of treaty reform.[95]

Of course, Tokyo too was a city of "national concern." It was, after all, this understanding of the city that had led to the creation of the TMP in 1874. However, until the 1880s the government, for the most part, held firm to the belief that local improvements should be financed at the local level, a stance that ignored the political and fiscal realities of Tokyo at the time, when many in the city were frustrated by what they felt were overly burdensome local taxes. The stalemate was broken in 1888 when the Home Ministry issued Imperial Ordinance 62. Known as the "Tokyo City Planning Ordinance" (*Tōkyō shiku kaisei jōrei*), it authorized the use of central government funds for broad infrastructure improvements in the capital. The following year an ambitious plan was drawn up to repair and rebuild streets, bridges, parks, sewers, and waterworks in the city.

W. K. Burton, a Scottish engineer hired in 1887 to teach "sanitary engineering" at the University of Tokyo was the central figure in the development of the waterworks project, although Palmer's plan was consulted as were experts from Belgian and German water bureaus. According to the final plan, the new water system would serve a population of 1.5 million residents, providing each household on average about 75 liters per day. This was to be accomplished by moving water from the Tama River through a new concrete channel to a new purifying plant. Areas of the city with higher elevation would be supplied with water via a new pressurized system, while gravity would be utilized to move water to supply stations in lower-lying areas of the city. From the supply stations, water would then be pressure-supplied to households. The project required the replacement of the antiquated wood piping with new cast-iron pipes.[96]

The plan for the new water system was submitted to the Home Ministry in 1890, along with a request for 6.5 million yen in support. During this process, however, cholera struck Tokyo again, providing, it might be imagined, a certain urgency to deliberations within the ministry. Nonetheless, in the end, it approved a grant of only 2.25 million yen, slightly more than a third of the requested amount.[97] To raise the remaining funds, the Tokyo City Council voted to issue municipal bonds. As the bond initiative got underway in 1892, some Tokyo residents responded by organizing the Tokyo Citizens Voluntary Association to protest the water improvement project, citing the high cost, the many other pressing public works projects, and concerns about whether the proposed technology was suited to the Tokyo environment, specifically whether the expensive cast-iron pipes could withstand earthquakes. The association organized a series of public lectures, some of which were banned by the TMP.[98] One of those who responded to the protests was Ban Naonosuke, a future railway developer who was then a member of the City Council representing Fukagawa Ward. In *An Opinion on Improving the Tokyo Waterworks,* he argued for the need to prioritize the project. The new water system would not only protect the health of Tokyo residents but also aid in fighting fires in the city, and both these results would contribute to Tokyo's economic development. Ban also justified the use of municipal bonds to finance the project and provided a lengthy explanation of how the proceeds from water fees would reward investors over the long term.[99]

Ultimately, the bond initiative continued, but other problems delayed construction. The purchase of the necessary land for the planned water purification plant in Yodobashi Village and the supply facilities in Shiba and Hongō proved contentious, requiring lengthy negotiations between city officials and landowners. Even more problematic was the sourcing of the cast-iron pipes required for the project.[100] The Yokohama project had relied on pipes purchased abroad, but in anticipation of the project, in 1890 Amemiya Keijirō (later known as the "king of speculators") created the Japan Cast Iron Company and lobbied the city to purchase the pipes locally, citing the need to develop a domestic cast-iron industry. Amemiya and his investors undertook an intensive public relations campaign that criticized those who advocated buying pipes from established European producers as unpatriotic, while extolling the economic benefits of using crude iron from the Kamino Mine in Iwate, which was processed in the newly established factory on Tsukishima, the island that lay in the mouth of Sumida River. In 1893, following three years of debate, the City Council agreed to purchase the pipes from Amemiya's company, but it was later exposed not only that the pipes were of poor quality and hence unusable but also that the company had resorted to bribing council members to gain their cooperation. As a result, the requisite iron pipes had to be acquired from manufacturers in Belgium and Britain, slowing progress and adding to the cost of the project.[101]

On December 17, 1899, a grand ceremony, attended by the mayor and prefectural governor, as well as members of the Tokyo City Council, the Diet, the nobility, and the various ministries was held at the Yodobashi Purification Plant to celebrate the completion of the first stage of the new waterworks.[102] These festivities notwithstanding it would take another twelve years to complete the project. A study conducted by Tōyama Chinkichi, the director of the Tokyo Municipal Sanitation Laboratory, and published in 1905 is revealing of the mixed results of the slow pace of completing the waterworks project. He found that 23,103 groundwater wells were still in use in Tokyo and that only 1.3 percent of these had acceptable levels of bacteria. He noted that on average the water supplied by the wells had 188 times the level of bacteria in the water supplied by the new system. This did not mean, however, that the purified water was free of contamination. Tōyama noted that while it was in the acceptable range, Tokyo's new water system supplied water that was inferior to that of Osaka and Yokohama.[103]

There were other problems as well. Many within the city balked at the high cost of accessing the new water supply. Until this time, landlords and property owners were responsible for payment of the water tax, but now individual users were billed based on their usage. This raised the cost of water for many, and businesses like bathhouses that used large amounts of water were particularly hard-hit. The latter responded by raising their fees, with bathhouse owners in Asakusa reportedly raising the cost of a bath from three sen to five sen.[104] There were also concerns about the quality of the water supplied. As the new system began functioning, newspapers reported that leaches, frogs, and other aquatic creatures were being found in the water supply.[105] Tōyama dismissed these accounts as baseless rumors, but whether true or not, they contributed to suspicion surrounding the new waterworks and an apparently unwillingness of some residents to pay a high price for what was perceived to be poor-quality water.[106]

These issues paled, however, in relation to the biggest problem: the system was obsolete by the time it was completed. As noted above, the water supply system was intended to serve a population of 1.5 million, but the population of Tokyo had grown to 2.2 million by 1910 and the area of the city too had expanded, exceeding the geographic coverage envisioned by the 1890 plan. As a result, many city residents had no option but to rely on water sellers or well water to supplement water from the new system.

The urban historian Ishizuka Hiromichi argues that the limited scale of the project reflected the competing priorities undertaken within the framework of the "Tokyo City Planning Ordinance." He notes that 80 percent of the total expenditure was spent on roads, bridges, and parks, and only 21 percent on the water supply.[107] A study of Tokyo slums published in 1921, a decade after the completion of the new waterworks, reveals the results of prioritizing what might be termed "visible infrastructure," or in Mishima's words, "the face of the city." It examined 497 households in four impoverished neighborhoods, two in Fukagawa, one in Asakusa, and one in Yotsuya, and found that a third were not connected to the modern water system.[108]

Public Health and Private Spaces

The failure to fully address the infrastructure deficits of the growing city reveal the tensions that plagued the public health and medical modernization efforts from the 1870s. The tensions between the central government and local government, the local government and the TMP, private capital and the public interest had shaped responses to syphilis and mental illness, even before the danger of cholera was fully recognized. But cholera evoked new levels of fear, anxiety, and frustration. While syphilis and mental illness could be viewed as problems of marginalized "others" within the city, the specter of *Vibrio cholerae* moving unseen through the degrading subterranean pipes of the city, connecting the toilets and wells of the wealthy, the poor, and those in between made it an issue for all Tokyo residents and ushered in a new need to grapple with the central logic of public health: the requirement that one accept and comply with new restrictions ostensibly for the larger public good.

In 1895 the popular author Ozaki Kōyō examined the personal and ethical tensions involved in the interiorization of this logic in a lightly fictionalized work of reportage serialized in the *Yomiuri* newspaper titled *Green Grapes* (*Aobudō*).[109] As the story opens, Ozaki is living with his family and literary apprentices in a large home in Tokyo when one of his students comes down with a suspected case of cholera. Narrating in the first person, he describes the sense of fear that pervades the household when his student "K" begins to experience intestinal distress. Ozaki first seeks the advice of several private physicians, but each confirms that "K" is suffering from cholera, and they instruct him that the illness must be reported to the local authorities. At issue of course is that the notification will lead to the transfer of the young man from the home to a quarantine hospital, unless Ozaki is willing to disrupt his household to provide care at home. The meaning attached to the hospital is apparent when the patient, apologizing for the trouble he has caused, asks that he be taken to the hospital, a request that evokes the following response from the author: "When he said the word 'hospital,' it was a metaphor for 'kill me.'"[110]

The decision to report "K" to the hygiene police is thus presented as an ethical dilemma. Should one submit to the regulatory regime of cholera prevention, even if it means the death of the infected person, or protect the afflicted person within the home, possibly endangering, certainly inconveniencing other household members? In *Green Grapes*, the path toward resolution is explored via the negotiations that ensue between Ozaki and two representatives of the TMP. The first is an ordinary police officer who, Ozaki writes, "gazed upon the outer walls of my home as though he was staring at the site of a crime. . . . And when I thought about it, I was a criminal . . . I was the master of a household that had not only inconvenienced *society* but had also troubled the *government* by becoming infected with a contagious disease."[111] Elsewhere in his account, Ozaki describes his discomfort about the social effects of the case of cholera within his home, which required that traffic in the neighborhood be stopped or diverted and the homes of neighbors be inspected.

Respite from the conflicting emotions of this situation arrives in the figure of the hygiene officer, described as a chubby, kindly old man wearing a Panama hat. According to Ozaki, the man's appearance and manner were at odds with his image of the doctor-inspector whom he imagined would be an "arrogant, unkind, and bureaucratic" man in his early forties wearing Western clothes, gold-rimmed spectacles, and an expedition hat like that worn by Henry Stanley, and the kind of person "who knew no second-person pronoun other than *omae*"—the form of address that characterized the superior-inferior relation of official to ordinary citizen. The seemingly benevolent figure who arrived made it possible for Ozaki to revise his view of the quarantine hospital. Congenial and familiar, the officer put a kindly face on the requirement for quarantine, and Ozaki revised his thinking, deciding that "the notion that sending someone to the hospital means seven or eight times out of ten that their life is at an end is nothing more than unreasonable superstition."[112] Ozaki thus exposed how members of Tokyo's middle class became complicit in the cruel choices demanded in the name of public health. And complicity is revealed to have its own rewards: the narrative ends as "K" is transported by the police to the quarantine hospital, while the author looks on from the restored privacy and safety of his home. Ironically, it is later revealed that "K" in fact did not have cholera, but nothing more serious than an upset stomach, the result of eating too many of the titular "green grapes."

The Afterlife of Cholera

Ozaki's response to a case of cholera in his household can be compared to that of Horii Tsunejirō sixteen years before. Ozaki, no less than Horii, resisted reporting the disease to the police and—initially, at least—resented their intrusion into the home. But Ozaki was later able to rationalize his compliance, while Horii submitted in despair only after seeing his family decimated by the disease. By the end of the nineteenth century, the phrase "cholera is the mother of public health" was well known.[113] In its narrow sense, it referred to the rapid rise of a public health administration to control cholera, but more important perhaps was the outcome that Ozaki exposed, the acceptance that bodily health was a legitimate object of governmental concern and control. Fear of cholera became a justification for governmental action, but it also propelled a new willingness of Tokyo residents to view the new web of regulations and the danger posed by the quarantine hospitals as in their best interest. As we have seen, however, there were other options. The prefecture, city, and central governments could have acted earlier to improve Tokyo's water supply and could have provided more support for home-based care. The decision to avoid the expense of infrastructure reforms and to focus cholera prevention on the regulation of daily life and the quarantine of city residents was a deliberate one.

But cholera exposed more than the problematic priorities of the state at all levels, it also revealed the social, economic, and material inequities that shaped urban life. Poor and working-class residents who lived in Tokyo's eastern wards were disproportionately vulnerable to cholera because of circumstances beyond their control, including their lack of access to clean water and sanitation, and they were also disproportionately affected by the onerous quarantine policy. Nonetheless, they and the spaces where they lived and worked were stigmatized as a danger to the city. Ironically, there is little evidence that the quarantine hospitals and other aspects of cholera prevention, which proved so divisive, played a meaningful role in controlling the spread of waterborne diseases in Tokyo. While cases of cholera gradually declined, outbreaks of waterborne diseases such as typhoid and shigellosis continued to plague Tokyo well into the twentieth century, until the construction of an adequate water system and improvements in sanitation finally became effective.

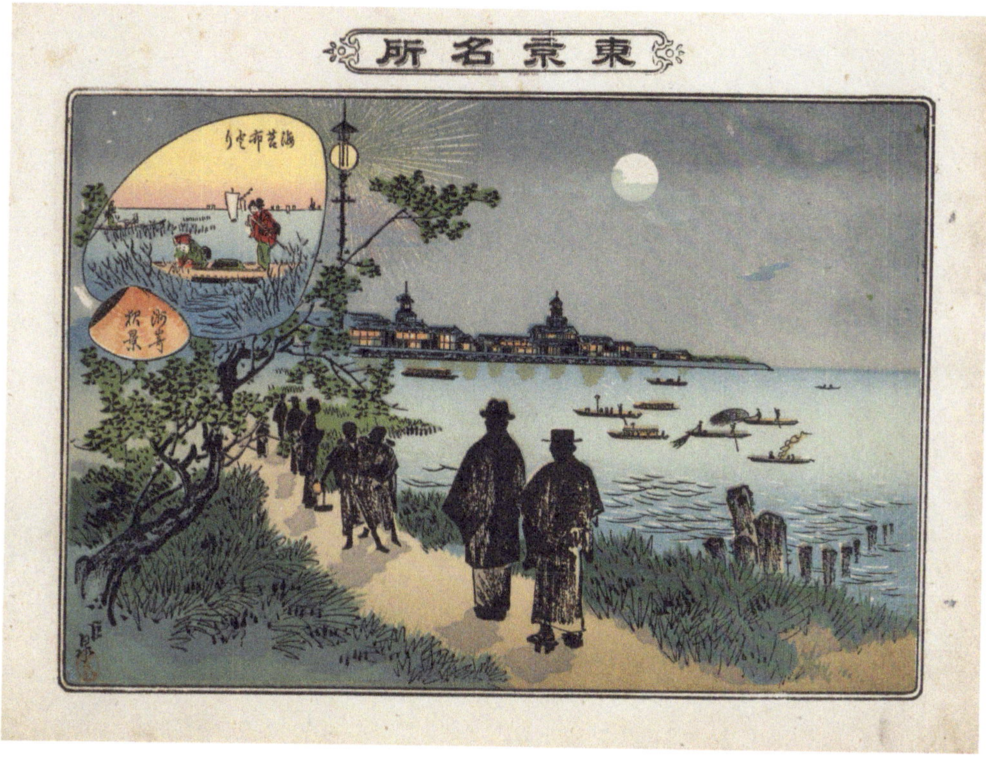

Plate 13. Susaki Brothel District at night, 1898. Kawasaki Kyosen, *Tōkyō meisho Susaki yakei* (1898). From the Edo-Tokyo Museum Digital Archive. Used with permission.

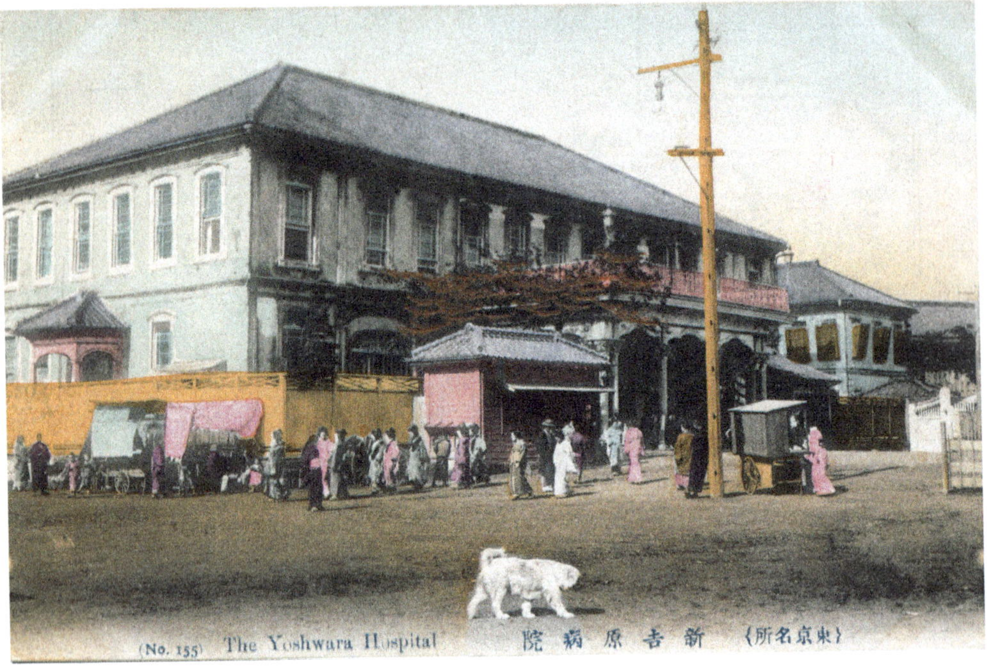

Plate 14. Picture postcard of New Yoshwara [*sic*] Hospital. Used with permission from Imagenet gallery.com.

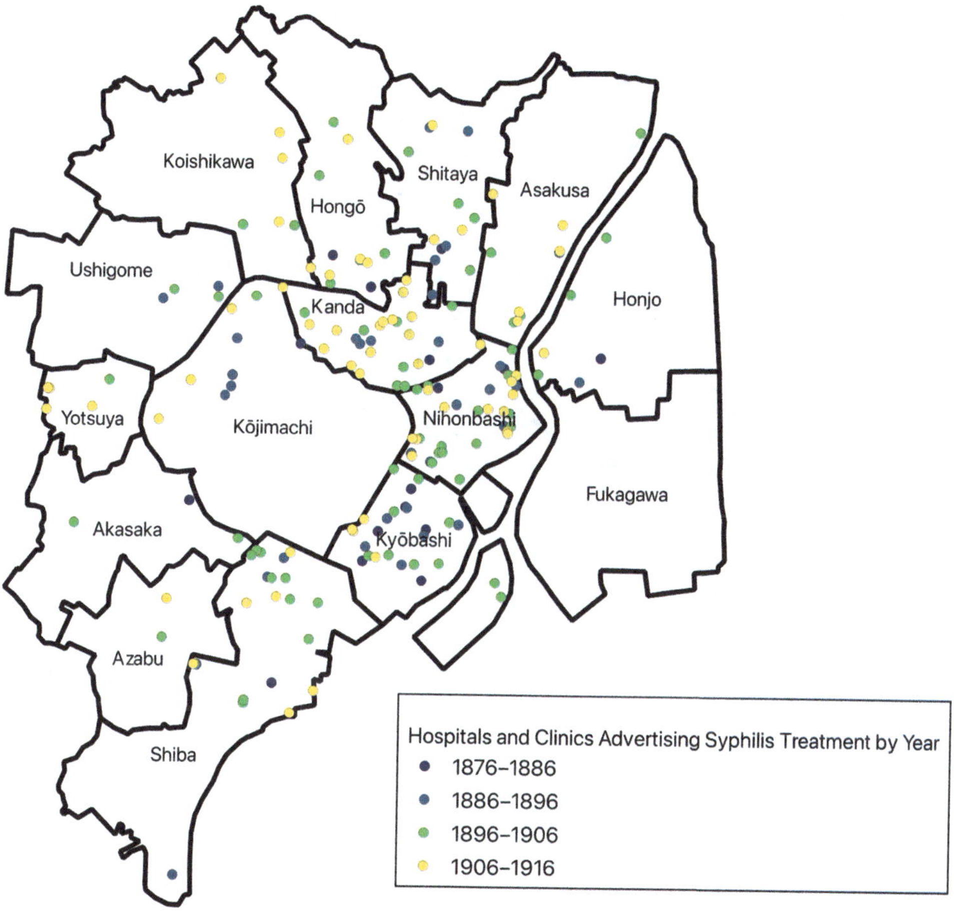

Plate 15. Hospitals and clinics that advertised treatment for syphilis in the *Asahi shinbun* and *Yomiuri shinbun* from 1876–1916.

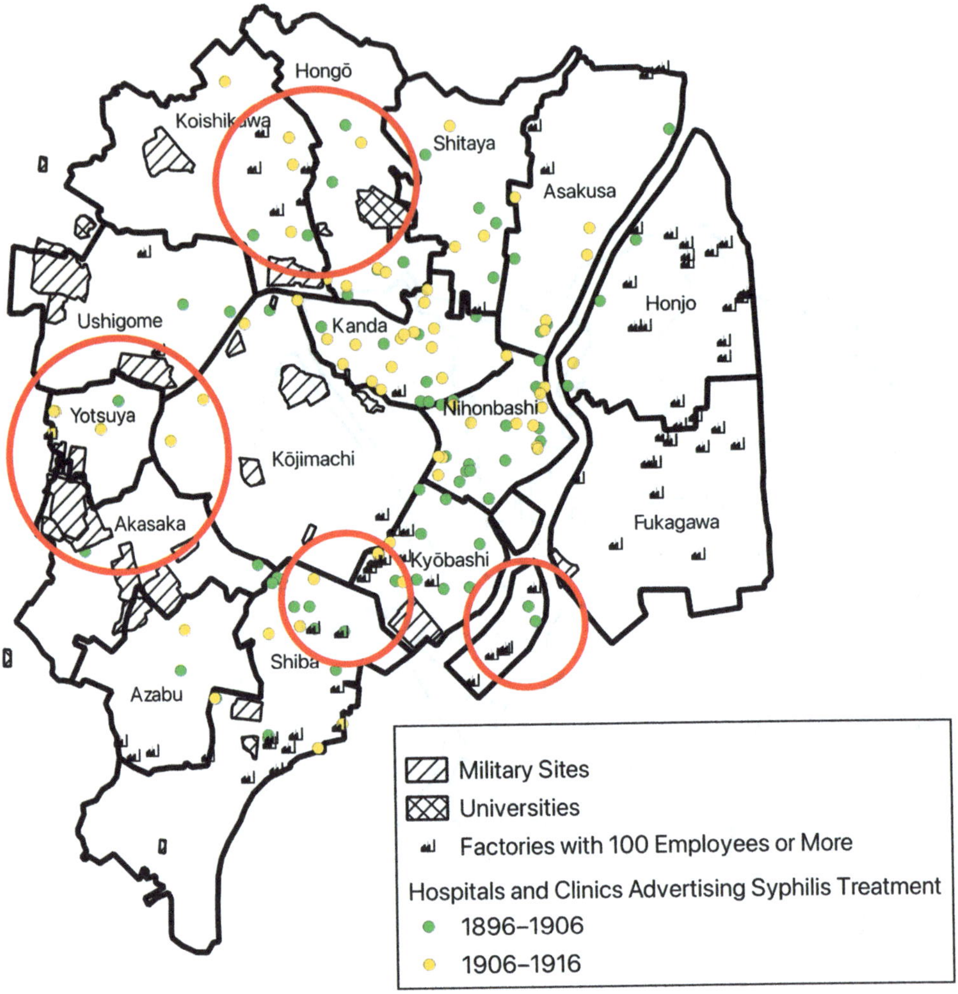

Plate 16. The location of syphilis hospitals and clinics advertising treatment for syphilis in relation to military facilities, universities, and factories. Data on the location of factories are from Tōkyō-fu, ed., *Taishō 3-nen Tōkyō-fu kōjō tōkeisho.*

Plate 17 (*opposite page*). Street sign for Dokumetsu, depicting the trademark, an image of Otto von Bismarck. From the collection of the Naitō Museum of Pharmaceutical Science and Industry, Gifu, Japan. Used with permission.

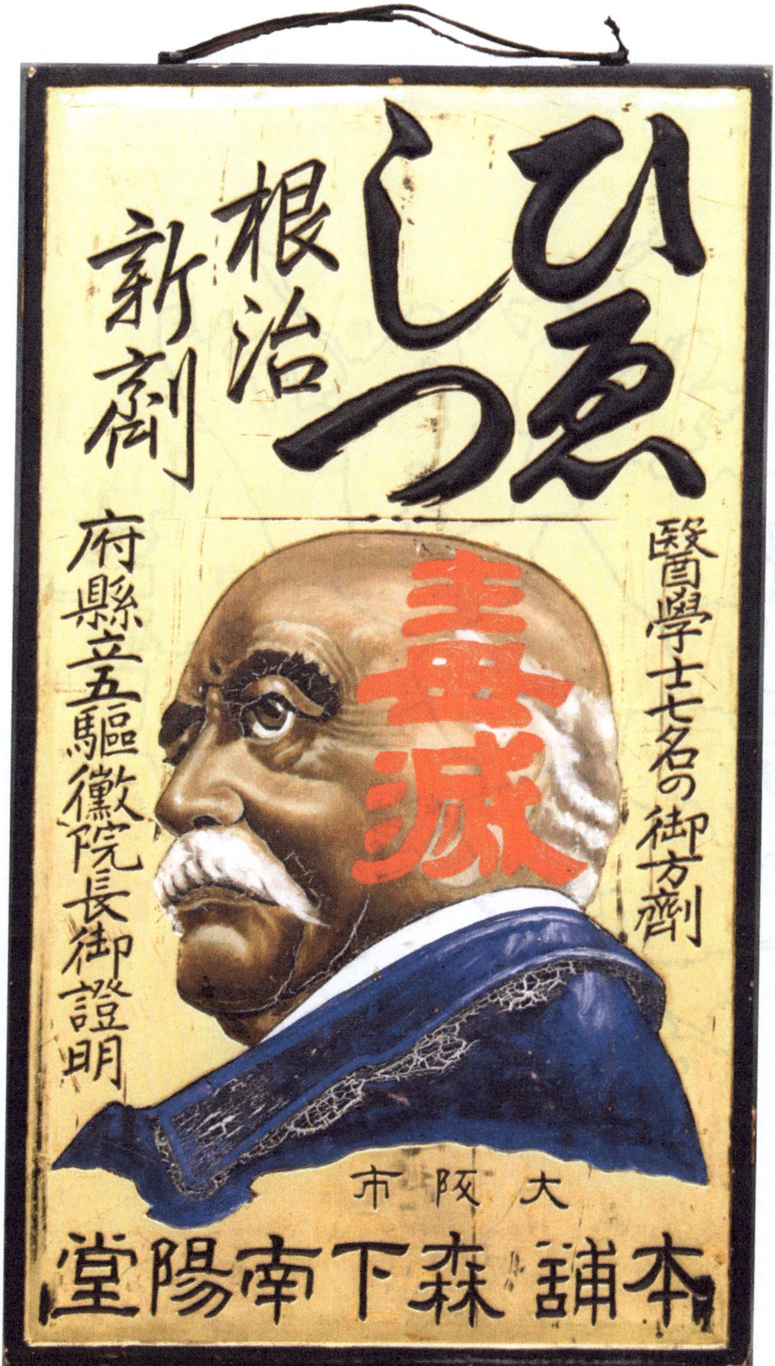
ひぜん
しつ
根治
新劑
醫學士七名の御方劑
毒滅
府縣立五驅黴院長御證明
大阪市
本舗　森下南陽堂

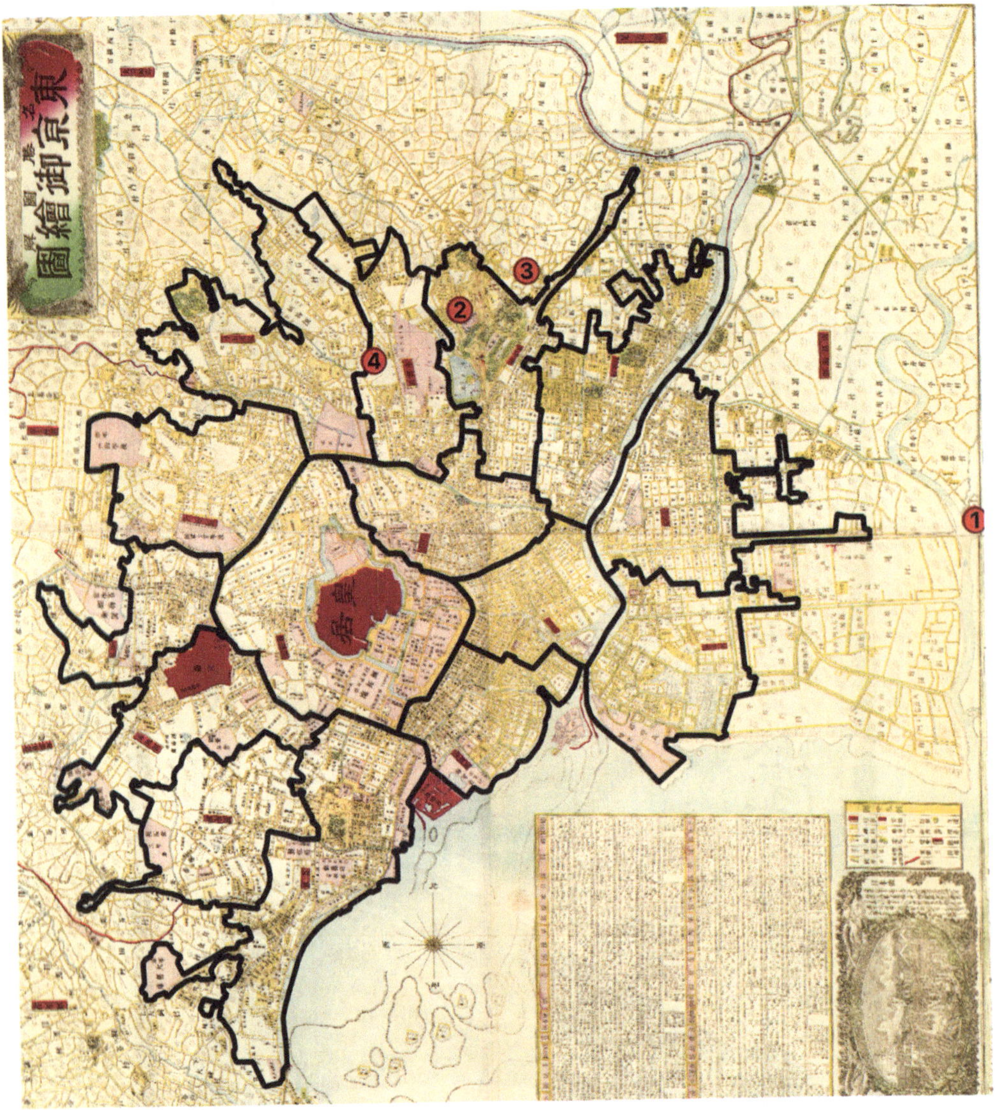

Plate 18. The Prefectural Asylum and Private Asylums, ca. 1880: (1) Komatsugawa Asylum, (2) Provisional Prefectural Asylum, (3) Negishi Hospital, and (4) Katō Asylum. The base map is from Itō Seisai, *Meishō zukai Tōkyō on ezu* (Tokyo: Kodama Yashichi, 1881). International Center for Japanese Studies (Nichibunken) Digital Map Collection, https://lapis.nichibun.ac.jp/chizu/map_detail.php?id=002147361. Used with permission.

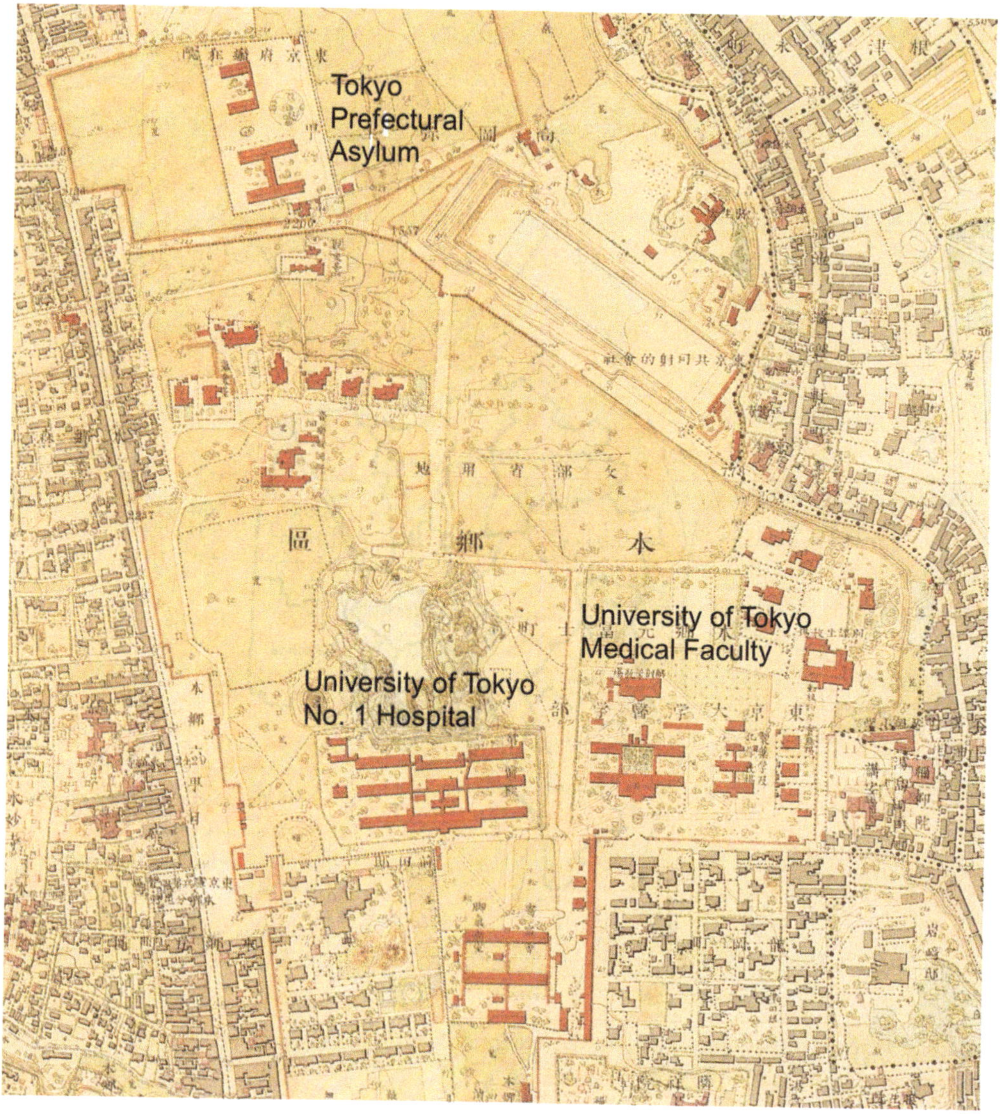

Plate 19. The environs of the Prefectural Asylum in Hongō. Detail from *Gosenbun no ichi Tōkyō-zu sokuryō genzu Tōkyō-fu Musashi no kuni Hongō-ku Motofuji-chō kinbō* (Tokyo: Sanbō honbu rikugunbu sokuryōkyoku, 1883). International Center for Japanese Studies (Nichibunken) Digital Map Collection, https://lapis.nichibun.ac.jp/chizu/map_detail.php?id=002275675-0013. Used with permission.

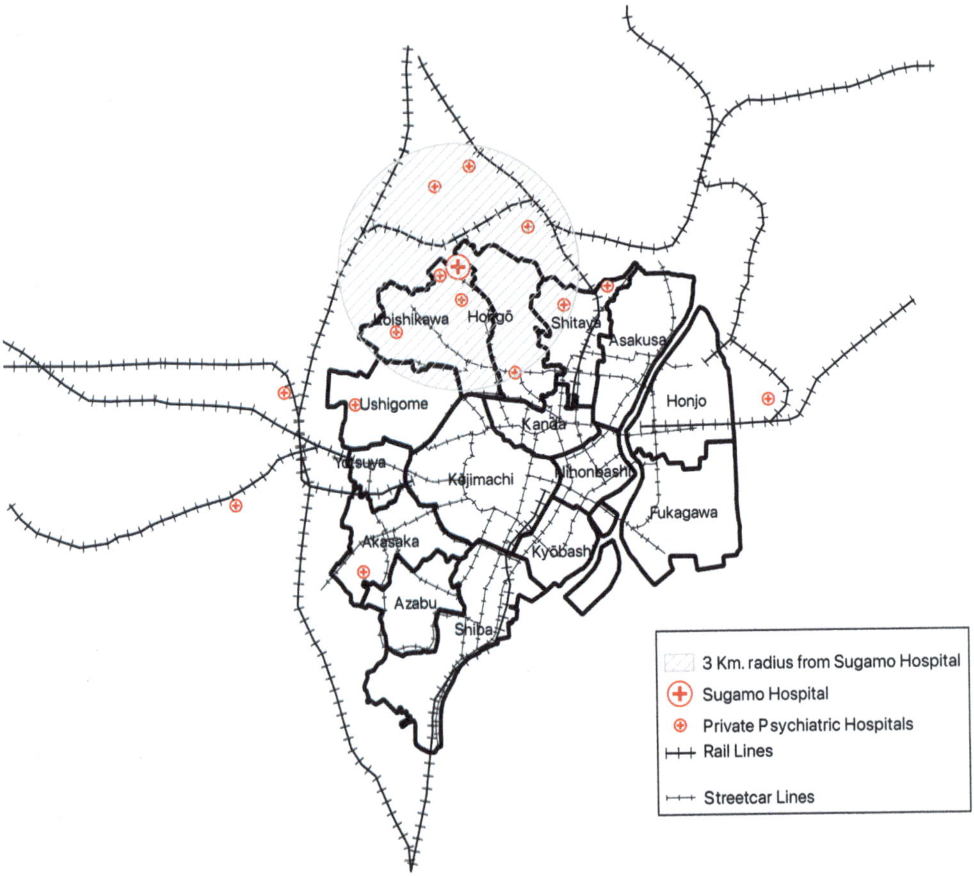

Plate 20. Psychiatric hospitals in and near Tokyo, ca, 1912. Information on the location of hospitals is from Imamichi, *Seishin byōsha kanchi tetsuzuki*.

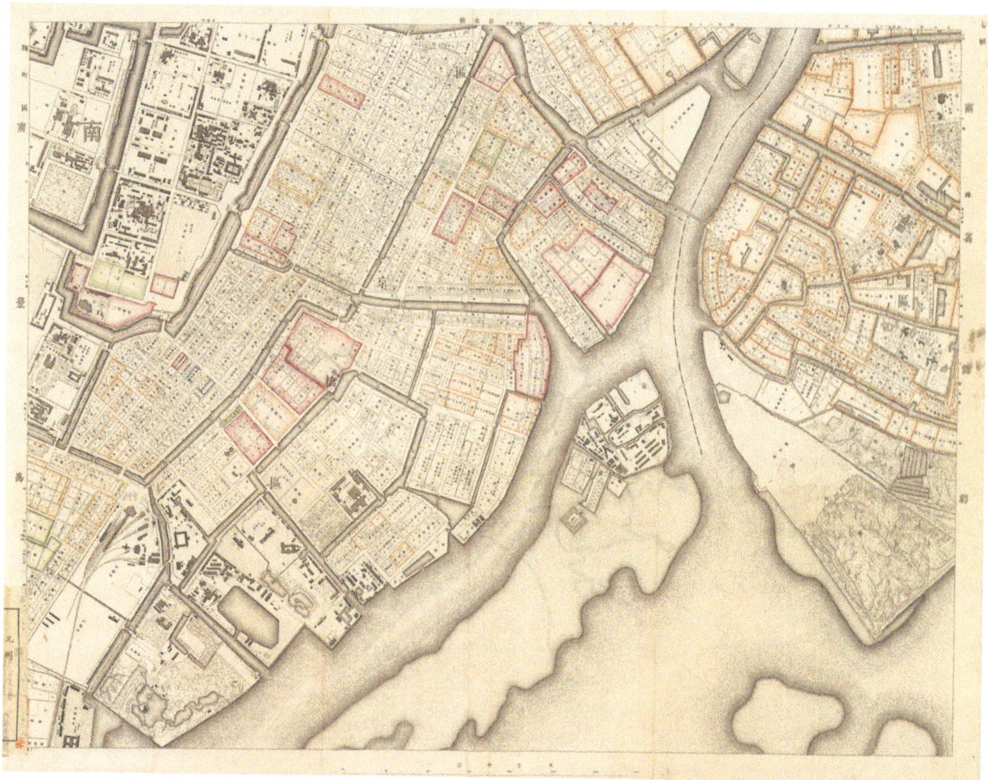

Plate 21. Map prepared by Tawara Yoshizumi showing the water quality of wells in Nihonbashi and Fukagawa. Red shading indicates poor water quality, and orangish-tan is used to indicate extreme levels of contamination. Courtesy of Tokyo Waterworks Historical Museum Digital Archive, https://www.ro-da.jp/suidorekishida/map/list?genre=2009&offset=0&limit=20.

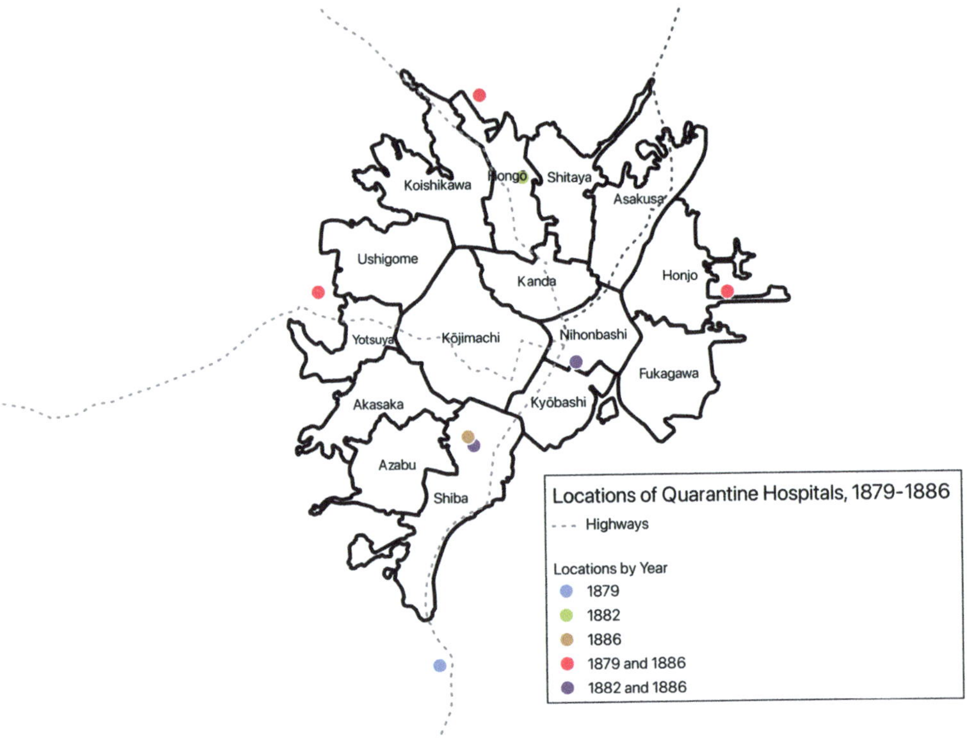

Plate 22. Quarantine hospitals established in 1879, 1882, and 1886. Information on locations from Tōkyō-fu, ed., *Tōkyō-fu shi, Gyōsei hen*, 6:666, 673–74.

Conclusion

Medical Modernity and Its Contradictions

This book has explored the process of medical modernization and the establishment of a public health regime in Tokyo in the first five decades of the modern era. Beginning in 1868, following the fall of the Tokugawa shogunate, bureaucrats associated with the new emperor-centered state began to call for medical reform. They viewed medicine, connected as it is to people's concerns about their own health, well-being, and longevity, as an important means to establish a new relationship between the emperor and his people. Measures to improve and safeguard the health of the Japanese people were initially intended to demonstrate the benevolence of the new state toward its subjects. The Medical Policy promulgated in 1874 set forth an ambitious template for reform that aimed to dismantle the laissez-faire medical marketplace of the early modern era. It called for a new system of education and licensing for medical professionals, the establishment of new medical institutions that would make modern medical care widely available, and the creation of a new administrative system that stretched from the central government in Tokyo to the grassroots level. Ordinary doctors had a crucial role to play in the medical system that was envisioned. They were to compile demographic data related to health, track outbreaks of infectious disease, and surveil the local environment for factors that might have an impact on health.

While the plan was national in scope, the new government made Tokyo a testing ground for the Medical Policy. There was a logic in this choice: Tokyo was the new capital, the most populous city, and the "face" of Japan for a growing number of international residents and visitors. These features distinguished it from Osaka and Kyoto, two other cities that were instructed to experiment with the Medical Policy, and they soon led to profound tensions between national and local interests that the other municipalities escaped. Nagayo Sensai, one of the architects of the Medical Policy, asserted that within the framework of national guidelines and goals, local communities should have autonomy to implement the medical reforms. In Tokyo, however, the creation of the Tokyo Metropolitan Police (TMP) under the Home Ministry complicated this stance, as did the chaotic conditions in the city in the 1870s: the result of population loss followed by an influx of migrants, the dissolution of the institutions of local governance, and the profound economic and social dislocations that accompanied the fall of the shogunate and the establishment of the new government.

Viewed from the vantage point of the late 1910s, it might seem that the medical reforms were successful. Over the course of half a century, medical care in Tokyo was transformed. Doctors of Sino-Japanese medicine had largely disappeared and were replaced by those trained in modern medical schools: some prestigious, some not. Hospitals and clinics, large and small, humble and grand, supplanted home-based care—at least for those who could afford their fees. For those who could not, over-the-counter medicines, both modern pharmaceuticals and traditional herbal medicines, promised relief from symptoms and even hope for a return to health. Walking down a street in Kanda, Nihonbashi, or Kyōbashi, or alighting from a streetcar in the city center, one would have been hard-pressed to avoid the visual evidence of the new healthscape, in the form of the hospitals, clinics, and pharmacies themselves as well as the ubiquitous advertisements for medical services and products that appeared on storefronts, telephone poles, and even as billboards, towering above the still low-lying city.

This visual evidence of medical modernity concealed the struggles that accompanied the reform process and the abandonment of key aspects of the original reform plan. As the TMP gradually assumed control of public health, the ethos of "protecting health" gave way to a new emphasis on "policing health," and concern for demonstrating benevolence was replaced by a new concern for "population," in the Foucauldian sense of the term. In other words, the aim of demonstrating the new state's legitimacy gave way to a new interest in improving statistical indexes of health, even if individuals and groups suffered under the weight of new policies. Under the TMP, prostitutes infected with syphilis were forcibly confined in police hospitals, the mentally ill were warehoused in the shabby communal rooms of private and public psychiatric hospitals, and cholera victims were transferred to quarantine hospitals where death rates could be as high as 70 percent.

Journalistic reportage and literary works offer some insight into how Tokyo residents negotiated the new meanings attached to health and disease. We have seen, for example, the resistance of the young prostitutes who lobbed sexually tinged insults at TMP physicians to protest the mandated syphilis exams, and the refusal of Horii Tsunejirō to allow the removal of his cholera-stricken children from his home. But equally telling were the works by Ishikawa Takuboku and Ozaki Kōyō. While the rules of the University of Tokyo Hospital made Ishikawa a useful case for teaching and research within the university hospital, he himself embraced his hospital stay as a retreat from the mundane yet burdensome constraints of work and family. In contrast, Ozaki's work reveals the complicated emotions that accompanied the embrace of the TMP's policing of health. The first person narrator of *Green Grapes* cycled from humiliation and anxiety at the presence of infectious disease within his household to a profound sense of relief when he decided to comply with public health regulations.

The contentious relationship between private physicians and prefectural authorities also shaped the medical system that emerged. The Medical Policy had imagined that private practice doctors would be the docile foot soldiers of medical reform, but Tokyo doctors responded by organizing to resist the prefecture's efforts to make health care available even to impoverished city residents via its system of ward doctors, "charitable care tickets," and the prefectural hospital. With the aim of protecting their financial interests, they lobbied effectively against the prefecture's efforts, characterizing it as an illegitimate extension of governmental power that undermined their livelihoods and exploited the taxpaying residents of the city. This exercise in self-interest came as the central government itself was attempting to shift responsibility for social welfare down to the localities so that it could focus on other national priorities. The resulting collapse of the ambitious and progressive prefectural system of accessible health care fundamentally altered the nature of the new medical culture, leaving poor and working-class residents of Tokyo to rely on the fragile safety net offered by a handful of charitable institutions and individuals.

As for-profit care became the norm, it ordered the distribution of medical providers and institutions around the city, limiting access to those who lived in the poorer wards, with Honjo and Fukagawa as notable examples. But the process of medical modernization, entangled as it was with medical capitalism and the extension of state power, reshaped the city in other ways as well. Concerns about syphilis and the identification of prostitutes as the nexus of infection led to the relocation of the Nezu brothels to Susaki in Fukagawa, an area known for its poor water supply and at times dangerous coastal conditions. Even before this change took place, the public clamor surrounding the examination of the prostitutes had rendered the syphilis hospitals attached to brothel areas as a new and uniquely modern kind of "famous place." With the aid of the TMP, these ostensibly medical institutions became the site of urban spectacles where the unfortunate women at the center of syphilis prevention efforts became objects of a sexualized gaze that simultaneously eroticized and degraded them.

Meanwhile, private syphilis clinics and hospitals, although widely dispersed around the city, were particularly prominent in sites associated with heightened concern for male health, including military installations, elite institutions of higher education, and factories. Largely ignored as the new gendered economy of syphilis treatment was inscribed in urban space were women like Nakajima Yoshi, with whose story I began chapter 4. For this twenty-year-old woman, the booming business of syphilis care apparently offered no hope of return to health and an ordinary life, leaving her to feel, it seems, that the waters of the Kanda River were her only option.

The rise of psychiatric medicine too left its traces on the cityscape. The relocation of the prefectural asylum first from Ueno and then from Hongō reveals the evolving priorities of local and national government officials. As Ueno was reimagined as the site of edifying leisure and Hongō as the home of elite higher education, it was deemed necessary to transfer the city's mentally ill to the margins of the city proper. By the early twentieth century, the northern part of Koishikawa Ward, formerly a patchwork of wet and dry fields, had become a center of psychiatric care not only for Tokyo but for the whole country. Hidden behind the walls and gates of Sugamo Hospital and the private psychiatric facilities that clustered around it was a complex and multitiered system of confinement that housed a heterogeneous population of patients, from the unruly members of the city's floating population of homeless people to members of the upper class exhausted by the exigencies of modern life, and many in between.

Cholera, the great scourge of nineteenth-century Japan, had the greatest impact on the built environment of the city and the lives of those within it. If syphilis and mental illness could be dismissed as problems of marginalized "others," cholera threatened all the city's residents. When waste and water were identified as the cause of the frequent epidemics, the city's toilets and wells were transformed from necessary aspects of everyday life to objects of fear and suspicion, precisely because they revealed the interconnectedness of the city's residents. That it took decades to address the dangers posed by the city's aging water system was a reflection on the strained finances of the new state but also a lack of political will to invest in social welfare. Ultimately, it was the poor of the city who bore the brunt of the repeated outbreaks of cholera. In the name of cholera prevention, poor neighborhoods were razed and new restrictions imposed on work and property. Worst of all, while those of means could escape the horrors of the quarantine hospitals, the poor could not.

The Janus-faced nature of medical modernization would shape life in Tokyo and Japan more generally well beyond the period explored in this work. The police control of public health established in Tokyo beginning in the 1870s, albeit with considerable contestation, became national policy in 1893 as part of a larger strategy of local government reform. Responding to this shift, Nagayo Sensai, reflecting the gender norms of the day, stated, "Giving the police complete control over public health is like a household that consists only of men with no women. This may seem to be very comfortable but [such a household] lacks real harmony and attentive care and in the end, this is not a path toward family fortune and longevity."[1] As this extended metaphor suggests, Nagayo regarded civic involvement in public health as necessary to curb police authority and bring about compliance and cooperation on the part of the public. Such concerns notwithstanding, the police-centered approach to public health was not only instituted in Japan but also simultaneously exported to the formal and informal colonies, often with devastating results for colonial subjects.[2]

Similarly, the limits of medical capitalism we observed in Tokyo were a precursor to developments nationwide. As we have seen, in the absence of policies designed to ensure access to health care, physicians in Tokyo established their clinics and hospitals in the more prosperous parts of the city. By the early 1920s, medical capitalism had led to the uneven distribution of doctors and clinics around the country and the proliferation of "doctorless villages." In 1923 a Home Ministry survey estimated that 25 percent of towns and villages in Japan lacked a single doctor. By 1936 it was reported that even in Tokyo Prefecture, despite its proximity to the center of modern medical education, at least twenty-one villages were doctorless.[3]

Like doctors in Tokyo who eschewed the poorer neighborhoods of the city, physicians around the country showed little interest in working in poor villages, leading to a cascade of problems that created growing disparities between urban and rural health, including higher rates of chronic disease, higher infant and maternal mortality, and shorter lifespans in the rural sector. Although this situation attracted considerable attention from bureaucrats, physicians, and others, the number of publicly funded medical facilities remained small. In 1935, for example, there were 3,002 hospitals in Japan, but more than 96 percent of these were private, for-profit, institutions.[4] Ironically, the choice of physicians to cluster in cities and larger towns led to extreme competition between them for patients, and as a result, significant numbers chose to leave Japan. Some sought their fortunes in the expanding empire while others followed Japanese migrants to Hawaii, the west coast of the US, Latin America, and elsewhere.[5]

It was only with the outbreak of war in 1937 that efforts were made to improve access to health care, driven by statist needs to expand the military and populate the empire. The passage of the Public Health Center Law in 1937, which funded a system of free public health clinics (*hokenjo*) in cities (including Tokyo), towns, and villages, was one such effort, as was the establishment of the Ministry of Health and Welfare (Kōseishō) and the passage of the National Health Insurance Law the follow year. While these developments arguably furthered the central government's powers over matters of medicine and public health, ultimately their effects on the health of ordinary citizens were constrained by exigencies of the war that contributed to the growth of health-care disparities. Real change came only in the postwar era as economic prosperity and universal access to high-quality health care increased life expectancy from forty-seven years in 1935, its prewar height, to almost eighty-five years by 2020.

Today only a few material traces of the healthscape of early twentieth-century Tokyo remain. Kanda is still a center of medical care with eight hospitals and 105 clinics, reflecting an association with medical institutions that dates to the early modern period.[6] Similarly, the four infectious disease hospitals established in 1886 to overcome the stigma and fear associated with the cholera-era quarantine hospitals are now general hospitals funded by the metropolitan government of Tokyo (Tōkyō-to). They still operate on their original sites, which were once Shibuya Village, Komagome, Honjo, and

Ōkubo. The establishment of the modern Tokyo waterworks in 1898 to aid in the fight against cholera is now memorialized in a metropolitan museum that tells a story of technological achievement. The celebratory tone of its exhibits conceals the dark history of water and waste in the city and the lack of political will that led to the deaths of thousands of people.[7] Sugamo Hospital was moved to what is now Setagaya Ward in 1919 and was renamed Matsuzawa Hospital. But the conditions that led private hospitals to cluster around the public psychiatric hospital in Koishikawa remained. Today Setagaya Ward is a psychiatric center within metropolitan Tokyo with forty-eight hospitals that offer specialized psychiatric care and more than a hundred outpatient clinics.[8]

The case of Tokyo in the first half-century of the modern era was both a bellwether and a cautionary lesson, albeit one that went largely unacknowledged and unaddressed by officials at every level. And today Tokyo again hints at an approaching medical crisis. A report issued by the Japanese Medical Association's Research Institute in 2012 on the "current status and future of local medical delivery systems" included a section on metropolitan Tokyo that detailed the peculiar situation. It noted that while Tokyo had the greatest concentration of doctors and hospitals in the country, they were clustered in the central and western wards, while the northeastern and eastern parts of the city, including Adachi, Katsushika, Arakawa, Sumida, Kōtō, and Edogawa had significantly fewer. The situation in the western and southern parts of the Tama region was even more dire.

This spatial disparity was not the only issue the city faced at the end of the first decade of the twenty-first century. The aging of the Japanese population notwithstanding, there was a critical scarcity of care facilities for the elderly, and a lack of other supporting medical personnel, including nurses, respiratory and physical therapists, among others.[9] Since 2012, such reports have continued, with the COVID pandemic prompting considerable hand-wringing over the lack of sufficient hospital beds in Tokyo.[10] A report issued by Tokyo's metropolitan health department in early 2024 noted the need for more obstetricians, gynecologists, pediatricians, and emergency care doctors and confirmed the spatial disparities within the greater metropolitan area.[11] In spite of the vast changes Tokyo has undergone in the past century and a half, the creation of a medical system that serves all its residents continues to be an elusive goal.

NOTES

Introduction: Medical Modernization and the Healthscaping of Tokyo

1. Galea, cited in Gharipour and DeClercq, *Epidemic Urbanism*, xxi.

2. Agostoni, *Monuments of Progress*; Molina, *Fit to Be Citizens?*; Armus, *Ailing City*; Risse, *Plague, Fear, and Politics*; Kerr, *Contagion, Isolation, and Biopolitics*; and Nakajima, *Body, Society, and Nation.*

3. Johnston, *Modern Epidemic*; Bay, *Beriberi in Modern Japan*; and Burns, *Kingdom of the Sick.*

4. Seidensticker, *Low City, High City*; Seidensticker, *Tokyo Rising*; Packard, *Old Tokyo*; and Mansfield, *Tokyo.*

5. Washington, *Church Space and the Capital*; Aso, *Public Properties*; Miller, *Nature of the Beasts.*

6. Hastings, *Neighborhood and Nation.*

7. Campbell, "Changing Role."

8. Kasahara, *Nihon no iryō gyōsei*; Kojima, *Nagayo Sensai*; and Kasahara and Kojima, *Meijiki iryō.*

9. Ishizuka, *Nihon kindai toshi iron*; and Kitahara, *Toshi to hinkon.*

10. Kobayashi Takehiro, *Kindai Nihon to kōshū eisei.*

11. Tōkyō-fu, *Tōkyō-fu tōkeisho Meiji 15-nen.*

12. On the limitations of the reliance on administrative units, see Rainham et al., "Conceptualizing the Healthscape," 669.

13. N. A., "Kyūmin ibun," *Kokumin shinbun*, June 15–16, 18, 20, 1890. Reprinted in Nakagawa Kiyoshi, *Meiji Tōkyō kasō seikatsushi*, 31–36. Kure Ayatoshi, "Tōkyō-fuka hinmin no jōkyō," *Sutachisuchikku zasshi* 57 (1891). Reprinted in Nakagawa Kiyoshi, *Meiji Tōkyō kasō seikatsushi*, 77–89.

14. Rainham et al., "Conceptualizing the Healthscape," 669.

15. Gottdiener, *Social Production of Urban Space.*

16. Clark, "From the Rise of Medicine," 105. Many thanks to Marta Hanson for introducing me to the concept of the "healthscape."

17. Gesler, "Therapeutic Landscapes."

18. *Healthscaping: Bio-Power, Space, and Society, 1200–1500* (ERC grant no. 724114). https://healthscapes.humanities.uva.nl/the-team/.

19. Geltner, "Healthscaping a Medieval City," 396. See also Geltner and Coomans, "Healthscaping Approach."

20. Porter, "Patient's View."

21. Weiner, *Citizen-Patient.*

22. Gilman, *Disease and Representation*, 7.

23. Rogaski, *Hygienic Modernity*.

Chapter 1. Medical Edo

1. Hanley, *Everyday Life*, 187–88.

2. Murakoshi Kazunori, "Daimyō no nyūji shibō ritsu." The focus on the warrior elite was born of necessity, since few population records for the commoners of the city have survived.

3. Masai, "Nimanbun no ichi," 15.

4. Masai, "Nimanbun no ichi," 11.

5. Calculated from information in Kōda Shigetomo, *Kōda Shigetomo chosakushū*, 263. See also Naitō, *Edo to Edo jō*.

6. Sippell, "Japan's First Urban Water Disaster."

7. Kuroki, *Edo no kaji*.

8. Fujikawa, *Nihon shippei shi*, 110, 182–287.

9. Kasai et al., "Research and Control of Parasitic Diseases, 230–35.

10. Slack, "Responses to Plague," 409–10.

11. On the work of the town magistrates, see Ishii, *Edo no machi bugyō*.

12. H. D. Smith, "Edo-Tokyo Transition," 368–69.

13. Ishigami, "Iseki kara mita toshi Edo no jōge suidō no kanri."

14. Suzuki, *Edo no hayari yamai*, 76–78.

15. Uramoto, *Edo Tōkyō*, 93, 99.

16. Uramoto, *Edo Tōkyō*, 100; Itahara and Kuwahara, "Edo jidai kōki . . . 5," 4.

17. Takayanagi, *Edo jidai hisabetsu mibunsō*, 59–60; and Ishii, *Edo no keibatsu*, 185–86.

18. Nishiyama M., *Edo chōnin no kenkyū*, 171.

19. N. A., "Yōjōsho no shimatsu," 72.

20. Tōkyō-shi, *Tōkyō shikō: Kyūsai*, 1:364–65.

21. Minami, *Edo no shakai kōzō*, 297.

22. Minami, *Edo no shakai kōzō*, 349–51, 355.

23. Minami, *Edo no shakai kōzō*, 300.

24. Ueda and Miura, *Nihon yakuenshi no rekishi*, 48–50.

25. Fukuhama, "Koishikawa Yōjōsho," 5.

26. Tōkyō-shi, *Tōkyō shikō: Kyūsai*, 1:350–51. See also Report submitted to Arima Ujinori dated June 24, 1723, in Juntendō Daigaku Komonjo Kenkyūkai, "Hinmin yōjōsho kiroku," 19. This is a collection of transcribed documents related to the Yōjōsho dated from 1722 to 1739.

27. Memorandum to the town magistrates, March 28, 1723, in Juntendō Daigaku Komonjo Kenkyūkai, "Hinmin yōjōsho kiroku," 23.

28. Orders to the *machi* headman regarding the Yōjōsho, dated July 3, 1723, in Juntendō Daigaku Komonjo Kenkyūkai, "Hinmin yōjōsho kiroku," 23; Memorandum to the town magistrates, dated March 28, 1873, in Juntendō Daigaku Komonjo Kenkyūkai, "Hinmin yōjōsho kiroku," 23.

29. Juntendō Daigaku Komonjo Kenkyūkai, "Hinmin yōjōsho kiroku," 29.

30. Tōkyō-shi, *Tōkyō shikō: Kyūsai*, 1:405.

31. Minami, *Edo no shakai kōzō*, 311.

32. Tode, "Igakukan ni okeru . . . (1)," 4.

33. Machi, "Igakukan no gakumon keisei 1," 351.

34. Machi, "Igakukan no gakumon keisei 1," 352.

35. Quoted in Tode, "Igakukan ni okeru . . . (1), 6.

36. Machi, "Igakukan no gakumon keisei 1," 348–49, 351.

37. Iwabuchi, "Kansei-Tempō," 48–49.

38. Machi, "Edo Igakukan," 18.

39. Machi, "Edo Igakukan," 20.

40. Machi, "Edo Igakukan," 19, 26.

41. On the historiography of the "medical marketplace," see Jenner and Wallis, *Medicine and the Market*, 1–23.

42. Takei and Inaba, *Edo kinsei ika jinmeiroku* (1819); Shiratsuchi, *Ika jinmeiroku* (1820); and Takei and Inaba, *Edo kinsei ika jinmeiroku* (1825).

43. Matsuzaki, "Sugita Genpaku," 15–16.

44. Sugita et al., *Kaitai shinsho*.

45. Matsuzaki, "Sugita Genpaku," 16–17.

46. Umihara, "Edo no rangakusha," 92.

47. Umihara, "Edo no rangakusha," 93–94.

48. For references to modes of transportation, see Sugi, *Sugita Genpaku zenshū*, vol. 1, "Isai nichiroku," 29, 68, 73.

49. Umihara, "Edo no rangakusha," 95.

50. On the early modern medicine trade, see Burns, "Marketing Health and Beauty."

51. Nakagawa and Katsushika, *Edo kaimono hitori annai*, vol. 2. In analyzing this text, I have made use of National Museum of Japanese History, "Database of Edo Merchants and Artisans."

52. For more on health care within Bakin's family, see Young, "Family Matters."

53. Nakayama, "Bakumatsu Edo," 282–84, 300.

54. Nakamura, "Mura to iryō," 37–38.

55. Minami, *Edo no shakai kōzō*, 310–11, 338.

56. Fukuhama, "Koishikawa Yōjōsho," 23.

57. Andō Yūichirō, *Edo no yōjōsho*, 178–80.

58. Fukuhama, "Koishikawa Yōjōsho," 17–18.

59. Minami, *Edo no shakai kōzō*, 305, 323–24.

60. Mori, "Tenpō kaikaku," 71–72.

61. Mori, "Tenpō kaikaku," 73–74.

62. Jannetta and Nakamura, "Translating Medical Knowledge."

63. Mori, "Tenpō kaikaku," 74–75.

64. Jannetta, *Vaccinators*, 132, 139–43.

65. Jannetta, *Vaccinators*, 159. On vaccination as a point of origin for public health, see, for example, Ehlers, *Give and Take*, 253–54.

66. Jannetta, *Vaccinators*, 161–62.

67. Yamamoto, *Nihon korera shi*, 14.

68. Yamamoto, *Nihon korera shi*, 6–7.

69. Singleton et al., "Effects of Temperature."

70. Kanagaki, *Ansei korori ryūkōki*, 11

71. Kanagaki, *Ansei korori ryūkōki*, 11–12, 14.

72. On the difficulty in calculating the number of deaths, see Yamaguchi, *Hasegawa Tai*, 19–23.

73. Yamazaki, "Otamagaike Shutōjo, 2," 188.

74. Yamazaki, "Otamagaike Shutōjo, 3," 205–7.

75. H. D. Smith, "Edo-Tokyo Transition," 348–53.

76. Naimushō, *Eiseikyoku nenpō*, 71.

77. H. D. Smith, "Edo-Tokyo Transition," 347.

78. Siddall, *Surgical Experiences*, 3.

79. Tōkyō Daigaku Igakubu Sōritsu Hyakunen Kinenkai and Tōkyō Daigaku Igakubu Hyakunenshi Henshū Iinkai, *Tōkyō Daigaku Igakubu hyakunenshi* , 96–98.

80. Siddall, *Surgical Experiences*, 4.

Chapter 2. The Medical Policy of 1874

1. Kōseishō Imukyoku, *Isei hyakunenshi*, 2:19.

2. Hochman, *Sanitation of Brazil*, 2.

3. McCrea, *Diseased Relations*, 4. On the case of Argentina, see Dimas, *Poisoned Eden*. On Ecuador, see A. K. Clark, *Conjuring the State*.

4. Nakano, *Nihon iji dainenpyō*, 196.

5. On Sagara, see Shinoda, *Shiroi gekiryū*.

6. Ozaki, "Meiji 'isei' saikō," 23.

7. Toyama, *Iryō fukushi*.

8. Kojima, *Nagayo Sensai*, 4–6.

9. On the history of the concept of "hygiene," see Mantovani and Marques, "Hygiene as Individual Practice."

10. Ogawa and Sakai, *Matsumoto Jun jiden*, 133–34.

11. Sugiura, "'Kenkō' to iu go." See also Kitazawa, *Kenkō no Nihonshi*, and Kano, *Kenkō-kan ni miru kindai*.

12. Quoted in Sugiura, "'Kenkō' to iu go," 249–50. Ogata, *Byōgaku tsūron*, 1.

13. Ogawa and Sakai, *Matsumoto Jun jiden*, 139. Johnston, *Modern Epidemic*, 179.

14. Quoted in Kasahara, "Kindai Nihon," 63.

15. Ozaki, "Meiji 'isei' saikō," 27.

16. Kōseishō Imukyoku, *Isei hyakunenshi*, 2:36. The parenthetical page numbers in the text are from this source.

17. Ueno, "Kishū han," 2–3.
18. Kōseishō Imukyoku, *Isei hyakunenshi*, 2:92–93.
19. Kōseishō Imukyoku, *Isei hyakunenshi*, 44.
20. Kōseishō Imukyoku, *Isei hyakunenshi*, 44.
21. Fujitani, *Splendid Monarchy*, 38.
22. Quoted in Shiomi, *Hinmin no teito*, 38.
23. Porter, "Meiji shoki Tōkyō," 170.
24. *Tōkyō-fu nisshi*, October 1, 1870.
25. Tōkyō Hyakunenshi Henshū Iinkai, *Tōkyō hyakunenshi*, 1:107.
26. Tōkyō-fu, ed., *Tōkyō-fu shi: Gyōseihen*, 1:877–78.
27. For an interesting study of the repurposing of warrior lands in early Meiji that makes use of GIS technology, see Yunoki, "Meiji shoki," 6, 21.
28. Ushigome,"Gojūkusei."
29. Matsukawa Yūsaku, "'Daiku shōku sei,'" 17–18.
30. Ushigome, "Tōkyō-fu ni okeru daiku shōku," 69–72.
31. Quoted in Kasahara, "Kindai Nihon," 63.
32. Ushigome, "Tōkyō-fu ni okeru daiku shōku," 68–69.
33. Westney, "Emulation of Western Organizations," 315–16.
34. *Yomiuri shinbun*, September 12, 1895, 5. For information on salaries, see Morinaga, *Bukka no bunkashi jiten*, 450.
35. See, for example, *Yomiuri shinbun*, July 23, 1885, 4; and *Yomiuri shinbun*, September 12, 1895, 5.
36. *Yomiuri shinbun*, June 8, 1877, 1; and *Yomiuri shinbun*, June 9, 1877, 1.
37. Kitahara, *Toshi to hinkon*, 336.
38. Fukuda, *Kaichū Tōkyō annai*, 11–12.
39. *Yomiuri shinbun*, December 15, 1878, 2.
40. Kitahara, *Toshi to hinkon*, 343–44; and Saiseikai, *Dai Nihon seyakuin shōshi*, 89.
41. *Yomiuri shinbun*, June 13, 1877, 1; and October 17, 1877, 1.
42. *Yomiuri shinbun*, May 18, 1880, 1.
43. Ishizuka, "Tōkyō no toshi suramu," 16.
44. *Yomiuri shinbun*, May 19, 1880, 1; and May 20, 1880, 1.
45. *Yomiuri shinbun*, July 10, 1881, 1.
46. *Yomiuri shinbun*, November 15, 1881, 2.
47. *Yomiuri shinbun*, June 11, 1903, 4.
48. *Yomiuri shinbun*, August 18, 1882, 1.
49. *Yomiuri shinbun*, March 31, 1894, 1; April 2, 1894, 2; April 6, 1894, 1; and May 2, 1895, 5.
50. *Yomiuri shinbun*, October 6, 1896, 5.
51. *Yomiuri shinbun*, October 3, 1895, 3.
52. *Yomiuri shinbun*, October 6, 1896, 5.
53. Burns, "In the Arena of the Courts."

54. *Yomiuri shinbun*, October 6, 1896, 5.
55. Burns, *Kingdom of the Sick*, 127–28.
56. Nakano, *Nihon iji dainenpyō*, 196.
57. *Yomiuri shinbun*, February 20, 1897, 3.
58. *Yomiuri shinbun*, April 1, 1887, 2.
59. Ikai, "Meiji-ki Nihon ni okeru," 50.
60. *Yomiuri shinbun*, February 25, 1897, 2; February 28, 1897, 5; and March 3, 1897, 5.

Chapter 3. Creating the Infrastructure of Medical Modernization

1. Nagao, *Aa ihei*, 50. Citations are from the reprint edition.
2. Fukazawa and Yasutake, "Nagasaki Kojima Yōjōsho," 1390–91.
3. Fukazawa and Yasutake, "Nagasaki Kojima Yōjōsho," 1391–92.
4. Kisacky, *Rise of the Modern Hospital*, 1, 9.
5. On nineteenth-century hospital architecture, see Taylor, *Hospital and Asylum Architecture*, 51–52; and Sugaya, *Nihon no byōin*, 18–19.
6. McFarlane, *Making of the Modern World*, 191.
7. Taylor, *Hospital and Asylum Architecture in England*, 54.
8. Fukunaga, *Nihon byōinshi*, 87–90; and Taylor, *Architect and the Pavilion Hospital*, 47–50.
9. Fukuzawa Yukichi, *Seiyō jijō*, 76–80.
10. I borrow the term "citizen-patient" from Weiner, *Citizen-Patient*. On hospitals in New York, see Opdyke, *No One Was Turned Away*, 19–23; on hospitals in London, see Waddington, *Charity and the London Hospitals*.
11. Kim, *Doctors of Empire*, 20–22.
12. Müller, "Tokio-Igaku."
13. Tōkyō Daigaku Igakubu Sōritsu Hyakunen Kinenkai and Tōkyō Daigaku Igakubu Hyakunenshi Henshū Iinkai, *Tōkyō Daigaku Igakubu hyakunenshi*, 232.
14. Müller, "Tokio-Igaku."324.
15. Teikoku Daigaku Ika Daigaku Dai Ichi Byōin, *Teikoku Daigaku Ika Daigaku iin ichiran Meiji 23 nen*, 11.
16. Tōkyō Daigaku Igakubu, *Tōkyō Daigaku Igakubu ichiran Meiji 16–17*, 123.
17. Morinaga, *Bukka no bunkashi jiten*, 398.
18. Tōkyō Daigaku Igakubu, *Tōkyō Daigaku Igakubu ichiran Meiji 13–14*, 178–79.
19. Kudō, ed., *Tōkyō iji tsūran*, 13.
20. Kudō, ed., *Tōkyō iji tsūran*, 13.
21. Kawakami, *Gendai Nihon iryōshi*, 26.
22. Nihon Shakai Jigyō Daigaku Kyūhin Seido Kenkyūkai, *Nihon no kyūhin seido*, 86.
23. Teikoku Daigaku Ika Daigaku Dai Ichi Byōin, *Teikoku Daigaku Ika Daigaku iin ichiran Meiji 23 nen*, 14–15.
24. Kawakami, *Gendai Nihon iryōshi*, 58.
25. Kawakami, *Gendai Nihon iryōshi*, 144–45.

26. Tōkyō-fu, *Tōkyō-fu tōkeisho Meiji 15-nen*, 23.

27. Tōkyō-fu, ed., *Tōkyō-fu shi: Gyōseihen*, 6:729.

28. Kawamoto and Fujisawa, *Tōkyō no hisabetsu buraku*, 119.

29. Takano, "Tōkyō ni okeru," 46, 56. Ishizuka, *Nihon kindai toshi ron*, 129.

30. Tokyo-fu, ed., *Tōkyō-fu shi: Gyōseihen*, 6:729.

31. Kitahara, *Toshi to hinkon*, 366–67.

32. On Hasegawa, see Yamaguchi, *Hasegawa Tai*; on Manning, see "Annotations: English Surgery in Japan," *Lancet* 116, no. 2974 (August 28, 1880), 349; on Beukema, see Umetani et al, *Oyatoi Gaikokujin*, 163–64.

33. See, for example, the announcements in *Yomiuri shinbun*, August 23, 1876, 4; August 30, 1876, 4; August 31, 1876, 4; September 6, 1876, 4; September 8, 1876, 4; September 11, 1876, 4; and September 14, 1876, 4.

34. See, for example, the advertisements in *Yomiuri shinbun*, August 4, 1876, 4; August 8, 1876, 4; August 12, 1876, 4; August 16, 1876, 4; August 21, 1876, 4; August 22, 1876, 4; and August 26, 1876, 4.

35. Tokyo-fu, ed., *Tōkyō-fu shi: Gyōseihen*, 6:730.

36. Tokyo-fu, ed., *Tōkyō-fu shi: Gyōseihen*, 6:730.

37. "Shinagawa ni Tōkyō-fu Byōin no bunkyoku wo setchi," *Yomiuri shinbun*, June 22, 1878.

38. "Koji no toriatsukai kata no kokoroe," *Yomiuri shinbun*, March 24, 1878, 3; and *Yomiuri shinbun*, March 25, 1878, 3; March 26, 1878, 3; March 27, 1878, 3; March 28, 1878, 3; March 29, 1878, 3; March 30, 1878, 3; March 31, 1878, 3; April 1, 1878, 3; April 2, 1878, 3; April 3, 1878, 3; April 4, 1878, 3; April 5, 1878, 3; April 6, 1878, 3

39. *Yomiuri shinbun*, January 19, 1879, 3.

40. *Yomiuri shinbun*, May 13, 1876, 1.

41. *Yomiuri shinbun*, February 7, 1875, 1.

42. Burns, "From 'Bad Karma' to 'Bad Blood': Medicalizing Rai in Early Modern Japan," chap. 2 in Burns, *Kingdom of the Sick*

43. Kawakami, *Gendai Nihon iryōshi*, 123–24.

44. Tōkyō-fu, *Tōkyō-fu tōkeisho Meiji 15-nen*, "Eisei," 7

45. Koishikawa-ku, *Koishikawa kukai shi*, 690–91.

46. Fukunaga, *Nihon byōninshi*, 220–23.

47. *Yomiuri shinbun*, March 3, 1878, 1.

48. *Yomiuri shinbun*, June 6, 1878, 3; December 3, 1878, 2.

49. Burns, "Body as Text."

50. Oyamada, "1890-nen ni kanritsu sanba gakkō setsuritsu sareru made no Tōkyō ni okeru sanba kyōiku," 102.

51. Takahashi, "Tōkyō-fu Byōin Sanba Kyōjujo no honmenjō sanba kyōiku ni kansuru kenkyū," 4–7.

52. Takahashi, "Shu-shi *Sanbaron* no hon'yaku to fuken e no kizō," 39–51.

53. *Yomiuri shinbun*, November 15, 1878, 2.

54. Tōkyō-fu, *Tōkyō-fu tōkeisho Taishō 1*, 3:47; *Tōkyō-fu tōkeisho Taishō 1*, 267–78; and *Tōkyō-fu tōkeisho Meiji 38-nen*, 224–25, 227–28.

55. *Yomiuri shinbun*, April 25, 1889, 2; August 3, 1882, 4; and September 5, 1883, 4.

56. See, for example, the advertisements in the *Yomiuri shinbun*, August 2, 1882, 4; August 8, 1882, 4; January 21, 1890, 4; and July 11, 1890, 4.

57. For example, the report of a man who was blinded by an acupuncture treatment was published in *Yomiuri shinbun*, February 25, 1875, 1.

58. *Yomiuri shinbun*, April 17, 1880, 1.

59. "Shinkyū eigyō torishimari kisoku aisadame," Tokyo Metropolitan Archive, doc. 614. B2. 02 (November 1885).

60. *Yomiuri shinbun*, November 23, 1907, 6.

61. Kōseishō Imukyoku, *Isei hyakunenshi*, 2:86–88.

62. Tōkyō-fu, *Tōkyō-fu tōkeisho Meiji 15-nen*.

63. Saiseikai, *Dai Nihon seyakuin shōshi*, 82.

64. Kitahara, *Toshi to hinkon*, 350.

65. *Yomiuri shinbun*, February 1, 1878, 3

66. *Yomiuri shinbun*, January 16, 1878, 3.

67. Tokyo Metropolitan Archives, doc. 610.C4.10 (1879).

68. Kitahara, *Toshi to hinkon*, 352–53.

69. Chūō Shakai Jigyō Kyōkai Shakai Jigyō Kenkyūkai, *Kindai iryō hogo*, 61.

70. Kitahara, *Toshi to hinkon*, 356.

71. Takaki, "Tōkyō seiikai iin igaku senmongakkō," in *Takaki Kanehiro den*, chap. 2; and "Tōkyō seiikai iin," in *Takaki Kanehiro den*, chap. 3.

72. Takaki, *Takaki Kanehiro den*, 125.

73. The petition is reproduced in Takaki, *Takaki Kanehiro den*, 126–27.

74. Chūō shakai jigyō shakai jigyō kenkyūkai, *Kindai iryo hogo*, 131–34.

75. Billings and Hurd, *Hospitals, Dispensaries, and Nursing*, 379–81.

76. The figures here and below are based on my analysis of the data from 1886 to 1898 in Tōkyō-fu, *Tōkyō-fu tōkeisho, Meiji 19-31*.

77. Billings and Hurd, *Hospitals, Dispensaries, and Nursing*, 380.

78. *Yomiuri shinbun*, March 27, 1893, 2; and March 29, 1893,1.

79. On Sano, see Miura, "Bakumatsu Pari banpaku"; and Tomita Hiroki, "Nihon Sekijūjisha."

80. Moorhead, *Dunant's Dream*, 23–29.

81. Tomita Hiroki, "Nihon Sekijūjisha."

82. Checkland, *Humanitarianism*, 30.

83. Nihon Sekijūjisha, *Nihon Sekijūjisha shikō*, 844–47.

84. *Yomiuri shinbun*, November 17, 1886, 2.

85. Nihon Sekijūjisha, *Nihon Sekijūjisha shikō*, 853–55.

86. Chūō Shakai Jigyō Kyōkai Shakai Jigyō Kenkyūkai, *Kindai iryō hogo*, 141–43.

87. Kudō, ed., *Tōkyō iji tsūran*, 54.

88. *Yomiuri shinbun*, July 7, 1888; February 24, 1890; March 13, 1890; March 14, 1893; and September 3, 1893.

89. Sōda, "Meiji shoki no igakkai jijō," 1277-83.

90. Tōkyō-fu, *Tōkyō-fu tōkeisho, vol. 5, Tōkyō-fu tōkeisho Meiji 19 nen*, 9–10.

91. See, for example, Satō, *Tōkyō hitori annai*; and Nagai, *Tōkyō hyakujiben*.

92. Gyōseisha, *Saikin chōsa Tōkyō iryō annai*.

93. Sōmuchō, Tōkeikyoku, and Nihon Tōkei Kyōkai, *Nihon Chōki Tōkei Sōran*, 228–30. Morinaga, *Bukka no bunkashi jiten*, 395.

94. Kudō, ed., *Nihon Tōkyō iji tsūran*, 71–75.

95. Kudō, ed., *Nihon Tōkyō iji tsūran*. The parenthetical page numbers in the text are from this source.

96. Kudō,ed., *Nihon Tōkyō iji tsūran*, 227–30; and Oyamada, "1890-nen ni kanritsu," 103.

97. Sugita Masayuki, *Saishin jitsuyō Tōkyō densha annai*, 155–68.

98. Gyōseisha, *Saikin chōsa Tōkyō iryō annai*, chap. 1: 28.

99. Quoted in Nagao, *Aa ihei*, 47.

100. Quoted in Nagao, *Aa ihei*, 47–48.

101. Okitsu et al., *Meiji Bungaku zenshū*, 333.

102. Tōkyō-fu, *Tōkyō-fu tōkeisho Meiji 15-nen*, 7.

103. Tōkyō-fu, *Tōkyō-fu tōkeisho Taishō 1*, 2–3, 47.

Chapter 4. Sex(ually Transmitted Diseases) and the City

1. *Yomiuri shinbun*, November 17, 1909, 3.

2. In Japanese, the term for syphilis is *baidoku* ("berry poison") and *baisō* ("berry rash"). The term *bai* is believed to derive from word for bayberry (*yōbai*), presumably because the small red fruit of this shrub resembles the syphilitic chancre. Colloquially, the disease was often simply termed *kasa* ("the pox").

3. Singh and Romanowski, "Syphilis."

4. Suzuki Noriko, "Edo jidai," 39.

5. Suzuki Noriko, "Edo jidai," 60–62.

6. Kariya, *Edo no seibyō*, 53.

7. Quoted in Tatsukawa, "Edo jidai," 30.

8. Takao Suzuki, *Palaeopathological and Palaeoepidemiological Study*, 40.

9. Kariya, *Edo no seibyō*, 33–34.

10. On the rise of "private" prostitution, see Stanley, *Selling Women*.

11. Quoted in Suzuki Noriko, "Edo jidai," 56.

12. Burns, "Bodies and Borders," 4–5.

13. On the use of mercury to treat syphilis, see O'Shea, "'Two Minutes with Venus.'" On syphilis treatments in early modern Japan, see Kariya, *Edo no seibyō*, 71–78. On the use of chinaroot in Europe, see Winterbottom, "Of the Chinaroot."

14. On the examination of prostitutes in Europe, see Garcia et al., *Selling Sex in the City*, chap. 5–7. On colonial India, see Levine, "Venereal Disease."

15. Ogawa and Sakai, *Matsumoto Jun jiden*, 42–43.

16. "Baidokuin toritate," Tokyo Metropolitan Archives, 605.A4.10, Item no. 000113330, and "Nezu Gongen keidai e baidokuin toritate no gi ni tsuki," National Archives of Japan, Ta 037509 (Tamon Yagura Monjo).

17. "Nezu monzen baidokuin toritatechō."

18. Ogawa and Sakai, *Matsumoto Jun jiden*, 45.

19. Yokohama-shi, *Yokohama-shi shikō fūzokuhen*, 410–11.

20. Ion, "Sexual Imperialism."

21. Harrison, "Health, Sovereignty and Imperialism," 51.

22. Ion, "Sexual Imperialism," 731.

23. "Tōkyō-fu yori kin 500 ryō jimugakusho, shutōkan, baidokuin, on'yakuen go-nyūyōkin haraitsukawasu," Tokyo Metropolitan Archives, 605.A6.14, Item no. 000114461.

24. "Goke Koto to segare Daikichi gi baidokuin tai'in ni tsuki," February 27, 1870. Tokyo Metropolitan Archives, 605.C4.15, Item no. 00019202.

25. "Tōkyō-fuka ni baidokuin wo kensetsusen koto wo kou," Japan Center for Asian Historical Records (JACAR) Ref. A15070668400, 2.

26. "Tōkyō-fuka ni baidokuin wo kensetsusen koto wo kou," 2.

27. "Tōkyō-fuka ni baidokuin wo kensetsusen koto wo kou," 2–3. On the value of currency in this period, see Asahi Shinbunsha Shūkan Asahi Henshūbu, *Sengo nedanshi nenpyō*.

28. "Tōkyō-fuka ni baidokuin wo kensetsusen koto wo kou," 3.

29. "Kinrai kakuchihō baita hanshoku ni tsuki baidoku densen shōgai no shisetsu sōritsu sashimu," Tokyo Metropolitan Archives, 632.B2.07, 632.C3.27, Item no. 000115475.

30. "Shinbun zasshi," no. 32 (February 1872), in Kimura and Meiji Bunka Kenkyūkai, *Bakumatsu Meiji shinbun zenshū*, vol. 6, part 2, 28.

31. Nakanishi and Higuchi, "Kyōkan Gijuku no kenkyū," 352–54. See also Yoshikawa, *Shin Yoshiwara*, 59.

32. Kawasaki, "Tsukiji iryūchi."

33. Nakanishi and Higuchi, "Kyōkan Gijuku no kenkyū," 350.

34. Nakanishi and Higuchi, "Kyōkan Gijuku no kenkyū," 347.

35. On the *Maria Luz* incident, see Howland, "*Maria Luz* Incident"; Botsman, "Freedom Without Slavery?"

36. Ikeda et al., eds., *Shiryō Nihon kindai hō*, 9.

37. Maki, *Kinsei Nihon no jinshin baibai*, 356–57.

38. Maki, *Kinsei Nihon no jinshin baibai*, 362–63.

39. *Tōkyō nichinichi shinbun*, October 10, 1872, 1.

40. "Tōkyō-fu chiji yori shizai kaku kuchō kochō e," Tokyo Metropolitan Archives, 606.B7.08 (66), Item no. 000111924.

41. Tōkyō-fu, ed., *Shōgi geigi kaihō shiryō*, 3,6, 8.

42. Tōkyō-fu, ed., *Shōgi geigi kaihō shiryō*, 3–4, 7–8.

43. Tōkyō-fu, ed., *Shōgi geigi kaihō shiryō*, 4–6.

44. Quoted in Tōkyō-fu, ed., *Tōkyō-fu shi: Gyōseihen*, 6:774.

45. Yamamoto, *Baishun seibyō shi*, 45–46.

46. *Yomiuri shinbun*, February 13, 1878, 1, and July 27, 1878, 3. Scott, *Weapons of the Weak*.

47. "Baidoku kensa no migiri haigyō mōshitate ni tsuki," Tokyo Metropolitan Archives, 606.A7.06, Item no. 000118218; "Shōgi kasegi no mono baidoku kensa no tame byōin kakari kan'in kata kakusho e shutchō torishirabe no setsu haigyō itashi mune mōshitate," Tokyo Metropolitan Archives, 606.B6.08, Item no. 000111917.

48. "Dai san daiku jū shōku Yotsuya Ōban-chō Miyahara Yuzō nijo Sen gi baidoku ni tsuki shōgi fukin menjo no ken"; "Daigo daiku yon shōku Kanda Kamezumi-chō Tsuruta Tetsugorō imo Kame baidoku ni tsuki shōgi fukin menjo no ken," Tokyo Metropolitan Archives, 607.B8.04, Item no. 000118250.

49. *Yomiuri shinbun* April 8, 1875, 1.

50. "Sangyō kaisha kisoku," Tokyo Metropolitan Archives, 607.B3.01, Item no. 000114654.

51. *Yomiuri shinbun*, May 2, 1875, 1.

52. See, for example, *Yomiuri shinbun*, January 28, 1875, 1; and February 25, 1875, 1.

53. Fukuda, *Kaichū Tōkyō annai*, 37.

54. *Yomiuri shinbun*, March 3, 1878, 3.

55. *Yomiuri shinbun*, April 19, 1878, 3.

56. Arai Shin, *Nihon keisatsu zensho*, 358–61.

57. *Yomiuri shinbun*, March 1, 1878, 2.

58. *Yomiuri shinbun*, April 19, 1878, 3.

59. *Yomiuri shinbun*, July 16, 1878, 1.

60. *Yomiuri shinbun*, June 5, 1878, 1; and June 28, 1883, 2.

61. *Yomiuri shinbun*, August 7, 1885, 1; November 27, 1885, 4; December 8, 1885, 2; July 27, 1886, 3; August 3, 1886, 3; and August 31, 1886, 4.

62. *Yomiuri shinbun*, February 10, 1889, 2.

63. *Kanayomi shinbun*, August 29, 1877, 1; and *Yomiuri shinbun*, September 1, 1877, 1.

64. *Yomiuri shinbun*, July 8, 1896, 3.

65. Ajioka, *Baidoku kensa no wake*, 132–35.

66. Suita Dōshi [Tajima Shōi], *Karyū jijō*, 1:55.

67. Suita Dōshi [Tajima Shōi], *Karyū jijō*, 1:33, 30–31.

68. Fujino Yutaka, "Baidoku byōin dai yonji nenpyō," in Yunomae and Akisada, *Baibaishun mondai*, 14:216.

69. Keishichō, ed., *Keishichō shikō*, 56–57.

70. *Yomiuri shinbun*, March 16, 1882, 1.

71. Katsuragi and Furusawa, *Yoshiwara yūkaku no uramen*, 281–82.

72. Kaneda, *Susaki no shiori*, 19–20.

73. *Yomiuri shinbun*, July 5, 1888, 3; and July 10, 188, 3.

74. *Yomiuri shinbun*, July 28, 1911, 3.

75. Suematsu Jun, ed., *Susaki Byōin*, 4–5.

76. Yamamotō, *Baishun seibyō shi*, 51.

77. Naimushō Eiseikyoku, *Karyūbyō chōsahyō*, 1.

78. Naimusho Eiseikyoku, *Karyūbyō chōsahyō*, 78, 84–87.

79. *Yomiuri shinbun*, March 1, 1893, 4; and *Asahi shinbun*, February 11, 1900, 4. For biographical information, see the Jinji Kōshinroku Database, https://jahis.law.nagoya-u.ac.jp/who/docs/who8-15003.

80. "Obituary: Keizo Dohi, MD, 1866–1931."

81. Rikugunshō, *Rikugun ni okeru*, 52–53.

82. *Yomiuri shinbun*, August 15, 1893, 2; and *Asahi shinbun*, August 15, 1893, 6.

83. *Asahi shinbun*, August 9, 1987, 8; July 4, 1889, 7; September 8, 1889, 8; April 1, 1900, 2; June 5, 1900, 7; and January 22, 1911, 7.

84. C. M. Smith, "Have the Early Claims of Salvarsan Been Realized?" 269.

85. For biographical information on Katō, see Takasu, "Katō Tokijirō ni tsuite," 417–19. *Yomiuri shinbun*, February 16, 1884, 4; December 17, 1887, 4; and March 26, 1886, 4.

86. *Yomiuri shinbun*, October 9, 1890, 4; and February 1, 1891, 2.

87. Takasu, "Katō Tokijirō ni tsuite," 419. *Yomiuri shinbun* May 13, 1885, 2; August 15, 1885; *Asahi shinbun* July 4, 1903, 3; and August 29, 1916, 5.

88. Information on fees is from Gyōseisha, *Saikin chōsa Tōkyō iryō annai* , chap. 2: 14–15, 21–22; chap. 8: 1–2.

89. Naito Pharmaceutical Museum, https://www.eisai.co.jp/museum/information/topics/topics14_12.html.

90. Information on pricing comes from an advertisement in *Yomiuri shinbun*, April 3, 1901, 6.

Chapter 5. Psychiatric Care in Tokyo

1. Kure, "Seishinbyō kanja" (1891).

2. Naimushō Eiseikyoku, *Seishin byōsha*, 2–3.

3. Okada Yasuo, "Kaidai," in Okada and Sakai, *Kindai shomin seikatsushi*, 588.

4. Itahara and Kuwahara, "Edo jidai kōki . . . 4," 82–83.

5. Hiruta, "Edo jidai ni okeru," 27.

6. Hiruta, "Edo jidai ni okeru," 27.

7. Itahara and Kuwahara, "Edo jidai kōki . . . 1," 42–47.

8. Yamazaki, "Seishin byōsha taigū."

9. Itahara and Kuwahara, "Edo jidai kōki . . . 2," 108–9.

10. Itahara and Kuwahara, "Edo jidai kōki . . . 2," 103.

11. Yamazaki, "Seishin byōsha taigū," 56.

12. Yamazaki, "Seishin byōsha taigū," 61.

13. Itahara and Kuwahara, "Edo jidai kōki . . . 4," 88.

14. Burns, "Relocating Psychiatric Knowledge."

15. Kobayashi Yasuhiko, "Edo jidai no seishin igaku 2."

16. Omata, *Seishin byōin no kigen*, 65–69. Kanegawa and Hori, *Seishin byōin no shakaishi*, 17–18.

17. Hiruta, "Edo jidai no seishin igaku," 41–43.

18. Tōkyo Seishin Byōin Kyōkai, *Tōkyō no shiritsu seishin byōin shi*, 33.

19. Narabayashi Makoto, "Kyūbaku jidai."

20. Fukuzawa, "Seiyō jijō," 309.

21. Kume, *Tokumei zenken taishi Bei-ō*, 115.

22. Brown and Hirota, *Diary of Kido Takayoshi*, 121

23. Kitahara, *Toshi to hinkon*, 264; and Kitahara, "Toshi ni okeru," 427.

24. Porter, "Meiji shoki Tōkyō," 166–67.

25. Buraku Kaihō Kenkyūjo, *Shiryōshū*, 355.

26. Tōkyō Yōikuin, *Yōikuin rokujūnenshi*, 45.

27. Tōkyō Yōikuin, *Yōikuin rokujūnenshi*, 42–45.

28. Shibusawa, *Tōkyō Yōikuin sōritsu gojūshūnen*, 4.

29. Tōkyō Yōikuin, *Yōikuin rokujūnenshi*, 52.

30. Tōkyō Yōikuin, *Yōikuin rokujūnenshi*, 55, 111.

31. Tōkyō Yōikuin, *Yōikuin rokujūnenshi*, 85.

32. Tomita Mikio, *Seishin byōin no teiryū*, 161–62.

33. Quoted in Okada et al., "Shitaku kanchi no unmei," 511.

34. Tōkyō Yōikuin, *Yōikuin rokujūnenshi*, 114–15.

35. Buraku kaihō kenkyūjo, *Shiryōshū*, 692.

36. Tōkyō Yōikuin, *Yōikuin rokujūnenshi*, 197–98, 201–2.

37. Kure and Kashida, *Waga kuni ni okeru seishinbyō*, 61.

38. *Yomiuri shinbun*, November 4, 1879, 3; May 12, 1880, 3; and November 28, 1880, 1.

39. *Yomiuri shinbun*, November 19, 1879, 1; and March 24, 1880, 2.

40. Kitahara, *Toshi to hinkon*, 326–27. The documents Kitahara examined, housed at the Tokyo Metropolitan Archives, were made inaccessible to researchers in 1995 due to privacy concerns.

41. Tōkyō Keishi Kangokusho, *Keishi honsho tasshi yōsan*, 896–97.

42. Tomita Mikio, *Seishin byōin no teiryū*, 162.

43. Tōkyō-fu, *Tōkyō-fu tōkeisho Meiji 15-nen*, 9.

44. *Yomiuri shinbun*, June 6, 1880, 4.

45. Tōkyo Seishin Byōin Kyōkai, *Tōkyō no shiritsu seishin byōin shi*, 42–43.

46. Kure, "Ko Ika Daigaku."

47. Sakaky, "Ueber das Irrenwesen in Japan," 148.

48. *Yomiuri shinbun*, June 6, 1882, 4; and March 25, 1881, 1.

49. Tōkyō-fu, *Tōkyō-fu tōkeisho Meiji 15-nen*,10; and *Tōkyō-fu tōkeisho Meiji 19-nen*, 272.

50. *Yomiuri shinbun*, October 11, 1889, 4; September 21, 1880, 4; and January 22, 1982, 4.

51. Kure and Kashida, *Waga kuni ni okeru seishinbyō*, 52; and Okada, *Shisetsu Matsuzawa Byōin shi*, 216.

52. Information on patient number is from *Tōkyō-fu tōkeisho* for the period 1882–92. For patient fees, see *Yomiuri shinbun*, August 15, 1882, 4.

53. Kure and Kashida, *Waga kuni ni okeru seishinbyō*, 62.

54. Kaneko, *Matsuzawa Byōin gaishi*, 67–68.

55. Kure and Kashida, *Waga kuni ni okeru seishinbyō*, 62, 66.

56. Kure and Kashida, *Waga kuni ni okeru seishinbyō*, 71–72.

57. Kure and Kashida, *Waga kuni ni okeru seishinbyō*, 98, 99.

58. Kure and Kashida, *Waga kuni ni okeru seishinbyō*, 97.

59. Bereridge and Renvoize, "Electricity"; and Shorter, *History of Psychiatry*, 120.

60. Ayabe, "Seishin shōgaisha shisetsu," 97.

61. Ayabe, "Seishin shōgaisha shisetsu," 97.

62. Kaneko, *Matsuzawa Byōin gaishi*, 50.

63. *Yomiuri shinbun*, April 27, 1878, 3.

64. Tōkyō Metropolitan Archives, folder 601.A4.13, ID no. 000113941, November 4 and December 21, 1881.

65. Sakaky, "Ueber das Irrenwesen in Japan," 147–48.

66. Ayabe, "Seishin shōgaisha shisetsu," 99.

67. Kure and Kashida, *Waga kuni ni okeru seishinbyō*, 27–28.

68. Tokyo Metropolitan Archives, folder 614.D7.12, ID no. 000116437, 1884.

69. Uchimura, "Sakaki Sensei to Tōkyō."

70. Sakaki, "Tōkyō-fu Tenkyōin no kanja."

71. Sakaki, "Tenkyōin setsuritsu no hitsuyō," 3.

72. Maudsley, *Seishinbyō yakusetsu*, 15.

73. I have not been able to identify Schūle's work. My translation is based on Eguchi, *Seishinbyōgaku*, 73.

74. Kure, *Seishinbyōgaku shūyō*, 1:86–87.

75. Kure and Kashida, *Waga kuni ni okeru seishinbyō*, 73. *Yomiuri shinbun*, March 28, 1885, 2.

76. Tōkyō-fu, *Tōkyō-fu tōkeisho Meiji 15-nen*, 65, 69.

77. Peterson, "Insane in Japan," 2–3.

78. Okada, *Shisetsu Matsuzawa Byōin shi*, 141.

79. Kure and Kashida, *Waga kuni ni okeru seishinbyō*, 153–56.

80. *Yomiuri shinbun*, July 9, 1890, 4.

81. Tanabe, "Seishin byōsha."

82. Kure, "Seishinbyō kanja jikken kiji."

83. Onodera, "Seishin byōsha . . . Tanjunsei yūutsu kyō"; and Onodera, "Seishin byōsha . . . Shusei chūdoku henshitsukyō."

84. Peterson, "Insane in Japan," 13–14.

85. Sōma Kyūshin Jimusho, *Sōma jitsuden*, 15.

86. Sōma Kyūshin Jimusho, *Sōma jitsuden*, 47.

87. Keishichō, ed., *Keishichōrei ruisan*, 5th ed., 409.

88. Keishichō, ed., *Keishichōrei ruisan*, 5th ed., 410–11.

89. Sōma Kyūshin Jimusho, *Sōma jitsuden*, 55–56.

90. Takahashi Tetsuo, *Shinsō Sōma jiken*, 34.

91. Kure and Kashida, *Waga kuni ni okeru seishinbyō*, 117–20.

92. Keishichō, ed., *Keishichōrei ruisan*, 5th ed., 739–40.

93. For the text of the law, see Kōseishō Imukyoku, *Isei hyakunenshi*, 2:262–66.

94. For more on the 1900 law and its impact until 1945, see Akihito Suzuki, "State, Family and the Insane."

95. See, for example, Kure and Kashida, *Seishin byōsha shitaku kanchi*, 138.

96. Nishikawa, *Nihon seishin shōgisha seisakushi*, 54.

97. Hashimoto, *Seishin byōsha to shitaku kanchi*, 151.

98. In identifying the hospitals, I have relied upon Kure and Kashida, *Waga kuni ni okeru seishinbyō*; Okada and Sakai, *Byōki eisei*, 183–223; and Tōkyo Seishin Byōin Kyōkai, *Tōkyō no shiritsu seishin byōin shi*.

99. *Yomiuri shinbun*, December 13, 1898, 4.

100. Nagao, *Aa ihei*, 38.

101. *Yomiuri shinbun*, October 29, 1889, 3; April 18, 1897, 4; April 15, 1902, 4; and September 22, 1907, 3.

102. Okada, *Shisetsu Matsuzawa Byōin shi*, 187.

103. Tōkyo Seishin Byōin Kyōkai, *Tōkyō no shiritsu seishin byōin shi*, 69–70. Information on his salary is from Okada, *Shisetsu Matsuzawa Byōin shi*, 214.

104. Okada, *Shisetsu Matsuzawa Byōin shi*, 214.

105. Kure and Kashida, *Waga kuni ni okeru seishinbyō*, 51–52. On the use of "rest homes" to describe psychiatric facilities, see Burns, "Reinvented Places."

106. Tōkyo Seishin Byōin Kyōkai, *Tōkyō no shiritsu seishin byōin shi*, 121–22, 125–26.

107. Tōkyo Seishin Byōin Kyōkai, *Tōkyō no shiritsu seishin byōin shi*, 110–12. *Yomiuri shinbun*, May 5, 1903, 4; and February 4, 1906, 4.

108. Yamada, "Meiji-ki no kaigyōi," 382–83.

109. Ishikawa, "Seishin byōsha no kanchi ni tsuite," 1, 5.

110. Ishikawa, "Seishin byōsha no kanchi ni tsuite," 2–4, 8.

111. "The Darkest World" was serialized from May 7 to June 20, 1903, page numbers here and below refer to the reprint in Okada and Sakai, *Kindai shomin seikatsushi*, 183–223.

112. Okada and Sakai, *Kindai shomin seikatsushi*, 221.

113. Kure and Kashida, *Waga kuni ni okeru seishinbyō*, 107; and Okada, *Shisetsu Matsuzawa Byōin*, 112.

114. Okada, *Shisetsu Matsuzawa Byōin*, 198–201.

115. Okada, *Shisetsu Matsuzawa Byōin*, 201–3, 206; and Kure and Kashida, *Waga kuni ni okeru seishinbyō*, 100–101.

116. *Fūzoku gahō*, no. 330 (December 10, 1908): 9–10, and no. 351 (October 25, 1906): 12. *Tōkyo kinkō meisho zue*, no. 3 (Tōyōdō, 1910), 2.

117. Muramatsu, "Fujin to seishin byōsha"; "Tōkyō Nōbyōin wo hōmon"; and Nagamatsu, "Fūten byōin ni nyūin."

118. Imamichi, *Seishin byōsha kanchi tetsuzuki*.

Chapter 6. Cholera in Tokyo

1. *Yomiuri shinbun*, August 9, 1879, 2.

2. Raw statistical data on cholera and population referenced here and below come from three sources, *Naimushō tōkeisho hōkokusho*, *Dai Nihon Naimushō tōkeisho hōkokusho*, *Tōkyō-fu tōkeisho*. All are available through the National Diet Library Digital Collection, Japan.

3. Tokyo-fu, ed., *Tōkyō-fu shi: Gyōseihen*, 6:682–84.

4. Tognotti, "Lessons," 258.

5. Nagayo, *Report of the Director*, 10.

6. Kōseishō Kōshū Eiseikyoku, *Ken'eki seido hyakunenshi*, 17–18.

7. Nagayo, *Report of the Director*, 4–5.

8. Harald Fuess, "Informal Imperialism."

9. Kōseishō Kōshū Eiseikyoku, *Ken'eki seido hyakunenshi*, 204–7.

10. Kōseirōdōshō, *Yokohama ken'eki*.

11. Yamamoto, *Nihon korera shi*, 64, 86–91.

12. There is a considerable literature on Snow's work: see, for example, Hempel, *Strange Case*.

13. Ishiguro, *Korera ron*.

14. *Yomiuri shinbun*, October 18, 1877, 4; October 19, 1877, 4; and October 21, 1877, 4.

15. Naikaku Kirokukyoku, *Hōki bunrui taizen*, 32:51.

16. *Yomiuri shinbun*, March 23, 1880, 3; October 6, 1880, 1; and November 19, 1880, 1.

17. Atkinson, "Water Supply of Tokio," 93.

18. Horikoshi, *Suidōno bunkashi*, 42–47.

19. Horikoshi, *Suidōno bunkashi*, 54.

20. Tōkyō Shiyakusho, ed., *Tōkyō-shi shikō Jōsuihen*, 2:392, 394.

21. Horikoshi, *Suidōno bunkashi*, 61–62.

22. Tōkyō-fu Suidō Kaisei Iin, *Tōkyō suidō kaisetsu gairyaku*, 36–38; "Nitrate and Nitrate in Drinking Water: Background Document for the Development of WHO Guidelines for Drinking Water Quality," https://www.who.int/docs/default-source/wash-documents/wash-chemicals/nitrate-nitrite-background-document.pdf.

23. Shiokawa, "Meiji zenhan," 21–22.

24. Moniwa, *Nihon suidōshi*, 267.

25. For information on the committee's calculation of the cost of modernizing the water system, see Tōkyō-fu Suidō Kaisei Iin, *Tōkyō suidō kaisetsu gairyaku*, 64–71. For information on the prefecture's tax revenue, see Naimubu Shomuka, ed., "Zeikin" in Tōkyō-fu, *Tōkyō-fu tōkeisho Meiji 15-nen*, 10.

26. Kosuge, *Development of Waterworks*, 14.

27. Horikoshi, *Suidōno bunkashi*, 63.

28. Atkinson, "Water Supply of Tokio," 95.

29. Atkinson, "Water Supply of Tokio," 98.

30. Korschelt, "Water Supply of Tōkio."
31. Shiokawa, "Meiji zenhan," 24.
32. Tawara, "Tōkyō-fu jōgesui shiken seiseki."
33. Tajima, "Marketing of Urban Human Waste," chap. 4.
34. Iwabuchi, "Kinsei toshi no toire," 48, 50.
35. Tōkyō-shi, ed., "Shinai shiyō chōsa sho" (1907), in Kingendai Shiryō Kankōkai, *Kindai toshi no eisei kankyō*, 39:33–34.
36. Keishichō, ed., *Tōkyō keishi honsho futatsu zensho*, 63–64.
37. Andō, "Tōkyō shiku kaisei izen," 199.
38. Andō, "Tōkyō shiku kaisei izen," 205.
39. Matsuyama and Itō, "Meiji ni okeru Yotsuya Samegabashi."
40. "Kanda-kunai shigai eiseijō jitchi chōsa," parts 1 and 2, in Tōkyō Shiyakusho, ed., *Tōkyō-shi shikō: Shigaihen*, 69:47–131.
41. Hein, "Shaping Tokyo."
42. Ishida, "1881-nen no Kanda Hashimoto-chō."
43. Nojima, "Kindai toshi kūkan no chitsujo," 442.
44. This document is available in Yamamoto, *Nihon korera shi*, 865–66.
45. Fukuzawa Shin-ichi, "Meiji shoki ni okeru," 283.
46. A chronology of the TMP's orders can be found in Naikaku Kirokukyoku, *Hōki bunrui taizen*, 32:206–40.
47. Fukuzawa Shin-ichi, "Meiji shoki ni okeru," 287–88.
48. Andō, "Shuto Tōkyō no kankyō," 54.
49. Keishichō, ed., *Keishichō shikō*, 195–96.
50. Yamaguchi, *Hasegawa Tai*, 870–80.
51. "Shigai sōji kisoku oyobi kawaya kōzō kisoku shinyō kumitori kisoku," National Archives of Japan, doc. tan 01304100.
52. Naikaku Kirokukyoku, *Hōki bunrui taizen*, 32:59.
53. Obinata, *Nihon kindai kokka*, 195.
54. Kasahara, "Kindai Nihon ni okeru eisei gyōsei no hen'yō," 64.
55. "Tōkyō chihō eiseikai kisoku," National Archives of Japan, doc. tai 00707100.
56. On the role of the TLSA in relation to quarantine hospitals, see Item ID 000119382, 000119389, 000118366; on its role in information gathering, see Item ID 000118750, and on relations with foreign consulates, Item ID 000116873, 000123169, Tokyo Metropolitan Archives.
57. Fukuzawa Shin-ichi, "Meiji shoki ni okeru," 290.
58. Yamaguchi, *Hasegawa Tai*, 874–75.
59. *Yomiuri shinbun*, September 21, 1881, 1; and September 22, 1881, 1.
60. Evans, *Death in Hamburg*, 244.
61. Rosenberg, *Cholera Years*, 29, 107–8.
62. Yamamoto, *Nihon korera shi*, 865.

63. Naikaku Kirokukyoku, *Hōki bunrui taizen*, 32:229, 230, 232, 234.

64. Yamamoto, *Nihon korera shi*, 431–32.

65. Keishichōrei dai kyūjō gō: Hibyōin kari kisoku (October 6, 1877), in Yamaguchi, *Hasegawa Tai*, 911–12.

66. Yamamoto, *Nihon korera shi*. 443. "Densen byōin shi."

67. Naikaku Kirokukyoku, *Hōki bunrui taizen*, 32:238–39.

68. *Yomiuri shinbun*, November 18, 1877, 3.

69. *Yomiuri shinbun*, July 26, 1879, 2; August 8, 1879, 2; and August 19, 1879, 2.

70. *Yomiuri shinbun*, August 8, 1879, 3.

71. *Yomiuri shinbun*, August 21, 1879, 3; and August 24, 1879, 3.

72. *Yomiuri shinbun*, September 12, 1979, 3.

73. *Eisei hōritsu kisoku*, 30–32.

74. "Shiba-ku Shiba Atago chō hibyōin onhaishi nangansho," Item ID 000116402, File no. 612. A6. 03, 66–68. Tokyo Metropolitan Archives.

75. "Shiba hibyōin rinchi kaiage negai," Item ID 000116402, File no. 612. A6. 03, 69–72. Tokyo Metropolitan Archives.

76. "Hibyōin kanja atsukaikata nado no gi ni tsuki kengen." Item ID 000116402, File no. 612. A6. 03, 36–37. Tokyo Metropolitan Archives

77. "Hibyōin shinsetsu no gi ni tsuki saido nangan negaitatematsuru." Item ID 000116402, File no.: 612. A6. 03, 73–78. Tokyo Metropolitan Archives

78. "Tōkyō chihō eisei kaigi jihitsu shoki dai 16 kai, Meiji 15-nen hachi-gatsu." Item ID 000116402, File no. 612. A6. 03, 93–94. Tokyo Metropolitan Archives.

79. See, for example, the advertisements in *Yomiuri shinbun* on July 25, 26, and 28, and August 6, 1882, during the 1882 epidemic.

80. "Meiji 15-nen hachigatsu kokonoka gogo dai-ichiji kaikai," Item ID 000116402, File no. 612. A6. 03, 99–100. Tokyo Metropolitan Archives.

81. "Meiji 15-nen hachigatsu kokonoka gogo dai-ichiji kaikai," 100, 103.

82. Tōkyō Shiyakusho, ed., *Tōkyō-shi shikō: Shigaihen*, 71:2–3.

83. Yamaguchi, *Hasegawa Tai*, 71.

84. Kudō, ed., *Nihon Tōkyō iji tsūran*, 94–95, 107, 111–12; Tokyo-fu, ed., *Tōkyō-fu shi: Gyōseihen*, 6:682–84.

85. Andō, "Tōkyō shiku kaisei izen," 213.

86. Hoshino, "Senzenki Tōkyō-shi ni okeru," 21–24.

87. Quoted in Gesuidō Tōkyō Hyakunenshi Iinkai, *Gesuidō Tōkyō 100-nenshi*, 118.

88. Gesuidō Tōkyō Hyakunenshi Iinkai, *Gesuidō Tōkyō 100-nenshi*, 119–20.

89. Tanaka, "Meiji 10-nendai," 110.

90. Tanaka, "Ichiren no nagaya kashitsu," 85–88.

91. Tanaka, "Meiji 19–20 nen," 90.

92. Cybriwsky, "From Castletown to Manhattan Town,", 63.

93. Tanaka, "Meiji 19–20 nen," 91.

94. Hardy, "Parish Pump to Private Pipes."

95. Horikoshi, *Suidōno bunkashi*, 14.

96. Kosuge, *Development of Waterworks*, 24.

97. Matsumoto, *Kindai suidō no seijishi*, 74.

98. On the municipal bond initiative, see *Yomiuri shinbun*, April 18, 1889, 1; August 22, 1890, 2; and September 23, 1890, 2. On the activities of the Tokyo Citizens Voluntary Association, see *Yomiuri shinbun* December 16, 1891, 4; March 16, 1892, 2; April 14, 1892, 3; and March 16, 1892, 1.

99. Ban, *Tōkyō-shi suidō kairyō iken*, 30–32.

100. Horikoshi, *Suidōno bunkashi*, 86–88.

101. Ishizuka, *Nihon kindai toshi ron*, 76–79. On the debates surrounding the sourcing issue, see *Yomiuri shinbun*, November 9, 1892, 2; November 11, 1892, 1; November 24, 1892, 2; December 4, 1892, 2; and December 12, 1892, 2. On the exposure of the bribery scandal, see *Yomiuri shinbun*, November 19, 1895–December 1, 1895.

102. *Yomiuri shinbun*, December 18, 1899, 1.

103. Tōyama, *Tōkyō-shi kairyō suidō*, 184–86.

104. *Fūzoku gahō*, no. 370 (September 15, 1907), 20.

105. See, for example, *Yomiuri shinbun*, May 19, 1901, 2; May 20, 1901, 3; May 24, 1901, 4; May 25, 1901, 4; and May 28, 1901, 3.

106. Tōyama, *Tōkyō-shi kairyō suidō*, 185.

107. Ishizuka, *Nihon kindai toshi ron*, 66.

108. Naimushō Eiseikyoku, *Saimin chōsa tōkeihyō*, 41.

109. This text was originally serialized in *Yomiuri shinbun* from September 16 to November 1, 1896. It is included in Ozaki and Honma, *Ozaki Kōyō zenshū*, 9:125–214.

110. Ozaki and Honma, *Ozaki Kōyō zenshū*, 9:168–169.

111. Ozaki and Honma, *Ozaki Kōyō zenshū*, 9:202. Emphasis added.

112. Ozaki and Honma, *Ozaki Kōyō zenshū*, 9:187.

113. On this phrase, see Tatsukawa, *Byōki no shakaishi*, 183–84.

Conclusion: Medical Modernity and Its Contradictions

1. Quoted in Kojima, *Nagayo Sensai*, 40.

2. On police involvement in colonial medicine, see Henry, *Assimilating Seoul*, chap. 4; Liu, *Prescribing Colonization*; and Yoo, *It's Madness*.

3. *Yomiuri shinbun*, July 31, 1923, 4; and *Yomiuri shinbun*, July 15, 1936, 2.

4. Naimushō, *Eiseikyoku nenpo* (1935), 218–30.

5. On migrant doctors see, Chen, "Cosmopolitan Medicine Nationalized"; T. Nishiyama, "Doctors for Frontier Expansion"; and Kim, "Disaggregating 'Japanese' Doctors."

6. This information comes from the website of the Kanda Medical Association, https://www.kanda-med.or.jp/.

7. See the museum's website at https://www.suidorekishi.jp/.

8. On psychiatric care in Setagaya, see https://nimohoukatsu.mhlw.go.jp/archive/share2023/146.pdf.

9. Takahashi Tai and Eguchi, "Chiiki iryō teikyō taisei."

10. See, for example, "Korona no saki e: Kiken no kyōkun," *Yomiuri shinbun*, May 1, 2023, 1.

11. Tōkyō-to Hoken Iryō Kyoku, "Ishi kakuho keikaku ni motozuku ishi kakuho taisaku," February 21, 2024, https://www.hokeniryo.metro.tokyo.lg.jp/iryo/sonota/tiikiiryoutaisaku/r5-2-chitaikyou.files/R5-2shiryou4-1.pdf.

BIBLIOGRAPHY

Archives, Serials, and Digital Collections

Asahi shinbun

Fūzoku gahō

Gotō Shinpei Kinenkan, ed. *Gotō Shinpei monjo* (microfilm collection)

International Research Center for Japanese Studies Map Collection

Japan Center for Asian Historical Records

Kanayomi shinbun

National Diet Library Digital Collection

Tōkyō kinkō meisho zue

Tokyo Metropolitan Archives

Tōkyō-fu nisshi

Yomiuri shinbun

Primary and Secondary Sources

Agostoni, Claudia. *Monuments of Progress: Modernization and Public Health in Mexico City, 1876–1910*. University of Calgary Press, 2002.

Ajioka Yasuke. *Baidoku kensa no wake*. Enjudō, 1879. In Yunomae and Akisada, *Baibaishun mondai shiryōshūsei*, 14:132–36.

Andō Yūichirō. *Edo no yōjōsho*. PHP Kenkyūjo, 2002.

Andō Yūichirō. "Shuto Tōkyō no kankyō eisei gyōsei: Shinyō shori shisutemu no henben to jōyaku kaisei." *Hikaku toshishi kenkyū* 22, no. 1 (2003): 47–70.

Andō Yūichirō. "Tōkyō shiku kaisei izen no shinyō shori taisaku: Ushigome-ku gaitō benjo sōjinin Nakamura Kametarō no dōkō wo chūshin ni." In *Kankyō to rekishi*, edited by Ishi Hiroyuki et al., 197–218. Shinseisha, 1999.

Arai Shin, ed. *Nihon keisatsu zensho kō hen*. Tokyo: Hakurakuho, 1878.

Arai Tōjirō, ed. *Tōkyō seikaku zuroku. Tokyo: Arai Tōjirō, 1885.*

Armus, Diego. *The Ailing City: Health, Tuberculosis, and Buenos Aires*. Duke University Press, 2011.

Asahi Shinbunsha Shūkan Asahi Henshūbu. *Sengo nedanshi nenpyō*. Asahi Shinbunsha, 1995.

Aso, Noriko. *Public Properties: Museums in Imperial Japan*. Duke University Press, 2014.

Atkinson, R. W. "The Water Supply of Tokio." *Transactions of the Asiatic Society of Japan* 6, part 1b (1878): 87–98.

Ayabe Yūko "Seishin shōgaisha shisetsu shogū zenshi: Tōkyō-fu Byōin kara Tōkyō Tenkyōin wo chūshin ni." *Seishin igakushi kenkyū* 10, no. 2 (2006): 92–102.

Ban Naonosuke. *Tōkyō-shi suidō kairyō iken*. Tokyo: Keizai Shinbunsha, 1892.

Bay, Alexander R. *Beriberi in Modern Japan: The Making of a National Disease*. University of Rochester Press, 2012.

Bereridge, A. B., and E. B. Renvoize. "Electricity: A History of Its Use in Britain in the Treatment of Mental Illness in the Second Half of the 19th Century." *British Journal of Psychiatry*, no. 153 (1988): 157–62.

Billings, John S., and Henry M. Hurd, eds. *Hospitals, Dispensaries, and Nursing: Papers and Discussions in the International Congress of Charities, Corrections, and Philanthropy, Section III, Chicago, June 12th to 17th, 1893*. Baltimore: Johns Hopkins Press, 1894.

Botsman, Daniel. "Freedom Without Slavery? 'Coolies,' Prostitutes, and Outcastes in Meiji Japan's 'Emancipation Moment.'" *American Historical Review* 116, no. 5 (2011): 1323–47.

Brown, Sydney DeVere, and Akiko Hirota, trans. *The Diary of Kido Takayoshi*. Vol. 2: *1871–1873*. University of Tokyo Press, 1981.

Buraku kaihō kenkyūjo, ed. *Shiryōshū: Meiji shoki hisabetsu buraku*. Kaihō Shuppansha, 1986.

Burns, Susan L. "Bodies and Borders: Syphilis, Prostitution, and the Nation." *US-Japan Women's Journal* 15 (1998): 3–30.

Burns, Susan L. "The Body as Text: Confucianism, Reproduction, and Gender in Early Modern Japan." In *Rethinking Confucianism: Past and Present in China, Japan, Korea and Vietnam*, edited by Benjamin Elman, Herman Ooms, and John Duncan, 178–219. UCLA Asia Pacific Monograph Series, 2002.

Burns, Susan L. "In the Arena of the Courts: The Prosecution of Abortion and Infanticide in Early Meiji Japan." In Burns and Brooks, *Gender and Law in the Japanese Imperium*, 81–108.

Burns, Susan L. *Kingdom of the Sick: A History of Leprosy and Japan*. University of Hawai'i Press, 2019.

Burns, Susan L. "Marketing Health and Beauty: Advertising, Medicine, and the Modern Body in Meiji-Taisho Japan." In *East Asian Visual Culture from the Treaty Ports to World War II*, edited by Hans Thomsen and Jennifer Purtle, 179–202. Paragon Books, 2009.

Burns, Susan L. "Reinvented Places: 'Tradition,' 'Family Care' and Psychiatric Institutions in Japan." *Social History of Medicine* 32, no. 1 (2019): 99–120.

Burns, Susan L. "Relocating Psychiatric Knowledge: Meiji Psychiatrists, Local Culture(s) and the Problem of Fox Possession." *Historia Scientarium* (Japan Society for the History of Science) 22, no. 2 (2012): 88–109.

Burns, Susan L., and Barbara Brooks, eds. *Gender and Law in the Japanese Imperium, 1868–1952*. University of Hawai'i Press, 2013.

Campbell, Scott. "The Changing Role of Capital Cities in the Global Era." Paper presented at the Annual Meeting of the Association of American Geographers, Pittsburgh, PA, April 4–8, 2000. https://public.websites.umich.edu/~sdcamp/workingpapers/URRC%2003-08.pdf.

Checkland, Olive. *Humanitarianism and the Emperor's Japan, 1877–1977*. St. Martin's Press, 1994.

Chen, Wei-ti. "Cosmopolitan Medicine Nationalized: The Making of Japanese State-Empire and Overseas Physicians in a Global World." PhD diss., University of Chicago, 2016.

Chūō Shakai Jigyō Kyōkai Shakai Jigyō Kenkyūjo, ed. *Kindai iryō hogo jigyō hattatsushi*. Nihon Hyōronsha, 1943.

Clark, A. Kim. *Conjuring the State: Public Health Encounters in Highland Ecuador, 1910–1945*. University of Pittsburgh Press, 2023.

Clark, Adele E. "From the Rise of Medicine to Biomedicalization: U.S. Healthscapes and Iconography, Circa 1890–Present." In *Biomedicalization: Technoscience, Health, and Illness in the U.S.*, edited by Adele E. Clark, Lauren Mamo et al. 104–46. Duke University Press, 2010.

Cybriwsky, Roman. "From Castletown to Manhattan Town with Suburbs: A Geographical Account of Tokyo's Landmarks and Symbolic Landscapes." In *The Japanese City*, edited by Pradyumna P. Karan and Kristin Stapleton, 56–78. University Press of Kentucky, 2015.

"Densen byōin shi." *Nihon densenbyō gakkai zasshi* 7, no. 4 (1932): 80–85.

Dimas, Carlos S. *Poisoned Eden: Cholera Epidemics, State-Building, and the Problem of Public Health in Tucumán, Argentina, 1865–1908*. University of Nebraska Press, 2022.

Eguchi Jo, trans. *Seishinbyōgaku*. Tokyo: Eirandō, 1887.

Ehlers, Maren A. *Give and Take: Poverty and the Status Order in Early Modern Japan*. Harvard University Asia Center, 2018.

Eisei hōritsu kisoku. Okayama: Saikinsha, 1891.

Evans, Richard J. *Death in Hamburg: Society and Politics in the Cholera Years, 1830–1910*. Clarendon Press, 1987.

Fuess, Harald. "Informal Imperialism and the 1879 'Hesperia' Incident: Containing Cholera and Challenging Extraterritoriality in Japan." *Japan Review*, no. 27 (2014): 103–40.

Fujikawa Yū. *Nihon shippei shi*. Heibonsha, 1969.

Fujitani, Takashi. *Splendid Monarchy: Power and Pageantry in Modern Japan*. University of California Press, 1996.

Fukazawa Megumi and Yasutake Atsuko. "Nagasaki Kojima Yōjōsho no keikaku jittai to Meiji shoki no Nihon no byōin kenchiku ni ataeta eikyō." *Nihon kenchiku gakkai hōkokusho* 27, no. 67 (2021): 1390–95.

Fukuda Eizō. *Kaichū Tōkyō annai*. 2nd ed. Tokyo: Dōmeisha Shuppan, 1877.

Fukuhama Yoshihiro. "Koishikawa Yōjōsho no ezumen wo chūshin to shita kenchikuteki shiryō no kentō to fukugenteki kōsatsu." *Tōkyō Daigaku shi kiyō*, no. 33 (2015): 1–37.

Fukunaga Hajime. *Nihon byōinshi*. Pillar Press, 2014.

Fukuzawa Shin'ichi. "Meiji shoki ni okeru gyōsei keisatsu no keisei to tenkai: Tōkyō-fu ni okeru korera taisaku no jirei wo chūshin to shite." *Hōgaku seijigaku ronkyū*, no. 37 (1986): 281–99.

Fukuzawa Yukichi. "Seiyō jijō." In *Fukuzawa Yukichi zenshū*. Vol. 1. Iwanami Shoten, 1958.

Garcia, Magaly Rodriguez, Lex Heerma van Voss, and Elise van Nederveen Meerkerk, eds. *Selling Sex in the City: A Global History of Prostitution, 1600s–2000s*. Brill, 2017.

Geltner, G. "Healthscaping a Medieval City: Lucca's *Curia viarum* and the Future of Public Health History." *Urban History* 40 (2013): 395–415.

Geltner, G., and Janna Coomans, "The Healthscaping Approach: Towards a Global History of Early Public Health." *Historical Methods: A Journal of Quantitative and Interdisciplinary History* 56 (2023): 18–33.

Gesler, Wilbert M. "Therapeutic Landscapes: Issues in Light of the New Cultural Geography." *Social Science Medicine* 34, no. 7 (1992): 735–46.

Gesuidō Tōkyō Hyakunenshi Iinkai, ed. *Gesuidō Tōkyō 100-nen-shi*. Tōkyō-to Gesuidō-kyoku, 1989.

Gharipour, Mohammed, and Caitlin DeClercq. *Epidemic Urbanism: Contagious Diseases in Global Cities*. Intellect, University of Chicago Press, 2021.

Gilman, Sander. *Disease and Representation: Images of Illness from Madness to AIDS*. Cornell University Press, 1988.

Goryūnen Ichinin et al. *Imayō shokuninzukushi uta-awase*. Edo: Shinsen'en Sagimaru, 1825.

Gottdiener, Mark. *The Social Production of Urban Space*. University of Texas Press, 1985.

Gyōseisha, ed. *Saikin chōsa Tōkyō iryō annai*. Gyōseisha, 1910.

Hanley, Susan. *Everyday Life in Premodern Japan*. University of California Press, 1997.

Hardy, Anne. "Parish Pump to Private Pipes: London's Water Supply in the Nineteenth Century." *Medical History*, Supplement no. 11 (1991): 76–93.

Harrison, Mark. "Health, Sovereignty and Imperialism: The Royal Navy and Infectious Disease in Japan's Treaty Ports." *Social Science Diliman* 14, no. 2 (2018): 49–75.

Hashimoto Akira. *Seishin byōsha to shitaku kanchi*. Rikka Shuppan, 2011.

Hastings, Sally A. *Neighborhood and Nation in Tokyo, 1905–1937*. University of Pittsburgh Press, 1995.

Hayakawa Masako. "Edo machikata ninbetsuchō dētabēsu." *Mejiro Daigaku sōgō kagaku kenkyū*, no. 10 (2014): 41–53.

Hein, Carola. "Shaping Tokyo: Land Development and Planning Practice in the Early Modern Japanese Metropolis." *Journal of Urban History* 36, no. 4 (2010): 447–84.

Hempel, Sandra. *The Strange Case of the Broad Street Pump: John Snow and the Mystery of Cholera*. University of California Press, 2007.

Henry, Todd A. *Assimilating Seoul: Japanese Rule and the Politics of Public Space in Colonial Korea, 1910–1945*. University of California Press, 2014.

Hiruta Genshirō. "Edo jidai ni okeru seishin igaku byōinron." *Seishin igaku kenkyū* 3, no. 3 (2000): 27–33.

Hiruta Genshirō. "Edo jidai no seishin igaku." *Rinshō seishin igaku* 11, no. 1 (1982): 39–47.

Hochman, Gilberto. *The Sanitation of Brazil: Nation, State, and Public Health, 1889–1930*. Translated by Diane Grosklaur Whitty. University of Illinois Press, 2016.

Horikoshi Masao. *Suidō no bunkashi: Edo no suidō, Tōkyō no suidō*. Kajima Shuppankai, 1981.

Hoshino Takanori. "Senzenki Tōkyō-shi ni okeru shinyō ryūtsūmō no saikeisei." *Rekishi to keizai* 56, no. 2 (2014): 15–29.

Howland, Douglas. "The *Maria Luz* Incident: Personal Rights and International Justice for Chinese Coolies and Japanese Prostitutes." In Burns and Brooks, *Gender and Law in the Japanese Imperium*, 21–47.

Ikai Shūhei. "Meiji-ki Nihon ni okeru kaigyōi shūdan no seiritsu: Senmon'i to ippan'i mibun bunri kōzō wo kaku Nihonteki ishi shūdan no genryū." *Ōhara Shakai Mondai Kenkyūjo zasshi*, no. 511 (2001): 31–57.

Ikeda Ryōji et al., eds. *Shiryō Nihon kindai hō*. Hōritsu Bunkasha, 1983.

Imamichi Kojūrō. *Seishin byōsha kanchi tetsuzuki: Seishin byōsha nyūin annai*. Tohōdō Shoten, 1912.

Ion, A. Hamish. "Sexual Imperialism on the China Station During the Meiji Restoration: The Control of Smallpox and Syphilis at Yokohama, 1868–1871. *International History Review* 31, no. 4 (2009): 711–39.

Ishida Yoshifusa. "1881-nen no Kanda Hashimoto-chō kairyō jigyō ni kansuru kenkyū." *Nihon kenchiku gakkai hōkokushū*, no. 288 (1980): 157–65.

Ishigami Hiroyuki. "Iseki kara mita toshi Edo no jōge suidō no kanri." In *Kinsei toshi no jōtai to hijōtai*, edited by Watanabe Kōichi and Matthew Davies, 71–92. Bensei Shuppan, 2020.

Ishiguro Tadanori. *Korera ron*. Tokyo: Shimamura Yarisuke, 1871.

Ishii Ryōsuke. *Edo no keibatsu*. Yoshikawa Kōbunkan, 2013.

Ishii Ryōsuke. *Edo no machi bugyō*. Akashi Shoten, 2012.

Ishikawa Teikichi. "Seishin byōsha no kanchi ni tsuite." *Kokka igakkai zasshi*, no. 236 (1906): 1–11.

Ishizuka Hiromichi. *Nihon kindai toshi ron: Tōkyō, 1868–1923*. Tōkyō Daigaku Shuppankai, 1991.

Ishizuka Hiromichi. "Tōkyō no toshi suramu to kōshū eisei mondai." *Kokuren Daigaku ningen to shakai no hattatsu puroguramu kenkyū hōkoku*. Kokuren Daigaku, 1981.

Itahara Kazuko and Kuwahara Haruo. "Edo jidai kōki ni okeru seishin shōgaisha no taigū 1." *Shakai mondai kenkyū* 48, no. 1 (1998): 41–59; "Edo jidai kōki ni okeru seishin shōgaisha no taigū 2." *Shakai mondai kenkyū* 49, no. 1 (1999): 93–111; "Edo jidai kōki ni okeru seishin shōgaisha no taigū 4." *Shakai mondai kenkyū* 50, no. 1 (2000): 79–84; "Edo jidai kōki ni okeru seishin shōgaisha no taigū 5." *Shakai mondai kenkyū* 50, no. 2 (2004): 1–45.

Itō Yōichi. *Edo jōsuidō no rekishi*. Yoshikawa Kōbunkan, 2010.

Iwabuchi Reiji. "Kinsei toshi no toire to shinyō shori no genkai." *Rekishi to chiri*, no. 484 (1995): 46–59.

Iwabuchi Yuriko. "Kansei-Tenpōki no Yōjōsho seisaku to bakufu Igakkan." *Ronshū kinsei*, no. 22 (2000): 40–61.

Jannetta, A., and E. Nakamura. "Translating Medical Knowledge: Japan's First Medical Journal—*Taisei meii ikō*." *Historia Scientiarum* 22 (2012): 68–87.

Jannetta, Ann Bowman. *The Vaccinators: Smallpox, Medical Knowledge and the "Opening" of Japan*. Stanford University Press, 2007.

Jenner, Mark S. R., and Patrick Wallis. *Medicine and the Market in England and Its Colonies, c. 1450–1850*. Palgrave Macmillan, 2007.

Johnston, William. *The Modern Epidemic: A History of Tuberculosis in Japan*. Harvard East Asian Monographs, 1995.

Juntendō Daigaku Komonjo Kenkyūkai, ed. "Hinmin Yōjōsho kiroku." *Nihon ishigaku kenkyū* 16, no. 1 (2016): 17–37.

Kanagaki Robun. *Ansei korori ryūkōki*. N.p.: Tenjudō, 1858.

Kaneda Eisuke. *Susaki no shiori*. Susaki sangyō kumiai, 1937.

Kanekawa Hideo and Hori Miyuki. *Seishin byōin no shakaishi*. Seikyūsha, 2009.

Kaneko Tsuguo. *Matsuzawa Byōin gaishi*. Nihon Hyōronsha, 1982.

Kano Masanao. *Kenkōkan ni miru kindai*. Asahi Sensho, 2001.

Kariya Haruo. *Edo no seibyō: Baidoku ryūkō jijō*. San'ichi Shobō, 1993.

Kasahara Hidehiko. "Kindai Nihon ni okeru eisei gyōsei no hen'yō: 'Jūkyūnen no tonza' no jissō." *Hōgaku kenkyū: Hōritsu, seiji, shakai* 73, no. 4 (2000): 63–84.

Kasahara Hidehiko. *Nihon no iryō gyōsei: Sono rekishi to kadai*. Keio University Press, 1999.

Kasahara Hidehiko and Kojima Kazutaka. *Meijiki iryō: Nagayo Sensai kara Gōtō Shinpei e*. Minerva Jinbun, 2011.

Kasai, T. et al. "Research and Control of Parasitic Diseases in Japan: Current Position and Future Perspectives." *Trends Parasitol* 23, no. 5 (2007): 230–35.

Katsuragi Tenka and Furusawa Kodō. *Yoshiwara yūkaku no uramen* (Daigakukan, 1903). In Yunomae and Akisada, *Baibaishun mondai shiryō shūsei*, 10:249–94.

Kawakami Takeshi. *Gendai Nihon iryōshi: Kaigyōisei no hensen*. Keisō Shobō, 1965.

Kawamoto Yoshikazu and Fujisawa Seisuke. *Tōkyō no hisabetsu buraku: Jittai, rekishi, genjō*. San'ichi Shobō, 1984.

Kawasaki Fusagorō, ed. "Tsukiji iryūchi." *Tosei kiyō* 4 (1956): 122–28.

Keishichō, ed. *Keishichōrei ruisan*. Keishichō, 2nd ed.1890; 5th ed. 1896.

Keishichō, ed. *Keishichō shikō*. Keishichō, 1894.

Keishichō, ed. *Tōkyō keishi honsho futatsu zensho, Meiji 11-nen*. Suhara Tetsuji, 1878.

Kerr, Matthew L. Newsome. *Contagion, Isolation, and Biopolitics in Victorian London*. Palgrave Macmillan, 2018.

Kim, Hoi-eun. "Disaggregating 'Japanese' Doctors in Colonial Korea: A Preliminary Prosopographical Analysis." Talk presented at Texas A&M University, February 20, 2019.

Kim, Hoi-eun. *Doctors of Empire: Medical and Cultural Encounters Between Imperial Germany and Meiji Japan*. University of Toronto Press, 2014.

Kimura Ki and Meiji Bunka Kenkyūkai. *Bakumatsu Meiji shinbun zenshū*. 6 vols. 2nd ed. Seikai Bunko, 1966.

Kingendai Shiryō Kankōkai, ed. *Kindai toshi no eisei kankyō (Tōkyō hen)*. 43 vols. Kingendai Shiryō Kankōkai, 2009.

Kisacky, Jeanne Susan. *Rise of the Modern Hospital: An Architectural History of Health and Healing, 1870–1940*. University of Pittsburgh Press, 2017.

Kitahara Itoko. "Toshi ni okeru bin'in and kyōki: Tōkyō-fu Tenkyōin no seiritsu wo megutte." In *Kinsei kokka no kaitai to kindai*, edited by Tsuda Hideo, 422–34. Hanawa Shobō, 1979.

Kitahara Itoko. *Toshi to hinkon no shakaishi: Edo kara Tōkyō e*. Yoshikawa Kōbunkan, 1995.

Kitazawa Kazutoshi. *Kenkō no Nihonshi*. Heibonsha, 2000.

Kobayashi Takehiro. *Kindai Nihon to kōshūeisei: Toshi shakaishi no kokoromi*. Yūzankaku, 2018.

Kobayashi Yasuhiko. "Edo jidai no seishin igaku 2: Chiryō hen." *Rinshō seishin igaku* 11, no. 1 (1982): 49–54.

Kōda Shigetomo. *Kōda Shigetomo chosakushū*. Vol. 2. Chūō Kōronsha, 1972.

Koishikawa-ku. *Koishikawa kukai shi*. Tōkyō-shi Koishikawa-ku, 1935.

Kojima Kazutaka. *Nagayo Sensai to Naimushō no eisei gyōsei*. Keiō Gijuku Daigaku Shuppankai, 2021.

Korschelt, O. "The Water Supply of Tōkio." *Transactions of the Asiatic Society of Japan* 12, part 3 (1883): 143–65.

Kōseirōdōshō. *Yokohama Ken'ekisho: Yokohama ken'ekishi ākaibu*. https://www.forth.go.jp/keneki/yokohama/museum/page2-1.html.

Kōseishō Imukyoku, ed. *Isei hyakunenshi*. 2 vols. Gyōsei, 1976.

Kōseishō Kōshū Eiseikyoku, ed. *Ken'eki seido hyakunenshi*. Gyōsei, 1980.

Kosuge, Nobuhiko. *The Development of Waterworks in Japan*. United Nations University, 1981.

Kudō Tetsuo, ed. *Tōkyō iji tsūran*. Nihon Iji Tsūran Hakkōjo, 1901.

Kume Kunitake. *Tokumei zenken taishi Bei-ō kairan jikki*. 5 vols. Iwanami Shoten, 1985.

Kure Shūzō. "Ko Ika Daigaku kyōju igaku hakushi Sakaki Hajime no den." *Tōkyō igakkai zasshi* 11, no. 5 (1897): 34–41.

Kure Shūzō. "Meiji 12-nen naishi 34-nen Tōkyō-fu Sugamo Byōin iji hōkoku." *Chūgai iji shinpō*, no. 682 (1908): 1086–87.

Kure Shūzo. "Seishinbyō kanja jikken kiji (Dai jūgo rei): Hisuteria." *Tōkyō igakkai zasshi* 4, no. 11 (1890): 39–47.

Kure Shūzō. "Seishinbyō kanja jikken kiji (Dai jūgo rei): Hisuteria." *Tōkyō igakkai zasshi* 5, no. 8 (1891): 44–47.

Kure Shūzō. *Seishinbyōgaku shūyō*. 2 vols. Tokyo: Tohōdō, 1894.

Kure Shūzō and Kashida Gorō. *Seishinbyōsha shitaku kanchi no jikkyō*. 1920. Repr., Seishin Igaku Shinkeigaku Koten Kankōkai, 1973.

Kure Shūzō and Kashida Gorō. *Waga kuni ni okeru seishinbyō ni kansuru saikin no shisetsu*. 1907. Repr., Seishin Igaku Shinkeigaku Koten Kankōkai, 1977.

Kuroki Takashi. *Edo no kaji*. Doseisha, 1999.

Levine, Philippa. "Venereal Disease, Prostitution, and the Politics of Empire: The Case of British India." *Journal of the History of Sexuality* 4, no. 4 (1994): 579–602.

Liu, Michael Shiyung. *Prescribing Colonization: The Role of Medical Practices and Policies in Japan-Ruled Taiwan, 1895–1945*. Association for Asian Studies, 2009.

Machi Senjurō. "Edo Igakukan ni okeru rinshō kyōiku." *Nihon ishigaku zasshi* 59, no. 1 (2013): 17–33.

Machi Senjurō. "Igakukan no gakumon keisei 1: Igakukan seiritsu zengo." *Nihon ishigaku zasshi* 45, no. 3 (1999): 339–72; "Igakukan no gakumon keisei 3: Bakumatsu kōshōgaku no isō." *Nihon ishigaku zasshi* 46, no. 1 (1999): 3–22.

Maki Hidemasa. *Kinsei Nihon no jinshin baibai no keifu*. Sōbunsha, 1970.

Mansfield, Stephen. *Tokyo: A Cultural and Literary History*. Signal Books, 2009.

Mantovani, Rafael, and Maria Cristina da Costa Marques. "Hygiene as Individual Practice and as an Instrument of the State." *História, ciências, saúde-Manguinhos* 27, no. 2 (2020): 337–54.

Marx, Otto M. "Wilhelm Griesinger and the History of Psychiatry: A Reassessment." *Bulletin of the History of Medicine* 46, no. 6 (1972): 519–44.

Masai Yasuo. "Nimanbun no ichi: 'Edo no toshiteki tochi riyōzu.'" *Chizu: Kūkan hyōgen no kagaku* 13, no. 1 (1975): 9–16.

Matsumoto Hiroyuki. *Kindai suidō no seijishi*. Yoshida Shoten, 2020.

Matsuyama Megumi and Itō Hirohisa. "Meiji ni okeru Yotsuya Samegabashi no toshi kūkan kōzō: Kinsei machikata basue to kindai 'suramu' no toshi kūkan ni okeru renzokusei to henshitsu katei—Yotsuya Samegabashi wo jirei ni." *Nihon kenchiku gakkai Kantō shibu kenkyū hōkokushū* (1998): 561–64.

Matsuzaki Kin'ichi. "Sugita Genpaku no 'Isai nichiroku' ni tsuite." *Shigaku* 49, no. 1 (1978): 1–43.

Matsuzawa Yūsaku. "'Daiku shōku sei' no keisei katei." *Rekishigaku kenkyū* 772 (2003): 17–34.

Maudsley, Henry. *Seishin byōsha yakusetsu*. Translated by Bun'ya Kanbe. Seishin Igaku Shinkeigaku Koten Kankōkai, 1973.

McCrea, Heather L. *Diseased Relations: Epidemics, Public Health, and State-Building in Yucatán, Mexico, 1847–1924*. University of New Mexico Press, 2010.

McFarlane, Alan. *The Making of the Modern World*. Palgrave, 2002.

Miller, Ian Jared. *The Nature of the Beasts: Empire and Exhibition at the Tokyo Imperial Zoo*. University of California Press, 2013.

Minami Kazuo. *Edo no shakai kōzō*. Hanawa Shobō, 1969.

Miura Hiroyuki. "Bakumatsu Pari banpaku shisestu haken to Sano Tsunetami." *Kokugakuin Daigaku kiyō* 50 (2012): 181–93.

Molina, Natalia. *Fit to Be Citizens? Public Health and Race in Los Angeles, 1879–1939*. University of California Press, 2006.

Moniwa Chūjirō. *Nihon suidōshi*. Nakajima Kōgaku Hakushi Kinen Jigyōkai, 1927.

Moorhead, Caroline. *Dunant's Dream: War, Switzerland and the History of the Red Cross*. Harper Collins, 1998.

Mori Mutsuhiko. "Tenpō kaikaku to Yōgakusho no shuppan: Toku ni Igakukan to no kankei ni tsuite." *Hōsei shigaku* 18 (1966): 71–80.

Morinaga Takurō. *Bukka no bunkashi jiten*. Tenbōsha, 2008.

Müller, Leopold. "Tokio-Igaku: Skizzen und Erinnerungen aus der Zeit des geistigen Umschwunges in Japan, 1871–1876." *Deutsche Rundschau Band* 57 (1888): 312–29.

Murakoshi Kazunori. "Daimyō no nyūji shibōritsu 1651–1850." *Jinkōgaku kenkyū* no. 24 (1999): 15–31.

Muramatsu Rakusui. "Fujin to seishin byōsha." *Jogaku sekai* 5, no. 7 (1905): 23–25.

Nagai Yoshitomo. *Tōkyō hyakujiben*. Tokyo: Sansan Bunbō, 1897.

Nagamatsu Aiko. "Fūten byōin ni nyūin seru fujin no fushigi na seikatsu." *Fujin sekai* 5, no. 6 (1910): 78–80.

Nagao Setsuzō. *Aa ihei*. Tohōdō, 1908. Repr., Shunjūsha, 1982.

Nagayo Sensai. *Report of the Director of the Central Sanitary Commission to His Excellency the Minister of the Home Department upon Cholera in the 12th Year of Meiji (1879)*. Tokyo: Naimushō Eiseikyoku, 1879.

Naikaku Kirokukyoku. *Hōki bunrui taizen*. 64 vols. Tokyo: Naikaku Kirokukyoku, 1889–1891.

Naimushō. *Eiseikyoku nenpō*. Tokyo: Naimushō Eiseikyoku, 1878–1935.

Naimushō Eiseikyoku, ed. *Karyūbyō chōsahyō*. Naimushō Eiseikyoku, 1918.

Naimushō Eiseikyoku, ed. *Saimin chōsa tōkeihyō*. Naimushō Shakaikyoku, 1910.

Naimushō Eiseikyoku, ed. *Seishin byōsha ni kansuru tōkei*. Naimushō eiseikyoku, 1911.

Naitō Akira. *Edo to Edo jō*. Kajima Kenkyūjo Shuppankai, 1967.

Nakagawa Hōzandō and Katsushika Hokusai, eds. *Edo kaimono hitori annai*. 2 vols. Kyoto: Namariya Yasubee, 1824.

Nakagawa Kiyoshi, ed. *Meiji Tōkyō kasō seikatsushi*. Iwanami Shoten, 1999.

Nakajima, Chieko. *Body, Society, and Nation: The Creation of Public Health and Urban Culture in Shanghai*. Harvard East Asia Center, 2018.

Nakamura Aya. "Mura to iryō: Shinano no kuni wo jirei to shite." *Rekishigaku kenkyū*, no. 639 (1992): 36–43.

Nakanishi Atsuo and Higuchi Teruo. "Kyōkan Gijuku no kenkyū: Tōkyō kenbaishi no hoi toshite." *Nihon ishigaku zasshi* 55, no. 3 (2009): 347–64.

Nakano Misao. *Nihon iji dainenpyō*. Shibunkaku, 1972.

Nakayama Manabu. "Bakumatsu Edo no byōke ni okeru iryō sentaku no jittai: Byōnin Takizawa Tarō no kaigo kirku wo tegakari to shite." In *Kantō kinseishi kenkyū ronshū*, edited by Nakayama Manabu et al. Vol. 2, *Geinō, shūkyō, iryō*, 279–305. Iwata Shoin, 2012.

Narabayashi Makoto. "Kyūbaku jidai no seishin byōin," *Nō* 1, no. 6 (1927): 50–54.

National Museum of Japanese History. "Database of Edo Merchants and Artisans." https://www.rekihaku.ac.jp/up-cgi/login.pl?p=param/edos/db_param.

National Museum of Japanese History. "Kinsei shokunin gazō database." https://www.www.rekihaku.ac.jp/up-cgi/login.pl?p=param/kins/db_param.

"Nezu monzen baidokuin toritatechō, Meiji gannen nigatsu." *Zakkenroku* 3, no. 2. National Diet Library Digital Collection. https://dl.ndl.go.jp/info:ndljp/pid/2609618.

Nihon Sekijūjisha, ed. *Nihon Sekijūjisha shikō*. Nihon Sekijūjisha, 1911.

Nihon Shakai Jigyō Daigaku Kyūhin Seido Kenkyūkai, ed. *Nihon no kyūhin seido*. Keisō Shobō, 1960.

Nishikawa Kaoru. *Nihon seishin shōgisha seisakushi: Senzenki wo chūshin to shite*. Kōkodō, 2010.

Nishiyama Matsunosuke. *Edo chōnin no kenkyū*. Vol. 4. Yoshikawa Kōbunkan, 1972.

Nishiyama, Takashi. "Doctors for Frontier Expansion: Japanese Physicians in Hawaii, 1868–1924." *East Asian Science, Technology and Society: An International Journal* 12, no. 3 (2018): 257–75.

Nojima Masakazu. "Kindai toshi kūkan no chitsujo keisei katei ni okeru eisei shisō to keisatsu." *Randosukēpu kenkyū* 65, no. 5 (1997): 441–46.

O'Shea, J. G. "'Two Minutes with Venus, Two Years with Mercury': Mercury as an Antisyphilitic Chemotherapeutic Agent." *Journal of the Royal Society of Medicine* 83 (June 1990): 392–95.

Obinata Sumio. *Naimushō tōkeisho*. San'ichi Shobō, 1984.

Obinata Sumio. *Nihon kindai kokka no seiritsu to keisatsu*. Azekura Shobō, 1992.

"Obituary: Keizo Dohi, MD, 1866–1931." *Archives of Dermatology and Syphilology* 25, no. 5 (1932): 940.

Ogata Kōan. *Byōgaku tsūron*. Vol. 2. Osaka: Kawachiya Usuke, 1849.

Ogawa Teizō and Sakai Shizu, eds. *Matsumoto Jun jiden, Nagayo Sensai jiden*. Heibonsha, 1980.

Okada Yasuo. *Shisetsu Matsuzawa Byōin shi*. Iwasaki Gakujutsu Shuppansha, 1981.

Okada Yasuo and Sakai Shizu, eds. *Kindai shomin seikatsushi*. Vol. 20, *Byōki eisei*. San'ichi Shobō, 1995.

Okada Yasuo, Kaneko Tsuguo, Yoshioka Shinji, and Hasegawa Gensuke. "Shitaku kanchi no unmei." *Seishin igaku* 7, no. 6 (1965): 510–16.

Okitsu Kaname et al., eds. *Meiji Bungaku Zenshū*. Vol. 52, *Ishikawa Takeboku*. Chikuma Shobō, 1977.

Omata Waichirō. *Seishin byōin no kigen*. Ōta Shuppan, 1998.

Onodera Yoshiaki. "Seishin byōsha jikken kiji (Dai jūsan rei): Shusei chūdoku henshitsukyō," *Tōkyō igakkai zasshi* 5, no. 14 (1891): 46–47.

Onodera Yoshiaki. "Seishin byōsha jikken kiji (Dai jūshi rei): Tanjunsei yūutsu kyō." *Tōkyō igakkai zasshi* 5, no. 6 (1891): 27–32.

Opdyke, Sandra. *No One Was Turned Away: The Role of Public Hospitals in New York City Since 1900*. Oxford University Press, 1999.

Oyamada Nobuko. "1890-nen ni kanritsu sanba gakkō setsuritsu sareru made no Tōkyō ni okeru sanba kyōiku." *Nihon sanba gakkai zasshi* 30, no. 1 (2016): 99–109.

Ozaki Kōji. "Meiji 'isei' saikō." *Ōtemae Daigaku ronshū*, no. 16 (2015): 15–53.

Ozaki Kōyō and Honma Hisao. *Ozaki Kōyō zenshū*. Chūō Kōron, 1942.

Packard, Keiko Imai. *Old Tokyo*. Oxford University Press, 2002.

Peterson, Frederick, "The Insane in Japan." *Studies in Psychiatry* 1, no. 9 (1912): 1–8.

Porter, John [Jyon Pōtā]. "Meiji shoki Tōkyō ni okeru machikaisho no kaitai to hinmin kyūsai tōsei." *Hisutoria*, no. 265 (2017): 163–88.

Porter, Roy. "The Patient's View: Doing Medical History from Below." *Theory and Society* 14, no. 2 (1985): 175–98.

Rainham, Daniel, Ian McDowell, Daniel Krewski, and Michael Sawada. "Conceptualizing the Healthscape: Contributions of Time, Geography, Location Technologies and Spatial Ecology to Place and Health Research." *Social Science Medicine* 70, no. 5 (2010): 668–76.

Reynolds, John Russell. *A System of Medicine*. 5 vols. London: Macmillan, 1866–1879.

Rikugunshō. *Rikugun ni okeru karyūbyō narabini chihō karyūbyō man'en no jōkyō chōsa*. Kobayashi Matashichi, 1906.

Risse, Guenter B. *Plague, Fear, and Politics in San Francisco's Chinatown*. Johns Hopkins University Press, 2012.

Rogaski, Ruth. *Hygienic Modernity: Meanings of Health and Disease in Treaty-Port China*. University of California Press, 2004.

Rosenberg, Charles E. *The Cholera Years: The United States In 1832, 1849, and 1866*. University of Chicago Press, 1987.

Saiseikai, ed. *Dai Nihon seyakuin shōshi*. Saiseikai, 1911.

Saitō Gesshin et al. *Tōto saijiki*. Edo: Suharaya Ihachi, 1838.

Sakaki Hajime. "Tenkyōin setsuritsu no hitsuyō wo ronsu." *Kokka igaku*, no. 1 (1892): 3–31.

Sakaki Hajime. "Tōkyō-fu Tenkyōin no kanja tōkeihyō oyobi seishinbyō gen'in no tsuika." *Tōkyō igakkai zasshi* 2 (1888), no. 17: 1–7; no. 19: 17–19; no. 20: 8–12; no. 21: 23–31.

Sakaky, Hasimé [Sakaki Hajime]. "Ueber das Irrenwesen in Japan: Nebst einer Karte der Irrenheilanstalt in Tokio." *Allgemeine Zeitschrift für Psychiatrie un psychisch-gerichtliche Medizin* 42 (1886): 144–53.

Satō Eikichi. *Tōkyō hitori annai*. Tokyo: Hirano Denkichi, 1881.

Scott, James. *Weapons of the Weak: Everyday Forms of Peasant Resistance*. Yale University Press, 1985.

Seidensticker, Edward. *Low City, High City: Tokyo from Edo to the Earthquake*. Knopf, 1983.

Seidensticker, Edward. *Tokyo Rising: The City Since the Great Earthquake*. Harvard University Press, 1991.

Shibusawa Eiichi. *Tōkyō Yōikuin sōritsu gojūsshūnen kinen kaiko gojūnen*. 1922. Repr., Heibunsha, 1988.

Shinoda Tatsuaki. *Shiroi gekiryū: Meiji no ikan Sagara Chian no shōgai*. Shin Jinbutsu Ōraisha, 1997.

Shiokawa Hisao. "Meiji zenhan ni okeru jōsui suishitsu bunseki ni tsuite." *Kagaku kenkyū* 6 (1977): 20–26.

Shiomi Sen'ichirō. *Hinmin no teito*. Bungei Shunjū, 2008.

Shiratsuchi Ryūhō, ed. *Ika jinmeiroku*. Edo: Ryūhō, 1820.

Shorter, Edward. *A History of Psychiatry: From the Era of the to the Age of Prozac*. Wiley, 1997.

Siddall, Joseph Bower. *Surgical Experiences in Military Hospitals in Japan*. Reprinted from *Reports of St. Thomas Hospital*. Vol. 5. London: J. E. Adlard, Bartholomew Close, 1875.

Sippell, Patricia. "Japan's First Urban Water Disaster: The Great Kanto Flood of 1742." *Gendai shi kenkyū* 10 (2014): 1–34.

Singh, A. E., and B. Romanowski. "Syphilis: A Review with Emphasis on Clinical, Epidemiologic, and Some Biologic Features." *Clinical Microbiological Review* 12, no. 2 (1999): 187–209.

Singleton, F. L. et al. "Effects of Temperature and Salinity on *Vibrio Cholerae* Growth." *Applied and Environmental Microbiology* 44, no. 5 (November 1982): 1047–58.

Slack, Paul. "Responses to Plague in Early Modern Europe: The Implications of Public Health." *Social Research: An International Quarterly* 87, no. 2 (2020): 433–53.

Smith, C. Morton. "Have the Early Claims of Salvarsan Been Realized?" *Boston Medical and Surgical Journal* 107, no. 9 (1914): 269–72.

Smith, Henry D. "The Edo-Tokyo Transition: In Search of Common Ground." In *Japan in Transition: From Tokugawa to Meiji*, edited by Marius B. Jansen and Gilbert Rozman, 347–74. Princeton University Press, 1986.

Sōda Hajime. "Meiji shoki no igakkai jijō, 3: Byōin shi wo megutte." *Ishigaku kenkyū* 26 (1967): 1277–83

Sōma Kyūshin Jimusho. *Sōma jitsuden: seiten hakujitsu*. Tokyo: Tashiro Tamenobu, 1893.

Sōmuchō Tōkeikyoku and Nihon Tōkei Kyōkai, eds. *Nihon chōki tōkei sōran*. Vol. 4. Nihon Tōkei Kyōkai, 1987.

Stanley, Amy. *Selling Women: Prostitution, Markets, and the Household in Early Modern Japan*. University of California Press, 2013.

Suematsu Jun, ed. *Susaki Byōin daiichiji nenpyō*. Tokyo: Susaki Byōin, 1895.

Sugaya Akira. *Nihon no byōin: Sono ayumi to mondaiten*. Chūō Kōronsha, 1981.

Sugi Yasusaburō. *Sugita Genpaku zenshū*. 11 vols. Seikatsusha, 1933.

Sugita Genpaku, Nakagawa Jun'an et al. *Kaitai shinsho*. Edo: Suharaya Ichibee, 1774.

Sugita Masayuki. *Saishin jitsuyō Tōkyō densha annai*. Sugita Masayuki, 1910.

Sugiura Morikuni. "'Kenkō' to iu go no sōshisha ni tsuite." *Nihon ishigaku zasshi* 43, no. 2 (1997): 249–54.

Suita Dōshi [Tajima Shōji]. *Karyū jijō*. 3 vols. Tokyo: Sawa Sayo, 1880.

Suzuki, Akihito. "The State, Family and the Insane in Japan, 1900–1945." In *The Confinement of the Insane: International Perspectives, 1800–1965*, edited by Roy Porter and David Wright, 193–225. Cambridge University Press, 2003.

Suzuki Noriko. "Edo jidai no igakusho ni miru baidokukan ni tsuite." In *Nihon baidokushi no kenkyū: iryō, shakai, kokka*, edited by Fukuda Mahito and Noriko Suzuki, 37–66. Shibunkaku Shuppan, 2005.

Suzuki Noriko. *Edo no hayari yamai: Hashika sōdō wa naze okotta no ka*. Yoshikawa Kōbunkan, 2012.

Suzuki, Takao. *Palaeopathological and Palaeoepidemiological Study of Osseous Syphilisin Skulls of the Edo Period*. University of Tokyo Press, 1984.

Tajima, Kayo. "The Marketing of Urban Human Waste in Edo/Tokyo Metropolitan Area, 1600–1935." PhD diss.. Tufts University, 2005.

Takahashi Miyako. "Shu-shi *Sanbaron* no hon'yaku to fuken e no kizō." *Chiba Daigaku Kangogakubu kiyō* 12 (1990): 39–51.

Takahashi Miyako. "Tōkyō-fu Byōin Sanba Kyōjujo no honmenjō sanba kyōiku ni kansuru kenkyū." *Kango kyōikugaku kenkyū* 2, no. 1 (1993): 1–13.

Takahashi Tai and Eguchi Narumi. "Chiiki iryō teikyō taisei no genjō to shōrai: Todōfuken betsu." Working Paper no. 269 (November 2, 2012). https://www.jmari.med.or.jp/download/wp269_data/13.pdf.

Takahashi Tetsuo. *Shinsō Sōma jiken*. Fukushima Minpōsha, 1992.

Takaki Yoshihiro. *Takaki Kanehiro den*. Takaki Yoshihiro, 1922; repr., Ōzorasha, 1998.

Takano Iwasaburō. "Tōkyō ni okeru 'Īsuto Rondon,'" edited and translated by Yamamoto Kiyoshi. *Ōhara Shakai Mondai Kenkyūjo zasshi* 634 (2012): 43–57.

Takasu Sachio. "Katō Tokijirō ni tsuite." *Nihon ishigaku zasshi* 60, no. 4 (2014): 417–19.

Takayanagi Kaneyoshi. *Edo jidai hisabetsu mibunsō no seikatsushi*. Asuka Shoten, 1979.

Takei Shūsaku and Inaba Katsudō. *Edo kinsei ika jinmeiroku*. Edo: Nishimura Sōshichi, 1819.

Takei Shūsaku and Inaba Katsudō. *Edo kinsei ika jinmeiroku*. Edo: Nishimura Sōshichi, 1825.

Tanabe Kōmin. "Seishin byōsha jikken kiji (Dai jūichi rei): Kyūsei mōsō kyō." *Tōkyō igakkai zasshi* 4, no. 20 (1890): 45–50.

Tanaka Yoshio. "Ichiren no nagaya kaoku kenchiku kisoku to chihō ni okeru sono seitei e no torikumi ni tsuite." *Nihon kenchiku gakkai keikakukei ronbun hōkokushū*, no. 399 (1989) : 85–92.

Tanaka Yoshio. "Meiji 10-nendai, Naimushō Eiseikyoku ni yoru kenchiku hōsei no suishin ni tsuite: ichiren no nagaya, kaoku kenchiku kisoku no seiritsu yōin." *Nihon kenchiku gakkai keigakakari ronbun hokokushū*, no. 405 (1989): 107–15.

Tanaka Yoshio. "Meiji 19-20-nen Tōkyō-fu ni yoru nagaya kenchiku kisokuan no fuseiritsu ni owaru keii to sono riyū ni tsuite." *Nihon kenchiku gakkai keikakukei ronbun hōkokushū*, no. 390 (1988): 86–94.

Tatsukawa Shōji. *Byōki no shakaishi: Bunmei ni saguru byōin*. Nihon Hōsō Shuppan Kyōkai, 1971.

Tatsukawa Shōji. "Edo jidai ni okeru baidoku kanja no jittai: 'Nihonjin no byōreki' oboegaki." *Nihon ishigaku zasshi* 22, no. 4 (1976): 360–76.

Tawara Yoshizumi. "Tōkyō-fu jōgesui shiken seiseki." *Eisei shiken ihō*, no. 3 (n.d.): 1–24.

Taylor, Jeremy. *The Architect and the Pavilion Hospital: Dialogue and Design Creativity in England 1850–1914*. Leicester University Press, 1997.

Taylor, Jeremy. *Hospital and Asylum Architecture in England, 1840–1914: Building for Health Care*. Mansell, 1991.

Teikoku Daigaku Ika Daigaku Dai-ichi Byōin, eds. *Teikoku Daigaku Ika Daigaku iin ichiran Meiji 23 nen*. Tokyo: Ika Daigaku Daiichi Iin, 1890.

Tode Ichirō. "Igakukan ni okeru igaku kōshi ni tsuite (1)." *Nihon ishigaku zasshi* 48, no. 1 (2002): 3–30; "Igakukan ni okeru igaku kōshi ni tsuite (2)." *Nihon ishigaku zasshi* 48, no. 2 (2002): 185–204.

Tognotti, E. "Lessons from the History of Quarantine, from Plague to Influenza A." *Emergent Infectious Diseases* 19, no. 2 (2013): 254–59.

Tōkyō Daigaku Igakubu, ed. *Tōkyō Daigaku Igakubu ichiran Meiji 13–14 nen*. Tokyo: Maruya Zenshichi, 1881.

Tōkyō Daigaku Igakubu, ed. *Tōkyō Daigaku Igakubu ichiran Meiji 16–17 nen*. Tokyo: Maruya Zenshichi, 1881.

Tōkyō Daigaku Igakubu Sōritsu Hyakunen Kinenkai and Tōkyō Daigaku Igakubu Hyakunenshi Henshū Iinkai, eds. *Tōkyō Daigaku Igakubu hyakunenshi*. Tōkyō Daigaku Shuppankai, 1967.

Tōkyō Hyakunenshi Henshū Iinkai. *Tōkyo̅ Hyakunenshi*. 6 vols. Tōkyō-to, 1972.

Tōkyō Keishi Kangokusho. Keishi honsho tasshi yōsan. Tōkyō Keishi Kangokusho, 1879.

"Tōkyō Nōbyōin wo hōmon shite fujin seishin byōsha wo kataru." *Fujin sekai* 4, no. 10 (1909).

Tōkyō Seishin Byōin Kyōkai, ed. *Tōkyō no shiritsu seishin byōin shi*. Makino Shuppan, 1978.

Tōkyō Yōikuin, ed. *Yōikuin rokujūnenshi*. 1928. Repr., Nihon Tosho Sentā, 2010.

Tōkyō-fu, ed. *Shōgi geigi kaihō shiryō*. Tōkyō-fu, 1873.

Tōkyō-fu, ed. *Taishō 3-nen Tōkyō-fu kōjō tōkeisho*. Tōkyō-fu, 1916.

Tōkyō-fu, ed. *Tōkyō-fu shi: Gyōseihen*. 6 vols. Tōkyō-fu, 1937.

Tōkyō-fu, ed. *Tōkyō-fu shi: Gyōseihen*. Vol. 6. Tōkyō-fu, 1936.

Tōkyō-fu, ed. *Tōkyō-fu tōkeisho Meiji 15-nen–43-nen*. Tōkyō-fu, 1884–1910.

Tōkyō-fu, ed. *Tōkyō-fu tōkeisho Meiji 19*. Tōkyō-fu, 1887.

Tōkyō-fu, ed. *Tōkyō-fu tōkeisho Meiji 44-nen-Taishō 15-nen*. Tōkyō-fu, 1911–1926.

Tōkyō-fu, ed. *Tōkyō-fu tōkeisho Taishō gannen*. Vol. 3. Tōkyō-fu, 1914.

Tōkyō-fu Suidō Kaisei Iin, ed. *Tōkyō suidō kaisetsu gairyaku*. Tōkyō-fu, 1877.

"Tōkyō-fuka ni baidoku byōin wo kensetsusen koto wo kou." Japan Center for Asian Historical Records (JACAR) Ref. A15070668400, pp. 1–4.

Tōkyō Shiyakusho, ed. *Tōkyō-shi shikō: Jōsuihen*. 4 vols. Tōkyō-shi, 1919–23.

Tōkyō Shiyakusho, ed. *Tōkyō-shi shikō: Kyūsaihen*. 4 vols. Tōkyō-shi, 1920–22.

Tōkyō Shiyakusho, ed. *Tōkyō-shi shikō: Shigaihen*. 73 vols. Tokyo: Rinsen, 1994–2004.

Tōkyō Shikai, ed. "Shinai shinyō chōsasho" (1907). In *Kindai toshi no eisei kankyō* (Tōkyō hen) 39:3–132. Kingendai Shiryō Kankōkai, 2009.

Tomita Hiroki. "Nihon Sekijūjisha no rekishi to katsudō 3: Nihon Sekijūjisha no sōsetsu to Sano Tsunetame." *Nihon byōinkai zasshi* 63, no. 3 (2016): 319–22.

Tomita Mikio. *Seishinbyōin no teiryū*. Seikyūsha, 1992.

Tōyama Chinkichi. *Tōkyō-shi kairyō suidō no eiseigakuteki kōsatsu*. Tōkyō-shi Eiseika, 1905.

Toyama Mikio. *Iryō fukushi no so Nagayo Sensai*. Shibunkaku, 2002.

Uchimura Yūshi. "Sakaki Sensei to Tōkyō Teikoku Daigaku Igakubu Seishinbyōgaku Kyōshitsu no sōsetsu." *Seishin shinkeigaku zasshi* 44 (1939): 63–79.

Ueda Sanpei and Miura Saburō. *Nihon yakuenshi no kenkyū*. Watanabe Shoten, 1972.

Ueno Kaneko. "Kishū han no iryō seisaku to chiiki shakai." *Mie shigaku*, no. 7 (2007): 1–20.

Umetani Noboru et al. *Oyatoi gaikokujin*. Vol. 9, *Igaku*. Kajima Kenkyūjo Shuppankai, 1969.

Umihara Ryō. "Edo no rangakusha: Bunsei-ki 'Ika jinmeiroku' no bunseki kara." *Kokuritsu Minzoku Rekishi Hakubutsukan kenkyū hōkoku*, no. 116 (2004): 91–108.

Uramoto Yoshifumi. *Edo Tōkyō no hisabetsu buraku no rekishi: Danzaemon to hisabetsu minshū*. Akashi Shoten, 2003.

Ushigome Tsutomu. "Gojūkusei no keisei to tenkai." *Rekishi hyōron*, no. 405 (1984): 5–20.

Ushigome Tsutomu. "Tōkyō-fu ni okeru daiku shōku sei no keisei no tenkai." *Chihōshi kenkyū* 43, no. 6 (1993): 67–82.

Waddington, Keir. *Charity and the London Hospitals, 1850–1898*. Boydell Press, 2000.

Washington, Garrett L. *Church Space and the Capital in Prewar Japan*. University of Hawai'i Press, 2022.

Weiner, Dora B. *The Citizen-Patient in Revolutionary and Imperial Paris*. Johns Hopkins University Press, 1993.

Westney, D. Eleanor. "The Emulation of Western Organizations in Meiji Japan: The Case of the Paris Prefecture of Police and the Keishi-chō." *Journal of Japanese Studies* 8, no. 2 (1982): 307–42.

Winterbottom, Anne E. "Of the Chinaroot: A Case Study of the Early Modern Circulation of *Materia Medica*." *Social History of Medicine* 28, no. 1 (2015): 22–44.

Yamada Mayumi. "Meiji-ki no kaigyōi: Kanō Kengo no shōgai: Zōki ryōhō no hakkensha kara shinkei suijaku no senmonka e." *Nihon ishigaku zasshi* 65, no. 3 (2019): 382–83.

Yamaguchi Gorō. *Hasegawa Tai sensei shoden*. Hasegawa Tai Sensei Ikōshū Kankōkai, 1935. Repr., Ōzorasha, 1994.

Yamamoto Shun'ichi. *Baishun seibyō shi*. Bunkōdō, 2002.

Yamamoto Shun'ichi. *Nihon korera shi*. Tōkyō Daigaku Shuppankai, 1982.

Yamazaki Tasuku. "Otamagaike Shutōjo, 2–3." *Nihon ishigaku zasshi*, no. 1330 (1944): 186–95; no. 1331 (1944): 203–9.

Yamazaki Tasuku. "Seishin byōsha taigū kō 4." *Shinkeigaku zasshi* 34, no. 4 (1932): 55–68.

"Yōjōsho no shimatsu." *Edo kaishi* 2, no. 4 (1889): 72–78.

Yokohama-shi, ed. *Yokohama-shi shikō fūzokuhen*. Rinsen Shoten, 1932.

Yoo, Theodore Jun. *It's Madness: The Politics of Mental Health in Colonial Korea*. University of California Press, 2016.

Yoshikawa Isaburō. *Shin Yoshiwara yūkaku ryakushi*. Shin Yoshiwara Sangyō Kumiai Torishimari Jimusho, 1936.

Young, William Evan. "Family Matters: Managing Illness in Late Tokugawa Japan, 1750–1868." PhD diss. Princeton University, 2015.

Yunoki Hanae. "Meiji shoki ni okeru bukechi no kōsakuchika ga kindai Tōkyō no shigaichi keisei ni ataeta eikyō." MA thesis, University of Tokyo, 2011.

Yunomae Tomoko and Akisada Yoshikazu. *Baibaishun mondai shiryō shūsei*. 32 vols. Henshū fukkokuban. Fuji Shuppan, 1997–2004.

INDEX

Note: *Italicized* page numbers indicate figures and illustrations.

Printed and bound by CPI Group (UK) Ltd, Croydon, CR0 4YY
16/09/2026
14963483-0001